Genetics and Genomics in Nursing

(Previously known as Human Genetics in Nursing)

(As per INC Syllabus)

Third Edition

Suresh K Sharma
PhD MSc (N) RN (USA)
Professor and Principal
College of Nursing
All India Institute of Medical Sciences (AIIMS)
Rishikesh, Uttarakhand, India

Foreword
Indarjit Walia

JAYPEE The Health Sciences Publisher
New Delhi | London | Panama | Philadelphia

Jaypee Brothers Medical Publishers (P) Ltd

Headquarters

Jaypee Brothers Medical Publishers (P) Ltd
4838/24, Ansari Road, Daryaganj
New Delhi 110 002, India
Phone: +91-11-43574357
Fax: +91-11-43574314
Email: jaypee@jaypeebrothers.com

Overseas Offices

J.P. Medical Ltd
83 Victoria Street, London
SW1H 0HW (UK)
Phone: +44 20 3170 8910
Fax: +44 (0)20 3008 6180
Email: info@jpmedpub.com

Jaypee Brothers Medical Publishers (P) Ltd
17/1-B Babar Road, Block-B, Shaymali
Mohammadpur, Dhaka-1207, Bangladesh
Mobile: +08801912003485
Email: jaypeedhaka@gmail.com

Jaypee-Highlights Medical Publishers Inc
City of Knowledge, Bld. 235, 2nd Floor, Clayton
Panama City, Panama
Phone: +1 507-301-0496
Fax: +1 507-301-0499
Email: cservice@jphmedical.com

Jaypee Brothers Medical Publishers (P) Ltd
Bhotahity, Kathmandu, Nepal
Phone +977-9741283608
Email: kathmandu@jaypeebrothers.com

Jaypee Medical Inc
325 Chestnut Street
Suite 412, Philadelphia, PA 19106, USA
Phone: +1 267-519-9789
Email: support@jpmedus.com

Website: www.jaypeebrothers.com
Website: www.jaypeedigital.com

Inquiries for bulk sales may be solicited at: jaypee@jaypeebrothers.com

Genetics and Genomics in Nursing

First Edition: **2007**

Second Edition: **2010**

Third Edition: **2016**

ISBN 978-93-85999-20-8

Printed at Rajkamal Electric Press, Plot No. 2, Phase-IV, Kundli, Haryana.

Dedicated to

Sweet memories

of my

Grandfather Late Shri Gularam Sharma

Foreword

Genetic nursing may seem like futuristic specialty healthcare, but along with managed care and evidence-based practice, a genetic science revolution is redefining basic nursing practice. Some revolutions are surprising because of the rapid pace of change that they create. The rapid and recent advances in techniques and knowledge in the field of human genetics have outpaced the transformation of professional education programs, leaving most postgraduate nurses and physicians lagging behind in knowledge of the essentials of practices in the new era of human genetics. This book offers the basics of genetics and genetic healthcare for the practice of every nurse and specialist.

The basic scientists have recently finished the work of sequencing a draft of the entire human genome. The much-publicized discovery of genes associated with specific diseases as this work progresses has the public demanding that this knowledge be used as the basis of their healthcare. What the public does not know is that genetic therapies are rare, whereas genetic testing poses immediate risks for individuals and their entire families in terms of discrimination and eugenics. There is also a misconception that every gene mutation will manifest as a disease. Actually, environmental factors, such as lifestyle and behavior, will determine disease manifestation for most gene mutations. This is an opportunity for the nurses to practice health promotion tailored to highly specific and uniquely personal predispositions. In other words, individualized health care nurses can offer care that protects patients and families from the risks associated with genetic information, including addressing family issues. Nurses are also needed to refer patients to genetic specialists and assist patients in making choices as a genetic healthcare. Every nurse is needed; do not miss the revolution.

I hope this book will serve all the above said purposes for the Indian nursing students and the practicing nurses.

Indarjit Walia PhD
Formerly Principal
National Institute of Nursing Education
PGIMER, Chandigarh, India

Preface to the Third Edition

This textbook retitled *Genetics and Genomics in Nursing* (previously known as *Human Genetics in Nursing*) is focused on nurses, which is covering the most desired areas of genetic and genomic nursing as prescribed in the nursing curriculum. This textbook is covering the following six broader domains of genetic and genomic nursing:

1. *Basic Concept of Molecular Genetics:* This chapter covers the entire breadth and depth of molecular genetics covering details on the basic introduction of genetics, basic terminology related to molecular genetics, review of cellular division, structure and characteristics of genes, DNA, RNA and chromosomes, protein synthesis, genetic code, chromosomal aberrations, gene mutation, mechanism of inheritance, laws of inheritance and patterns of inheritance, including autosomal dominant, autosomal recessive, sex-linked and nonmendelian patterns of inheritance, such as codominant pattern, mitochondrial pattern and multifactorial pattern of inheritance. It is also covering the details of multiple allots and blood groups, reduced penetrance, variable expressivity, anticipation, practical applications of genetics in nursing, impact of genetic conditions on families, factors influencing the impact of genetic conditions of families and role of nurses in managing the impact of genetic conditions on families.
2. *Emerging Paradigm of Genetics in Nursing:* This chapter enumerates the details on milestones achieved by genetic nursing, role of nurses in genetics, importance of genetics in nursing curriculum, barriers and approaches for the implementation of genetics in nursing and assumptions regarding genetics and healthcare in future.
3. *Maternal and Prenatal Genetics:* This chapter covers the content on areas related to maternal and prenatal genetics, such as maternal infections and fetal genetic consequences, genetic aspect of consanguinity, prenatal nutrition and food allergies in children, role of prenatal nutrition in the prevention of genetic disorders in children, genetic aspect of advanced maternal and parental

age, genetic effect of maternal drug therapy on pregnancy and fetus, genetic consequences of maternal exposure to radiation, chemical and illicit drugs, prenatal testing and diagnosis including ultrasound, fetal echocardiography, fetal radiology, amniocentesis, chorionic villus sampling, fetal blood sampling, maternal blood sampling, fetal tissue sampling, fetoscopy, and preimplantation and prenatal testing. This chapter also covers the infertility, spontaneous abortion, neural tube defect and Down's syndrome from genetic point of view. The role of nurses in each of the above mentioned maternal and prenatal genetic conditions and testing is precisely covered in this chapter.

4. *Genetic Testing in the Neonates and Children:* Many of the genetic disorders, if identified in newborns and early childhood, may prevent the individual from experiencing the symptoms of that particular genetic disease or complications with adaption of preventive measures. This chapter covers the meaning and purposes of neonatal screening/genetic testing, important elements of newborn screening, common disorders screened in newborns, approaches of genetic testing and screening in children. The meaning, genetic causes, tools and methods of genetic screening, medical management and nurses' role in congenital abnormalities, developmental delay and dysmorphism are also precisely covered in this chapter. This chapter also includes the role of nurses in genetic testing for neonates and children.
5. *Genetic Conditions of Adolescents and Adults:* Recently, many diseases were found to have genetic predisposition. However, this chapter has covered only selected core genetic conditions, such as cancer genetics—familial cancer, inborn errors of metabolism, hematological genetic disorders, genetic hemochromatosis, Huntington's disease and mental illnesses with genetic predisposition. It also covers the therapeutic approaches used for the medical management and nursing management in genetic disorders.
6. *Services Related to Genetics:* This chapter covers the details of genetic testing, different types of genetic testing, genetic test techniques, interpreting genetic test results, ethical, legal and social issues in genetic testing and role of nurses in genetic testing, human genome project, nursing and human genome

project, genomic era, gene therapy, role of nurses in gene therapy, eugenic movement, genetic counseling, role of nurses in genetic counseling and pharmacogenomics.

At the end of each chapter, the open-ended and multiple choice questions are also included, which have appeared differently in the undergraduate and postgraduate nursing examinations of different universities. I expect that the content covered in this textbook will be most suitable for the undergraduate and postgraduate nursing students and a reference book for the nursing faculty.

Suresh K Sharma

Preface to the First Edition

Understanding the molecular and clinical human genetic principles and concepts for nursing practice is relevant in assisting nurses to understand the disease, assess risk for the disease, provide a scientific foundation for the care they provide and promote health and wellness among the patients and their families. Today, a foundational knowledge of the principles, practices, and psychosocial implications of genetics is essential to basic nursing care.

This book is not intended to be exhaustive of the genetic issues important for nurses. Instead, it is meant to provide insight and food for thought into some of the human responses, care delivery, and professional issues nurses will be required to grapple with today and in the coming years. The edition begins with a brief overview of molecular human genetics. It is critical that each of us grasp this basic information because it is foundational to understanding human form and function, disease genesis and progression, health promotion, and disease prevention. As a nurse, you will be asked to explain it and relate it to personal and family health and illness. Because increasingly it is believed that all the diseases have a genetic component, and because nurses interact with those having diseases, we will be responsible for identifying the hereditary, familial, environmental, and lifestyle characteristics that increase family members' risk for disease and promoting behaviors that reduce such risks. A nurse's role in genetics extends across all age groups. Therefore, this book will serve the purpose of covering the prescribed syllabus of genetics for the graduate and postgraduate nurses, and it will also be useful to enhance the knowledge of nurses about genetics who are actively involved in nursing care for all age-group patients to understand genetic foundation of different diseases.

Suresh K Sharma

Acknowledgments

Writing a book needs many direct and indirect personal and professional inputs. I feel greatly delighted to acknowledge the active support and love of my grandmother (Smt GD Sharma), mother (Late Smt BD Sharma), father (Shri BN Sharma), brothers (Er KK Sharma and Shri Dinesh Sharma), sister-in-law (Smt Poonam Sharma), my sisters (Mrs Saroj Sharma and Mrs Sunita Sharma), and all other members of my family, without whom this attempt would not have been possible. The perseverance shown by my wife, Reena Sharma, daughter Simone and son Rishit during my overstretched working hours is greatly appreciated. Reena's critical analysis was very helpful in improving the quality of illustrations. I would like to thank my teachers, Dr Madan Mohan Sharma, Shri AP Chowdia, Dr Indarjit Walia, Dr Sandhya Ghai, Dr Sukpal Kaur, Mrs Gurmeet Bajwa and all my other teachers who taught me from day one till date for their blessings and encouragement in my academic development. It gives me immense pleasure to thank all my friends, colleagues, faculty of my college and other senior nursing faculty members of different nursing colleges from various states of India and abroad, who helped me to bring this edition.

I convey my sincere thanks to Jaypee Brothers Medical Publishers (P) Ltd, New Delhi, India for their efforts and suggestions, especially Shri Jitendar P Vij (Group Chairman), Mr Ankit Vij (Group President), Ms Chetna Malhotra Vohra (Associate Director), and Ms Payal Bharti (Project Manager) for helping me through my idea.

INC Syllabus

Placement: Second **Time:** Theory-15 hours

Course Description: This course is designed to enable students to acquire understanding of Genetics, its role in causation and management of defects and diseases.

Unit	Time (Hrs)	Objectives	Content	Teaching Learning Activities	Assessment methods	Chapter
1	3	• Explain nature, principles and perspectives of heredity	**Introduction:** • Practical application of genetics in Nursing • Impact of genetic condition on families • Review of cellular division mitosis and meiosis. • Characteristics and structure of genes • Chromosomal aberrations Patterns of inheritance – Mendelian theory of inheritance – Multiple allots and blood groups – Sex-linked inheritance – Mechanism of inheritance – Errors in transmission (Mutation)	• Lecture Discussion • Explain using charts, slides	• Short answers • Objective type	1
II	3	• Explain Maternal, prenatal and genetic influences on development of defects and diseases	**Maternal, prenatal and genetic influences on development of defects and diseases** • Conditions affecting the mother: Genetic and infections • Consanguinity atopy • Prenatal nutrition and food allergies • Maternal age • Maternal drug therapy • Prenatal testing and diagnosis	• Lecture Discussion • Explain using charts, slides	• Short answers • Objective type	3

Contd...

Contd...

Unit	Time (Hrs)	Objectives	Content	Teaching Learning Activities	Assessment methods	Chapter
			• Effect of Radiation, drugs and chemicals • Infertility • Spontaneous abortion			3
III	2	• Explain the screening methods for genetic defects and diseases in neonates and children	**Genetic testing in the neonates and children** • Screening for – Congenital abnormalities – Developmental delay – Dysmorphism	• Lecture Discussion • Explain using charts, slides	• Short answers • Objective type	4
IV	2	• Identify genetic disorders in adolescents and adults	**Genetic conditions of adolescents and adults** • Cancer genetics-Familial cancer • Inborn errors of metabolism • Blood group alleles and hematological disorders • Genetic hemochromatosis • Huntington's disease • Mental illness	• Lecture Discussion • Explain using charts, slides	• Short answers • Objective type	5
V	5	• Describe the role of nurse in genetic services and counseling	**Services related to Genetics** • Genetic testing • Human genome project • Gene therapy • The Eugenics movement • Genetic counselling • Legal and Ethical issues • Role of nurse	• Lecture Discussion	• Short answers • Objective type	6

Contents

Contents

Chapter

1 Basic Concept of Molecular Genetics

Learning Objectives

This chapter is designed to enable the reader to:

- Understand the concept of genetics and definition of basic genetic terms.
- Describe the practical applications of genetics in nursing and impact of genetic conditions on families.
- Discuss the review of cell division, chromosome, gene, DNA, RNA, protein synthesis, genetic code.
- Identify the chromosomal and gene mutations.
- Appraise the mechanism, law and patterns of inheritance
- Discuss the multiple allots and blood groups.
- Recognizes the reduced penetrance and variable expressivity.

Key Terms

- Genetics
- Gene
- Alleles
- Genotype
- Phenotype
- Cellular Division
- Mitosis
- Meiosis
- Deoxyribonucleic Acid
- Ribonucleic Acid
- Protein Biosynthesis
- Genetic Code
- Chromosome
- Chromosomal Aberrations
- Mechanism of Inheritance
- Laws of Inheritance
- Patterns of Inheritance
- Multiple Allots and Blood Groups
- Gene Mutations
- Reduced Penetrance
- Variable Expressivity

INTRODUCTION

In 1865, Gregor Mendal was the first to describe the elements of hereditary genes. His observation and analysis of the observable features of Pea led him to conclude that specific traits particulate factors were passed on unchanged from a parent plant to the next generation. Scientific discoveries during the last several decades have provided more information about how genes function and how they contribute to human health and disease. Currently more than 10,371 identified genetic disorders are known to be inherited in a predictable pattern in families. Nurses are at present in all health care setting and care for individuals who may have genetic conditions or predisposition. They also ensure that these individuals have access to the most current genetic information, genetic diagnosis, treatment and management therapeutics. With this knowledge, nurses can collect appropriate family information; provide current and appropriate information and support patients, families and communities as they integrate this new information and technology into their daily lives.

CONCEPT OF GENETICS

The term 'Genetics' was introduced by Bateson in 1906. It has been derived from the Greek word *'gene'*, which means *'to become'* or 'to grow into'. Therefore, genetics is the science of coming into being.

'Genetics is that branch of biological sciences which deals with the transmission of characteristics from parents to offspring'.

In other words 'Genetics is the study of inheritance of disease in families, mapping of disease genes to specific location on chromosomes, analysis of molecular mechanism through which genes cause disease and the diagnosis and treatment of genetic diseases'.

Traditionally genetics has been associated with childbearing decision-making and caring for children with genetic disorders. Medical genetics has focused on the inheritance of hereditary disorders affecting only a small portion of the population. Genetic services have been primarily associated with prenatal genetic counseling, identification of pediatric disorders associated with birth defects and dysmorphology, and in some cases rare adult onset single gene disorders. Recent genetic and technological advances are helping us to better understand how genetic changes impact human variation as well as the development of cancer, Alzheimer's, diabetes and other multifactorial diseases that are prevalent in adults.

The Human Genome Project, one of the most significant research endeavors of the twentieth century, deserves much of the credit for the discovery of these new applications of genetic information. Specifically, research from the Human Genome Project is providing a new and better understanding of the genetic contribution to disease, the development of targeted drug therapy (pharmacogenetics) and the development of genetic tests that identify those who may have or are at risk for genetic diseases. The results of this explosion of knowledge is a rapid paradigm shift from the 'old genetics' to the 'new genetics'. Under the 'new genetics' paradigm nearly all diseases have a genetic component. Now recognized is the fact that most common human diseases, such as myocardial infarction, cancer, mental illness, diabetes, and Alzheimer disease are a result of complex interactions between a number of factors including the influence of one or more genes and a variety of environmental exposures.

The influence of recent genetic advances on nursing practice is especially evident in oncology. Oncology nurses practicing in cancer prevention and control apply genetic principles to their daily clinical practice. For example, nurses assess hereditary and non hereditary cancer risk factors, take detailed family histories and construct pedigrees, identify individuals and families at risk for hereditary cancer syndromes, make recommendations for cancer risk reduction, surveillance, and management, and when appropriate, counsel and educate about the risks and benefits of genetic testing.

This genetic revolution and shift to the 'new genetics' has created a demand for health professionals in a number of clinical specialties who understand the genetic contribution to disease risk, the impact on disease management, and the genetic educational needs of patients and families. Nurses have risen to the challenge capitulating genetic nursing practice into a new era.

Basic Genetic Terms

- *Genes:* Genes are genetic material on a chromosome that code for a trait. For example, one person has a gene for eye color.

- *Alleles:* They are variations of genes. Means the two genes, which occur on the same locus in the two homologous chromosomes of an individual and control the expression of a character, are called alleles. For example, one person has the allele for brown eye color. Note that some alleles are *dominant* over others. That is, if a person inherits both the dominant and the *recessive* alleles, the dominant allele will be the one expressed.
- *Gene locus:* A particular portion or region of the chromosome representing a single gene is called locus. The alleles of gene occupy the same gene locus on the two homologous chromosomes.
- *Homologous Chromosomes:* Members of the chromosome pairs with same gene number and arrangement.
- *Dominant allele:* It is one of a pair of alleles, which can express itself whether present in homozygous or heterozygous state, e.g. the gene for tallness Tt and TT, where T is dominate alleles and person will be tall in both conditions.
- *Recessive allele:* The allele of an allelic or allelomophic pair, which is unable to express its effect in the presence of its contrasting alleles in a heterozygote is called recessive alleles. For example, one has alleles of eye 'Bb' (B- Brown, b-blue) here b is recessive allele therefore person will have brown eye not blue. The effect of recessive allele become known only when it is present in the homozygous state (bb), in this state person will have blue eye.
- *Codominant alleles:* The alleles, which do not show dominance-recessive relationship and are able to express themselves independently when present together are called codominant alleles. Here in heterozygous state both alleles express themselves. As a result, the heterozygous condition has a phenotype different from either homozygous genotypes. The joint character may appear to be intermediate between the ones produced by the two homozygous genotypes.
- *Heterozygous alleles:* One alleles of the same gene pair differs from the other. For example, for eye color Bb
- *Homozygous alleles: Alleles* that are identical or same in gene pair. For example, for eye color BB.

- *Hemizygous:* Having one copy of a particular gene. For example, for eye color only B is present.
- *Genotype:* It is the gene complement or genetic constitution of an individual with regard to one characters irrespective of whether the genes are expressed or not. For example, one has the genotype Bb since one have the allele for brown eye color (B) and the allele for blue eye color (b). An organism is said to be *homozygous* for a certain trait if both it carries two of the same alleles. It is *homozygous dominant* if it carries two dominant alleles and *homozygous recessive* if it carries two recessive alleles. The organism in above said example is *heterozygous* — it carries two different alleles.
- *Phenotype:* It is observable or measurable distinctive structure or functional characteristics of an individual with regard to one or more characters which is a result of gene products brought to expression in a given environment. The characteristics are visible to a person (e.g. height, color of eyes, etc.) or require special test for its identification (e.g. serological test for blood group). In other words it is the expression of a gene.
  For example, since one has the genotype Bb with one dominant and one recessive allele, the dominant allele (B) will mask the recessive allele (b) and one will have the phenotype for brown eyes. Phenotype can be modified by environment through genotype establishes the boundaries within which the environment can modify the phenotype. For example, a fair colored person can have tanned colored skin due to excessive exposure to skin.
- A *karyotype* is a picture showing the arrangement of a full set of human chromosomes.

PRACTICAL APPLICATIONS OF GENETICS IN NURSING

In last few years genetics gained several major developments and discoveries related to health and disease. Medical and nursing care practices are largely influenced with recent genetic advancements in health care. Recent advances in genetics knowledge and technology have impacted all areas of nursing practices. Application of genetics in nursing is very wide since:

- All nurses have role in the delivery of genetic services and management of genetic information.

- Nurses require genetic knowledge to identify, support, refer and care for persons affected by or at risk for genetic conditions.
- Nurses can offer care that protects patients and families from the risk associated with genetic information, including addressing family issues.
- Nurses are also needed to refer patients to genetic specialist and assist in making choice as a genetic health care.
- Genetic nursing is practiced in different environment, such as maternity, pediatrics, medical-surgical, psychiatric and community health nursing.
- Genetic nursing is a holistic practice that includes assessing, planning, implementing and evaluating the physical, spiritual, ethical and psychosocial aspects of patients and families who have genetic concerns.
- Genetic nursing includes following:
  - Client and family assessment to identify genetic risk factors. In assessment takes detailed family history and construct a pedigree, analyze the assessment data. In addition interpret information collected.
  - Planning and implementation of care during diagnosis and management of genetic disorders. In care, provide genetic education and develop and carryout a plan of care to address genetic concerns.
  - Information, counseling and support services to person affected by or at risk for genetic conditions.
  - Meeting referral needs.
  - Long-term follow-up.
- Advanced practice nurses may play direct roles in genetic counseling and in advanced assessment. They also may work within a particular specialty in which genetics plays a role, such as an oncology or cardiology clinic, as well as in long-term management of specific genetic disorders depending on the specialty area in which they are trained.

The past several years have transformed genetic nursing practice from an all but, hidden practice to a recognized nursing specialty with a visible contribution to the genetic and overall health of individuals and families. Nurses have been involved in managing genetic information since the 1960's, when nurses provided services to children with genetic disorders and their families. Although in some respects the nurse's role today in managing genetic information and caring for individuals and families at risk for or diagnosed with genetic diseases or conditions is similar to this traditional role, the scope of practice is much broader and more encompassing. What has also changed, according to Forsman, is the amount of genetic information available and the population to which this information may be applied. It is clear that genetic changes contribute to most, if not all diseases. Consequently, the scope of genetic knowledge application in nursing is limitless. 'Nursing can no longer ignore genetics. The time for meaningful action is now'. Major practical applications of genetics in nursing are as follows:

- *Understands genetic basis of disease:* With knowledge of genetics, nurses well understand that large proportion of total disease has genetic basis. In addition will learn about:
  - Role of different genes in causation of genetic disorders and defects.
  - Good or bad genes for health-illness continuum.
  - Role of gene and chromosomal mutation in health and illness.
  - Normal and abnormal cell division and its genetic regulation.
  - Mechanism of disease inheritance from one generation to next generation.
  - Basic mechanisms of inheritance and transmission of chromosomes and genes, including the concepts of variation and mutation.
  - Role of genetic factors in individual's health.
  - Genetic contribution towards different diseases, disorders and defects.
  - Genetic contributions to common and complex conditions, such as breast cancer, colorectal cancer, heart disease and hypercholesterolemia, mental illness, certain behavioral traits, and Alzheimer disease.
- *Early and effective diagnosis of genetic disorders:* Genetic knowledge of nurses will equip them with:
  - Information about genetic risk, genetic testing and screening, and the implications both positive and negative results.

- Interpretations of the results of genetic tests.
- Interpretation of genetic risks (i.e. how to explain the meaning of a I in 4 risk for having another child with Tay-Sachs disease).
- Awareness of the possibility of an inherited or genetic component for a client's condition and knowledge of cardinal features of familial predisposition, such as early age of disease onset, multiple family members with the same diagnosis, predisposing risk factors.
- Key information while collecting family history, construction and understanding pedigree.

- *Contribution towards health promotion with genetic aspect:* By learning about genetics nurses will enhance their understanding about:
  - Relationship of health and disease in respect to genetics, including how genetics and the environment interact and how genes interact with genes. This should lead to new ways of thinking about health promotion and disease prevention.
  - Creating a healthy prenatal environment by ensuring minimal or no risk of genetic defects among new-born's.
  - Environmental interaction of an individual is an important factor in reference to gene or chromosomal mutation, which may have positive or negative impact on health of an individual.
  - Learn about phamacogenomics, that every individual have unique genetic make-up therefore responds differently with same drug. For example, a drug 'A' may be very effective to cure an illness in an individual, but same drug may bring sever hypersensitive reaction for another person.
  - An understanding of genetic contributions to human diversity including concepts, such as discrimination and eugenics.
- *Prevention of genetic conditions:* Prevention is major principle of any medical discipline, similarly knowledge of genetics well enhance nurse's understanding that:
  - Several genetic disorders can be prevented with prompt and early diagnosis and treatment. For example, Phenylketonuria (PKU) related mental retardation can be

prevented with early newborn screening and diagnosis and diet management.
- The genetic disorders can be prevented by selected intervention. For example, risk of Neural Tube Defect can be minimized with administration of Folic acid in first trimester of pregnancy.

- *Management and care in genetic disorders:* Knowledge of genetics will empower the nurses to manage and care patients with genetic disorders in their routine health care practice by building up their understanding about:
  - Genetic approaches to the therapy of genetic and complex diseases.
  - Care management of adults with childhood genetic disorders
  - Care management of persons with adult genetic disorders, such as Huntington disease.
  - Ways in which genetic knowledge is used in diagnosis and treatment applications.
- *Genetic information and counseling:* Nurses are largely involved in providing genetic information and counseling to patients and families, who are at risk or experiencing genetic disorders. Therefore, knowledge of genetics well help them to:
  - Development of nonjudgmental attitudes about genetics and related disorders.
  - What information needs to be collected before providing genetic counseling.
  - What information needs to be provided to patient and family before offering genetic counseling.
  - Role of nurses in delivering genetic information and counseling.
  - Application of traditional nursing skills, such as patient education, confidentiality, and counseling about genetic information. The concept of nondirective counseling can be included.
- *Referral services:* In developing countries, there is less awareness about genetic disorders and health care facilities offering services for testing and management of genetic disorders. Nurses are the primary health care providers who can direct the patients and caregivers to right place for their diagnosis and

management. So that, genetic information will equip nurses to provide effective referral services to their genetic clients:
  - Services available to manage the genetic disorders in local or national level.
  - Knowledge about referral possibilities knowing not only who should be referred but also how and to whom it should be done.
  - Ways to access resources relating to genetics for patient and self-education and the need to keep updated with current available resources.
- *Social and ethical issues in genetics:* There are several social and ethical issues, which play important role in care of patients with genetic disorders. Therefore, study of genetic will make nurses to build:
  - An awareness of social, legal, and ethical issues related to genetics, including effects on individuals, groups, and societies, some of which are unique to genetic conditions.
  - An understanding of the social and ethical ramifications of possessing a particular genotype or genetic disorder in terms of societal issues, confidentiality, freedom of choice, and risks in terms of insurance and disclosure.

IMPACT OF GENETIC CONDITIONS ON FAMILIES

Genetic disorders or defects are chronic and long lasting, permanent, even after repair. A person in family with genetic problem if cause of the genetic disorder is said to be hereditary,the news can be seriously difficult for parents to accept. In many families,when they know that one of the family members is suffering from genetic problem, they may go into series of grief reactions like mourning, loss of hope and expections. The grieving, with all its feeling of anger, depression and intense sadness is not an uncommon phenomenon.

It is normal and natural reaction whenever a person experiences a loss, whether it be the any morbidity or mortality of a person in a family. Grieving is one dimension of emotional impact of genetic conditions on family. There are several other aspects of impact on family like cognitive, social, cultural, and economic impact of genetic conditions on families (Fig. 1.1).

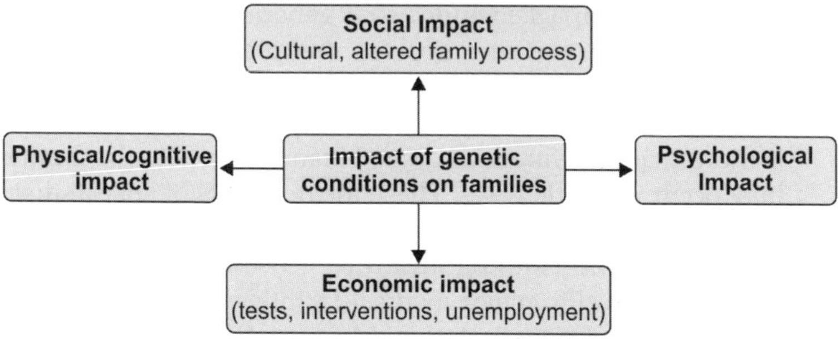

Fig. 1.1: Dimensions of impact of genetic conditions on families

- *Social impact:* Genetic conditions in a family may lead mild to serious level of social impact on the family. Some of them are:
  - Social stigma
  - Social discrimination
  - Decreased planned family size
  - Loss of geographical mobility
  - Decreased opportunities for siblings
  - Loss of family integrity
  - Social isolation
  - Lifestyle alterations
  - Reduction in contribution to their community by families
  - Disruption of husband-wife or partner relationship
  - Threatened family self-concept
  - Genetically affected persons are considered less than human being in society
  - Altered family process
  - Altered marriage and reproductive implications (infertility, abortions, defective child birth)
  - Prenatal conflicts (whether to get pregnant or not, whether to continue pregnancy or not)
  - Disruption in parent-child relationship
  - Marriage partner selection problems
  - Guilt regarding putting child in long-term care facilities
  - Difficult child rearing
  - Housing and living arrangement changes

  - Cultural impact includes that genetic screening are not allowed in certain cultures, people perceive genetic conditions a punishment of god for bad deeds.
- *Economic Impact:* The impact of burden of genetic conditions is more than just financial costs. Financial costs to the family may occur in subtle ways. These include costs of special diet, day care, household help, housing adaptations, buying special equipments and clothing and travel. If the family is not in large city, travel to major medical facilities means more than just expenses of transportation. Major economic impacts are:
  - Cost of genetic testing and screening
  - Cost of long-term genetic therapies and repeated surgeries and transfusions
  - Cost of institutionalization or long-term home of community care
  - Cost of bearing additional burden and needs of other family members
  - Other additional costs of care including travel and stay in city of health care facility. Moreover, job leave of family member accompanying for diagnosis and treatment.
  - Loss of carrier opportunities and job flexibility
  - In addition nonproductive life, job discrimination, insurance discrimination and financial dependence on family.
- *Psychological impact:* Psychological reactions include shock, disbelief, denial, guilt, grieving, mourning, hostility, anger, anxiety, bargaining, resentment, shame, sorrow, self-pity, and eventually adaptation and adjustment are very common psychological responses of a family who is having a person with genetic disorder. As discussed above a family with genetically affected person may experience wide variety of emotional trauma, some of the emotional concerns include:
  - Loss of self-esteem
  - Altered self- concept
  - Hopelessness
  - Helplessness
  - Stress and emotional threat because of uncertainty of future
  - Loss of dream and aspirations
  - Coping with intolerant public attitudes

- *Physical and cognitive impact:* Genetic disorders are responsible to cause variety of physical and cognitive manifestations; to mention a few:
  - Physical health problems
  - Individual's inability to get equal opportunity to learn
  - Mental retardation
  - Misunderstanding regarding implications of carrier state

Factors Influencing the Impact of Genetic Conditions on Families

There are various factors, which influence the impact of genetic conditions on the family and the way in which they cope. There are factors for individual families. Some of them are as follows:

- *The size, structure and stage of the development cycle of the family:* Families in which there is only one child born with congenital defects after six or seven normal ones, may be less disrupted because there are more hands to help with all that needs to be done. In general the most successful in coping are homes in which both the parents are present and they have matured in their marriage or relationship. Couples who have an affected first child early in their marriage have not yet developed their own interrelationships before having to cope with additional burden. The age of other children also determines family function. The sex of the affected children is also relevant. There is some evidence to show that father may have more difficulty in coping with severely affected sons.
- *Religious, ethnic and cultural beliefs and practices:* Some couples believe that a child who is mentally retarded or physically affected has been sent to them a special gift from God. Others, on such a discovery curse God and lose faith. If strong faith is present that comfort to family. It is also useful to know the cultural aspect of disease, disability, healing the body and death and how the individual's belief is to influence or be influenced by life event.
- *Availability of and relationship with extended family members or close friends:* Having many relatives available may mean more helping hands and loving support, if the relationships are positive ones. Sometimes friends may fill the gap of relatives.

- *The prior status of the relationship between parents:* It appears that those who had a satisfactory marital relationship prior to the genetic problem have the best chance of remaining intact.
- *Coping resources both tangible and intangibles:* Some communities are able to form a network that provides loving support for families. Some individuals learn to draw on deep resources that they did not realize they possessed. The nurse should make every effort to identify and mobilize support from parents group, private, public, government agencies and foundations.
- *The visibility and severity of the disorder and its meaning to the family:* In certain groups, superstitions associated with particular defect may cause the avoidance and rejection of the individual and family. Certain disorders have become more accepted than others, through the media and through the appearance of the affected person. Family may have more tolerance for a cute little girl with braces on her legs than for an 18 years adolescent who is mentally retarded and cannot control motion or drooling. Hidden disorders, such as congenital heart defects may cause burdens in the way of finances, care and concern but not in appearance. Craniofacial anomalies until they can be corrected may cause suffering that is related to the reaction of others. Many societies equate beauty with goodness and ugliness with evil. The meaning of the disorders to each parent should be explored, often separately.
- *Variable relating to individual family* members including personalities, past experience, view of roles, attitude toward child rearing, education, etc.
- *How the family function together and has dealt with previous crisis:* This ability may be assessed by observation, interview or the use of tools, such as the family APGAR or parenting stress Index.
- *The lifestyle and plans of the family:* A family who travel and couple extensively may have to modify such plans. If they have a child who cannot walk or who requires special food that cannot last for a long-time on trip. They can be helped to plan and modify activities in a way that may include everyone.
- *Other attributes of the disorders:* This includes the severity of the disease, its natural history, age of onset, type and frequency of treatment, the necessary for surgery or repeated hospitalization and the long-term outlook so that future planning can occur.

Role of Nurses in Managing the Impact of Genetic Conditions on Families

Nurse need to remember that the discovery of genetic disorder or anomaly is a shattering experience for a family. It can permanently and abruptly alter the life plans of a family. Nurses can promote an effective coping among family with following interventions:

- Recognize that different people cope with such a shock in different ways. Resist labeling parents as noncaring, rejecting, etc.
- Do not inject personal biases.
- Build a trusting and permissive atmosphere.
- Emphasize the legitimacy of parents feeling.
- Work with the family in identifying family strength, support, limitations and other concerns, such as time, financial obligations and other children.
- Build family strength.
- Raise the issues of pre-birth expectations and how these may be related to present feelings, the mother may need to verbally relive the pregnancy before she can go on.
- Identify willingness and ability of parents to cope.
- Special care procedure, such as moving the child with osteogenesis imperfecta or feeding the infant with cleft palate should be taught, help in such situation brings success in such endeavors helps to boost parents self-confidence, shows them that they can cope and gives them same sense of self-worth.
- Recognize that the emotions they are experiencing are exhausting and disorganizing. Decision-making may be difficult and may need to be postponed
- Observe and record the interaction of parents with each other and with child, family communication pattern, their concern, their needs, so that nursing plans and interventions are not repeated but are built on what have occurred previously.
- Help the father and mother to maintain open communication and plan for their role at home. Before discharge help parents, plan for what supplies and equipments will be needed and where they can be obtained.
- Ascertain the support system available to the family.
- Contact patient groups of person with similar affected children. These provide various type of assistance, from financial to

equipments, to telephone crisis lines, to friendly listening and sharing, to coping measures, to hospital visiting and more.

- Work with parents to plan a timetable that includes needs of normal sibling and for parents, tension-reducing activities.
- Often provide opportunities to ask questions and voice concern.
- Follow-up care and regularly scheduled session with the care coordinator is essential before parents leave the hospital.
- Obtain information and refer parents to respective advanced care facilities and programs.
- Plan for follow-up should include counseling for grief resolution, marital and family relationships, reproductive options discussion and genetic counseling.
- Help parents and family to rebuild self-esteem and feel that they are human beings worthy of being linked.
- Make it clear to family that you are willing to listen and talk and be sure that you are willing when called on.
- If the parents have not raised the issue, the nurse should ask the parents, if they have considered discussing the newly diagnosed disorder with others in family and outside.
- Be aware of some of the signs of successful adjustment, an intact family, the resumption of sexual relationship between partners, appropriate plans for future reproduction in light of genetic counseling and family goal, ability to help other parents, realistic plans for management of the affected child, retention of the family health practitioner and ability to relate to others are some measures that can be used.
- Remember to ask the parents how are they doing. This will give them feeling of concerned.

REVIEW OF CELLULAR DIVISION

Cell division is a process by which a cell, called the parent cell, divides into two or more cells, called *daughter cells*. Cell division is usually a small segment of a larger cell cycle. This type of cell division in eukaryotes is known as mitosis, and leaves the daughter cell capable of dividing again. The primary concern of cell division is the maintenance of the original cell's genome. Before division can occur, the genomic information which is stored in chromosomes must be replicated, and the duplicated genome separated cleanly between cells. A great deal of cellular infrastructure is involved in keeping genomic information consistent between 'generations'.

In another type of cell division present only in eukaryotes, called meiosis, a cell is permanently transformed into a gamete and cannot divide again until fertilization. As the cell division is the part of the cell cycle; where cell grow and divide. Therefore, it is wise to first understand about the cell cycle.

Cell Cycle

The cell cycle consists of four distinct phases: G1 phase, S phase, G2 phase (collectively known as interphase) and M phase. M phase is itself composed of two tightly coupled processes: mitosis, in which the cell's chromosomes are divided between the two daughter cells, and cytokinesis, in which the cell's cytoplasm divides forming distinct cells. Activation of each phase is dependent on the proper progression and completion of the previous one. Cells that have temporarily or reversibly stopped dividing are said to have entered a state of quiescence called G_0 phase (Fig. 1.2).

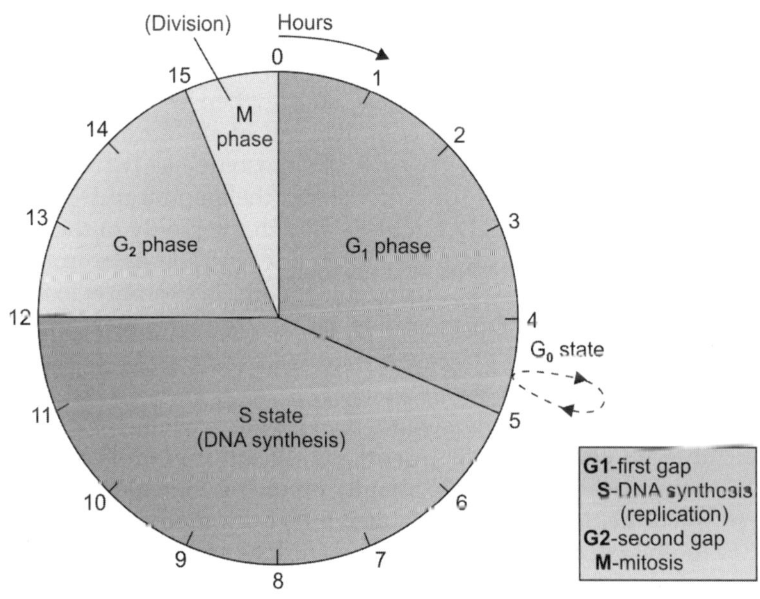

Fig. 1.2: Schematic presentation of the cell cycle

M Phase

The relatively brief M phase consists of nuclear division (mitosis) and cytoplasmic division (cytokinesis). Mitosis divides genetic information during cell division.

Interphase

After M phase, the daughter cells begin interphase of a new cycle. Although the various stages of interphase are not usually morphologically distinguishable, each phase of the cell cycle has a distinct set of specialized biochemical processes that prepare the cell for initiation of cell division. Interphase is a phase of the cell cycle, which includes:

- *G_1 Phase:* The first phase within interphase, from the end of the previous M phase till the beginning of DNA synthesis is called G1 (G indicating *gap* or *growth*). During this phase the biosynthetic activities of the cell, which had been considerably slowed down during M phase, resume at a high rate. This phase is marked by synthesis of various enzymes that are required in S phase, mainly those needed for DNA replication. Duration of G_1 is highly variable, even among different cells of the same species. The G_1 phase is a period in the cell cycle during interphase, after cytokinesis and before the S phase.
- *S Phase:* The ensuing S phase starts when DNA synthesis commences; when it is complete, all of the chromosomes have been replicated, i.e. each chromosome has two (sister) chromatids. Thus, during this phase, the amount of DNA in the cell has effectively doubled, though the ploidy of the cell remains the same. Rates of RNA transcription and protein synthesis are very low during this phase. An exception to this is histone production, most of which occurs during the S phase. The duration of S phase is relatively constant among cells of the same species.
- *G_2 Phase:* The cell then enters the G_2 phase, which lasts until the cell enters mitosis. Again, significant protein synthesis occurs during this phase, mainly involving the production of microtubules, which are required during the process of mitosis. Inhibition of protein synthesis during G_2 phase prevents the cell from undergoing mitosis. G_2 phase is a the 3rd and final subphase in interphase of the cell cycle.

G_0 Phase

The term 'postmitotic' is sometimes used to refer to both quiescent and senescent cells. Nonproliferative cells in multicellular eukaryotes generally enter the quiescent G_0 state from G_1 and may remain quiescent for long periods of time, possibly indefinitely (as is often the case for neurons). This is very common for cells that are fully differentiated. Cellular senescence is a state that occurs in response to DNA damage or degradation that would make a cell's progeny nonviable; it is often a biochemical alternative to the self-destruction of such a damaged cell by apoptosis. Some cell types in mature organisms, such as parenchymal cells of the liver and kidney, enter the G_0 phase semi-permanently and can only be induced to begin dividing again under very specific circumstances; other types, such as epithelial cells, continue to divide throughout an organism's life.

Considering the cell cycle in its entirely, the sequence of event is (Fig. 1.3):

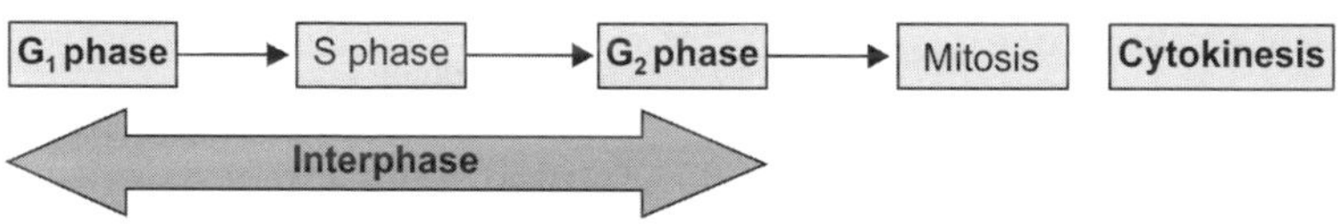

Fig 1.3: Events of cycle in somatic cell

Mitosis

Mitosis is the process in which a eukaryotic cell separates the chromosomes in its cell nucleus, into two identical sets in two daughter nuclei (Fig. 1.4). It is generally followed immediately by cytokinesis, which divides the nuclei, cytoplasm, organelles and cell membrane into two daughter cells containing roughly equal shares of these cellular components. Mitosis and cytokinesis together define the *mitotic (M) phase* of the cell cycle—the division of the mother cell into two daughter cells, genetically identical to each other and to their parent cell.

Mitosis occurs exclusively in eukaryotic cells, but occurs in different ways in different species. The process of mitosis is complex and highly regulated. The sequence of events is divided into phases, corresponding to the completion of one set of activities and the start of the next. These stages are prophase, prometaphase, metaphase, anaphase and telophase. During the process of mitosis the pairs of chromosomes condense and attach to fibers that pull the sister chromatids to opposite sides of the cell. The cell then divides in cytokinesis, to produce two identical daughter cells.

Because cytokinesis usually occurs in conjunction with mitosis, 'mitosis' is often used interchangeably with 'mitotic phase'. Errors in mitosis can either kill a cell through apoptosis or cause mutations that may lead to cancer.

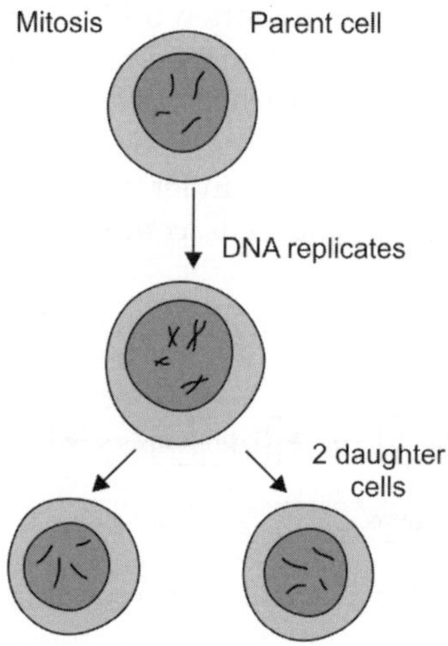

Fig 1.4: Mitosis

Phases of Mitosis

The mitotic phase is a relatively short period of the cell cycle. It alternates with the much longer *interphase*, where the cell prepares itself for cell division. Interphase is therefore not part of mitosis. Interphase is divided into three phases, G_1 (first gap), S (synthesis), and G_2 (second gap). During all three phases, the cell grows by producing proteins and cytoplasmic organelles. However, chromosomes are replicated only during the S phase. Thus, a cell grows (G_1), continues to grow as it duplicates its chromosomes (S), grows more and prepares for mitosis (G_2), and divides (M).

- *Prophase:* It is the first stage of mitosis. During early prophase, the chromatin fibers condense and shortened into chromosome that are visible under the light microscope. The condensation process may prevent entangling of the long DNA strands as they move during mitosis. Because DNA replication took place during the S phase of interphase, each prophase chromosome consists of a pair of identical, double-stranded chromatids. A constricted region called a centromere holds the chromatid pair together. At the outside of each centromere is a protein complex known as the *kinetochore*. Later in prophase, tubulins in the pericentriolar material of the centrosomes start to form the mitotic spindle, a football-shaped assembly of microtubules lengthen, they push the centrosomes to the poles (end) of the cell so that the spindle extends from pole to pole. The spindle is responsible for the separation of chromatids to opposite poles of the cell. Then, the nucleous disappears and the nuclear envelop breaks down (Fig. 1.5).

Schematic diagram	Brief description
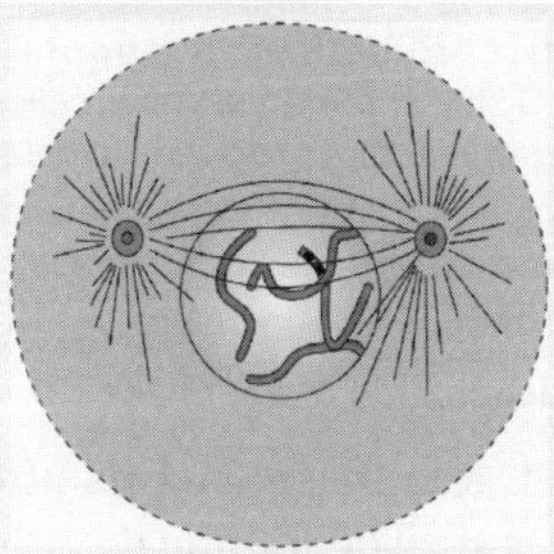	• The chromosomes condense and become visible • The centrioles form and move toward opposite ends of the cell ('the poles') • The nucleoli and nuclear membrane disappear • The mitotic spindle forms (from the centrioles in cells) • Spindle fibers from each centriole attach to each sister chromatid at the kinetochore.

Fig. 1.5: Schematic diagram and brief description of prophase

- *Metaphase:* During metaphase, the kinetochore microtubules align the centromeres of the chromatid pair at the exact center of the mitotic spindle. This midpoint region in called the metaphase plate (Fig. 1.6).

Schematic diagram	Brief description
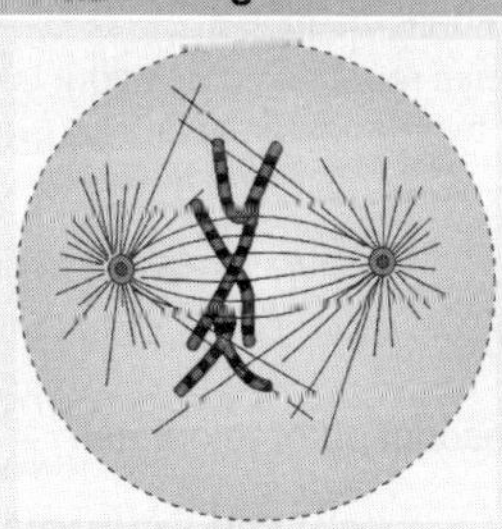	• The centrioles complete their migration to the poles • The chromosomes align across the equator of the spindle fiber (middle of the cell) at its centromere.

Fig. 1.6: Schematic diagram and brief description of metaphase

- *Anaphase:* During anaphase, the centromeres split, separating the two members of each chromatid pair, which move toward opposite poles of the cell (Fig. 1.7). Once separated, the chromatids are termed as chromosomes. As the chromosomes are pulled by the kinetochore microtubules lead the way, dragging the trailing arms of the chromosomes towards the pole.

Schematic diagram	Brief description
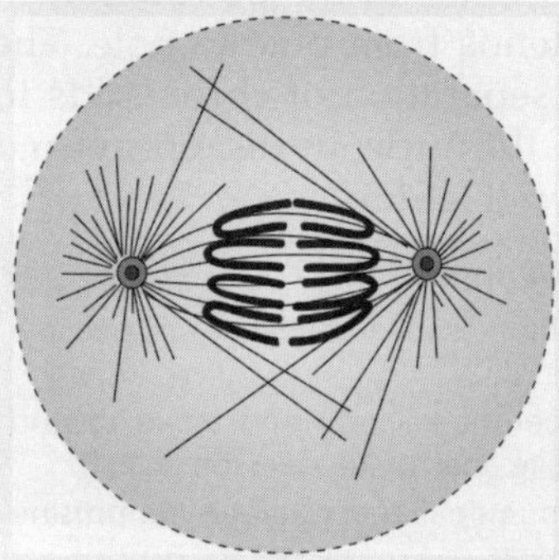	• Spindles attached to kinetochores begin to shorten • This exerts a force on the sister chromatids that pulls them apart. Each centromere splits, thereby detaching two chromatids • Spindle fibers continue to shorten, pulling chromatids to opposite poles. Sister chromatids (now called chromosomes) move to opposite poles • This ensures that each daughter cell gets identical sets of chromosomes.

Fig. 1.7: Schematic diagram and brief description of anaphase

- *Telophase:* The final stage of mitosis, telophase, begins after chromosomal movement stops (Fig. 1.8). The identical sets of chromosomes now at opposite poles of the cell, unicoil and forms around each chromatin mass, nucleoli reappear in the daughter nuclei and the mitotic spindle disappears.

Schematic diagram	Brief description
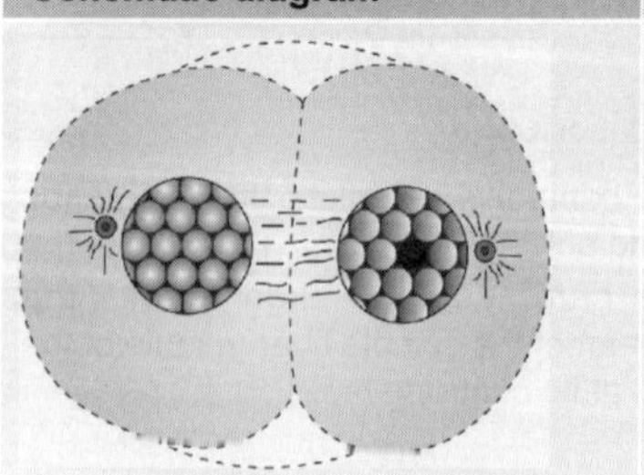	• The chromosomes decondense • The nuclear envelope forms • Spindle fibers disappear • Cytokinesis reaches completion, creating two daughter cells.

Fig. 1.8: Schematic diagram and brief description of telophase

Cytoplasmic division/Cytokinesis: Division of a parent cell's cytoplasm and organelles into two daughter cells is called *cytokinesis*. This process begins in late anaphase or early telophase with formation of a cleavage furrow, a slight indention of the plasma membrane. The cleavage furrow usually appears midway because the centrosomes extends around the periphery of the cell (Fig. 1.9). Actin microfilaments that lie just inside the plasma membrane progressively inward. The ring constructs the center of the cell, like tightening a belt around the waist and ultimately pinches it in two. Because the plane of the cleavage furrow is always perpendicular to the mitotic spindle, the two sets of chromosomes end up in separate daughter cells. When cytokinesis is complete, interphase begins.

Schematic diagram	Brief description
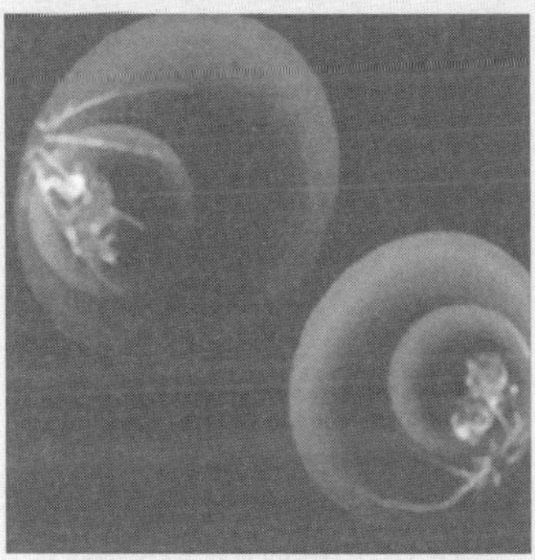	• First, a cleavage furrow appears – Cleavage furrow = shallow groove near the location of the old metaphase plate • A contractile ring of actin microfilaments in association with myosin, a protein – Actin and myosin are also involved in muscle contraction and other movement functions • The contraction of a the dividing cell's ring of microfilaments is like the pulling of drawstrings – The cell is pinched in two.

Fig. 1.9: Schematic diagram and brief description of cytokinesis

Meiosis

In biology or life science, ***meiosis*** (pronounced my-oh-sis) is a process of reductional division in which the number of chromosomes per cell is cut in half. In animals, meiosis always results in the formation of gametes (Fig. 1.10).

During meiosis, the genome of a diploid germ cell, which is composed of long segments of DNA packaged into chromosomes, undergoes DNA replication followed by two rounds of division, resulting in four haploid cells. Each of these cells contain one complete set of chromosomes, or half of the genetic content of the original cell. If meiosis produces gametes, these cells must fuse during fertilization to create a new diploid cell, or zygote before any new growth can occur. Thus, the division mechanism of meiosis is a reciprocal process to the joining of two genomes that

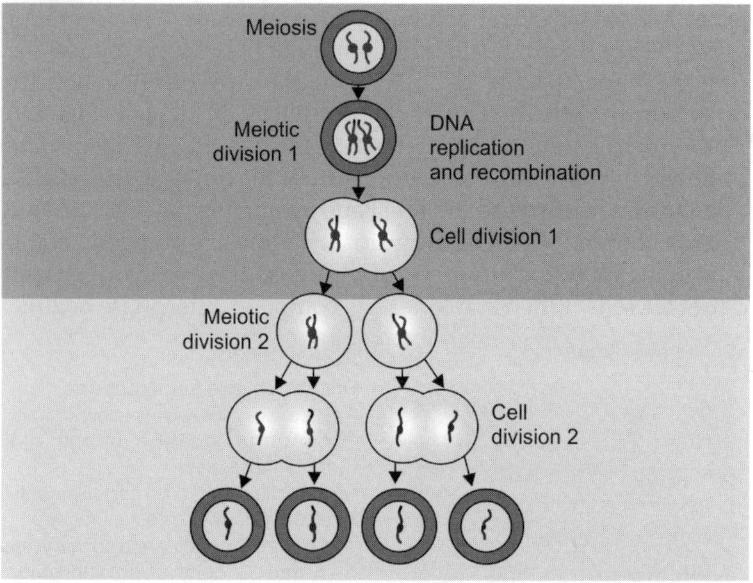

Fig. 1.10: Meiosis

occurs at fertilization. Because the chromosomes of each parent undergo genetic recombination during meiosis, each gamete, and thus each zygote, will have a unique genetic *blueprint* encoded in its DNA. Together, meiosis and fertilization constitute sexuality in the eukaryotes, and generate genetically distinct individuals in populations.

Meiosis uses many of the same biochemical mechanisms employed during mitosis to accomplish the redistribution of chromosomes. There are several features unique to meiosis, most importantly the pairing and genetic recombination between homologous chromosomes.

Process

Because meiosis is a 'one-way' process, it cannot be said to engage in a cell cycle as mitosis does. However, the preparatory steps that lead up to meiosis are identical in pattern and name to the interphase of the mitotic cell cycle.

Interphase is divided into three phases:

1. *Gap 1 (G_1) phase:* This is a very active period, where the cell synthesizes its vast array of proteins, including the enzymes

and structural proteins it will need for growth. In G1 stage each of the chromosomes consists of a single (very long) molecule of DNA. In humans, at this point cells are *46 chromosomes, 2N,* identical to somatic cells.

2. *Synthesis (S) phase:* The genetic material is replicated: Each of its chromosomes duplicates, producing 46 chromosomes each made-up of two sister chromatids. The cell is still considered diploid because it still contains the same number of centromeres. The identical sister chromatids have not yet condensed into the densely packaged chromosomes visible with the light microscope. This will take place during prophase I in meiosis.
3. *Gap 2 (G_2) phase:* G2 phase is absent in Meiosis. *Interphase* is followed by meiosis I and then meiosis II. Meiosis I consists of separating the pairs of homologous chromosome, each made-up of two sister chromatids, into two cells. One entire haploid content of chromosomes is contained in each of the resulting daughter cells; the first meiotic division therefore reduces the ploidy of the original cell by a factor of 2. Meiosis II consists of decoupling each chromosome's sister strands (chromatids), and segregating the individual chromatids into haploid daughter cells. The two cells resulting from meiosis I divide during meiosis II, creating 4 haploid daughter cells. Meiosis I and II are each divided into prophase, metaphase, anaphase, and telophase stages, similar in purpose to their analogous subphases in the mitotic cell cycle. Therefore, meiosis includes the stages of meiosis I (prophase I, metaphase I, anaphase I, telophase I), and meiosis II (prophase II, metaphase II, anaphase II, telophase II).

Meiosis generates genetic diversity in two ways: (1) independent alignment and subsequent separation of homologous chromosome pairs during the first meiotic division allows a random and independent selection of each chromosome segregates into each gamete; and (2) physical exchange of homologous chromosomal regions by recombination during prophase I results in new genetic combinations within chromosomes.

Meiosis Phases

Meiosis I: In meiosis I, the homologous pairs in a diploid cell separate, producing two haploid cells *(23 chromosomes, N* in humans), so meiosis I is referred to as a *reductional division.* A regular diploid human cell contains 46 chromosomes and is considered 2N because it contains 23 pairs of homologous chromosomes. However, after meiosis I, although the cell contains 46 chromosomes it is only considered N because later in anaphase I the sister chromatids will remain together as the spindle pulls the pair toward the pole of the new cell. In meiosis II, an *equational division* similar to mitosis will occur whereby the sister chromatids are finally split, creating a total of 4 haploid cells *(23 chromosomes, N)* per daughter cell from the first division.

Prophase I: Homologous chromosomes pair (or synapse) and crossing over (or recombination) occurs a step unique in meiosis. The paired and replicated chromosomes are called bivalents or tetrads, which have two chromosomes and four chromatids, with one chromosome coming from each parent. At this stage, non-sister chromatids may cross-over at points called chiasmata (plural; singular chiasma) (Fig. 1.11).

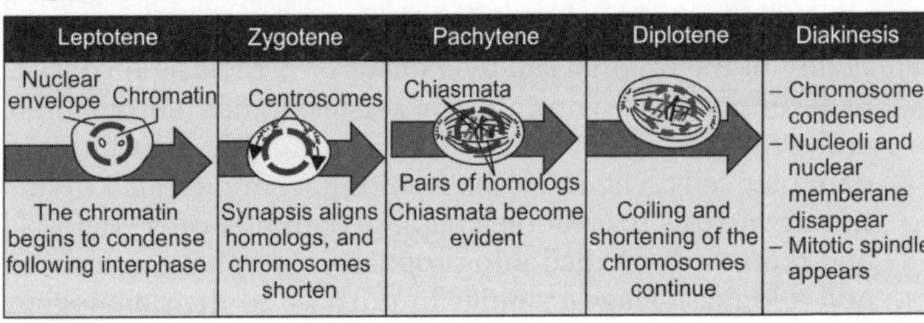

Fig. 1.11: Substages of prophase I

Leptotene: The first stage of prophase I is the *leptotene* stage, also known as *leptonema,* from Greek words meaning 'thin threads'. During this stage, individual chromosomes begin to condense into long strands within the nucleus. However the two sister chromatids are still so tightly bound that they are indistinguishable from one another. The chromosomes in the leptotene stage show a specific arrangement where the telomeres are oriented towards the nuclear membrane. Hence, this stage is called 'bouquet stage' (Fig. 1.11)

***Zygotene*:** The *zygotene* stage, also known as *zygonema,* from Greek words meaning 'paired threads'. We have seen that the 46 chromosomes in each cell consist of 23 pairs (the X and Y chromosomes of the male being taken pair). The two chromosomes of each comes to lie parallel to each other, and are closely apposed. This pairing chromosomes also reffered to as synopsis or conjugation. Two chromosomes together constitute a bivalent (Fig. 1.11).

Pachytene: The *pachytene* stage, also known as *pachynema,* from Greek words meaning 'thick threads', contains the following chromosomal crossover. The two chromatids of each chromosomes together become distinct. The biovalent now has four chromatids in it and is called a tetrad. There are two central and two peripheral chromatids, one from each chromosome. An important event now takes place. The two central chromatids (one belonging to each chromosome of the bivalent) become coiled over each other so that they cross at a number of points. This is called crossing over. At the site where the chromatids cross they become adherent; the point of adhesion are called chiasmata (Fig. 1.11).

Nonsister chromatids of homologous chromosomes randomly exchange segments of genetic information over regions of homology. (Sex chromosomes, however, are not wholly identical, and only exchange information over a small region of homology.) Exchange takes place at sites where *recombination nodules* (the aforementioned chiasmata) have formed (Fig. 1.12). The exchange of information between the non-sister chromatids results in a recombination of information; each chromosome has the complete set of information it had before, and there are no gaps formed as a result of the process. Because the chromosomes cannot be distinguished in the synaptonemal complex, the actual act of crossing over is not perceivable through the microscope.

Diplotene: During the *diplotene* stage, also known as *diplonema,* from Greek words meaning 'two threads', the synaptonemal complex degrades and homologous chromosomes separate from one another a little. The chromosomes themselves uncoil a bit, allowing some transcription of DNA. However, the homologous chromosomes of each bivalent remain tightly bound at chiasmata, the regions where crossing-over occurred. The chiasmata remain on the chromosomes until they are severed in Anaphase I (Fig. 1.13).

In human fetal oogenesis all developing oocytes develop to this stage and stop before birth. This suspended state is referred to as

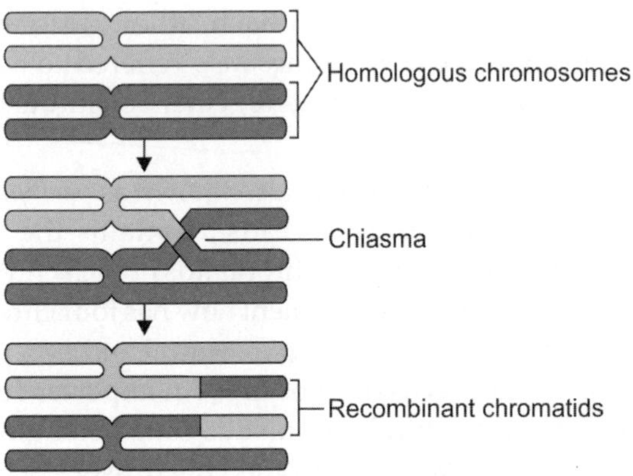

Fig. 1.12: Crossing-over (Recombination)

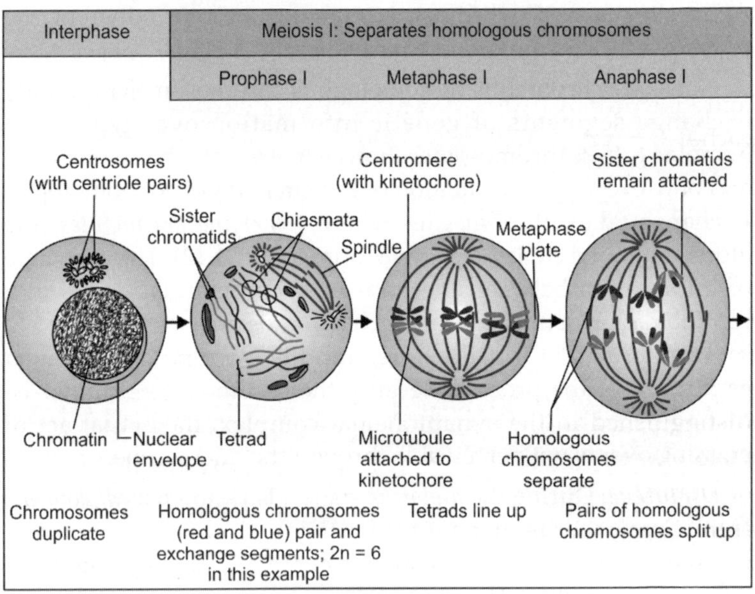

Fig. 1.13: Meiosis I

the *dictyotene stage* and remains so until puberty. In males, only spermatogonia exist until meiosis begins at puberty.

Diakinesis: Chromosomes condense further during the *diakinesis* stage, from Greek words meaning 'moving through'. This is the first point in meiosis where the four parts of the tetrads are actually visible. Sites of crossing over entangle together, effectively overlapping, making chiasmata clearly visible. Other than this observation, the rest of the stage closely resembles prometaphase of mitosis; the nucleoli disappear, the nuclear membrane disintegrates into vesicles, and the meiotic spindle begins to form (Fig. 1.11).

Synchronous Processes

During these stages, two centrosomes, containing a pair of centrioles in animal cells, migrate to the two poles of the cell. These centrosomes, which were duplicated during S-phase, function as microtubule organizing centers nucleating microtubules, which are essentially cellular ropes and poles. The microtubules invade the nuclear region after the nuclear envelope disintegrates, attaching to the chromosomes at the kinetochore. The kinetochore functions as a motor, pulling the chromosome along the attached microtubule toward the originating centriole, like a train on a track. There are four kinetochores on each tetrad, but the pair of kinetochores on each sister chromatid fuses and functions as a unit during meiosis I.

Microtubules that attach to the kinetochores are known as *kinetochore microtubules*. Other microtubules will interact with microtubules from the opposite centriole: these are called *nonkinetochore microtubules* or *polar microtubules*. A third type of microtubules, the aster microtubules, radiates from the centrosome into the cytoplasm or contacts components of the membrane skeleton.

Metaphase I: Homologous pairs move together along the metaphase plate: As *kinetochore microtubules* from both centrioles attach to their respective kinetochores, the homologous chromosomes align along an equatorial plane that bisects the spindle, due to continuous counterbalancing forces exerted on the bivalents by the microtubules emanating from the two kinetochores of homologous chromosomes. The physical basis of the independent assortment of chromosomes is the random orientation of each bivalent along the metaphase plate, with respect to the orientation of the other bivalents along the same equatorial line.

Anaphase I: Kinetochore microtubules shorten, severing the recombination nodules and pulling homologous chromosomes apart. Since each chromosome has only one functional unit of a pair of kinetochores, whole chromosomes are pulled toward opposing poles, forming two haploid sets. Each chromosome still contains a pair of sister chromatids. Nonkinetochore microtubules lengthen, pushing the centrioles farther apart. The cell elongates in preparation for division down the center.

Telophase I: The last meiotic division effectively ends when the chromosomes arrive at the poles. Each daughter cell now has half the number of chromosomes but each chromosome consists of a pair of chromatids. The microtubules that make-up the spindle network disappear, and a new nuclear membrane surrounds each haploid set. The chromosomes uncoil back into chromatin. Cytokinesis, the pinching of the cell membrane in animal cells or the formation of the cell wall in plant cells, occurs, completing the creation of two daughter cells. Sister chromatids remain attached during telophase I.

Cells may enter a period of rest known as interkinesis or interphase II. No DNA replication occurs during this stage.

Meiosis II

Meiosis II is the second part of the meiotic process. Much of the process is similar to mitosis (Fig. 1.14). The end result is production of four haploid cells (*23 chromosomes, 1N* in humans) from the two haploid cells (*23 chromosomes, 1N*, each of the chromosomes consisting of two sister chromatids) produced in meiosis I.

Prophase II takes an inversely proportional time compared to telophase I. In this prophase we see the disappearance of the nucleoli and the nuclear envelope again as well as the shortening and thickening of the chromatids. Centrioles move to the polar regions and arrange spindle fibers for the second meiotic division.

In **metaphase II**, the centromeres contain two kinetochores, that attach to spindle fibers from the centrosomes (centrioles) at each pole. The new equatorial metaphase plate is rotated by 90 degrees when compared to meiosis I, perpendicular to the previous plate.

This is followed by **anaphase II**, where the centromeres are cleaved, allowing microtubules attached to the kinetochores to pull the sister chromatids apart. The sister chromatids by convention

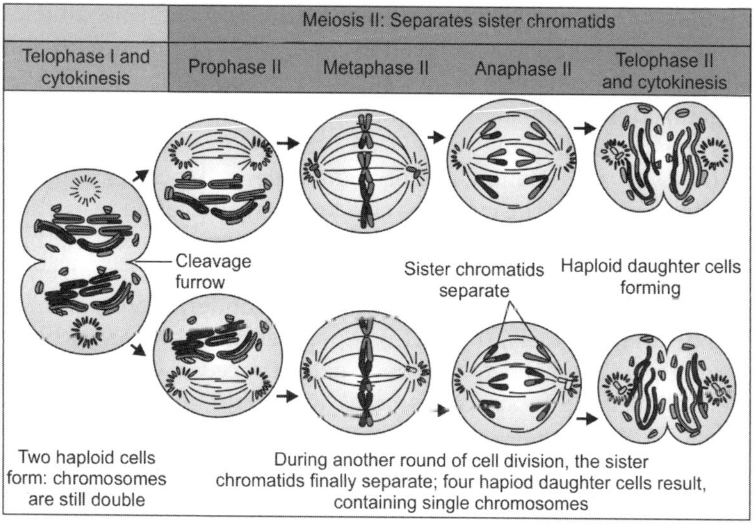

Fig. 1.14: Meiosis II

Table 1.1: Comparison of mitosis and meiosis

Mitosis	Meiosis
Function is for growth and repair	Function is for gamete formation
Happens in most somatic cells	Happens in testes and ovary to form gametes
Proceeded by replication of chromosomes	Proceeded by replication of chromosomes
Has one cell division	Has two cell divisions
Result in two diploid daughter cells	Results in four haploid daughter cells
Daughter cells chromosome number is same as parent cell (2N, diploid)	Daughter cells chromosome number is half of the parent cell (N, haploid)
Daughter cells normally genetically identical	Daughter cells are genetically not the same

are now called sister chromosomes as they move toward opposing poles.

The process ends with **telophase II**, which is similar to telophase I, and is marked by uncoiling and lengthening of the chromosomes and the disappearance of the spindle. Nuclear envelopes reform and cleavage or cell wall formation eventually produces a total of four daughter cells, each with a haploid set of chromosomes. Meiosis is now complete.

Regulation of Cell Division and Growth

A variety of genes are involved in the control of cell growth and division. The cell cycle is the cell's way of replicating itself in an organized, step-by-step fashion. Tight regulation of this process ensures that a dividing cell's DNA is copied properly, any errors in the DNA are repaired, and each daughter cell receives a full set of chromosomes. The cycle has checkpoints (also called restriction points), which allow certain genes to check for mistakes and halt the cycle for repairs if something goes wrong. If a cell has an error in its DNA that cannot be repaired, it may undergo programmed cell death (apoptosis) (Fig. 1.15). Apoptosis is a common process throughout life that helps the body get rid of cells it does not need. Cells that undergo apoptosis break apart and are recycled by a type of white blood cell called a macrophage (Fig. 1.16). Apoptosis protects the body by removing genetically damaged cells that could lead to cancer, and it plays an important role in the development of the embryo and the maintenance of adult tissues.

Cancer results from a disruption of the normal regulation of the cell cycle. When the cycle proceeds without control, cells can divide without order and accumulate genetic defects that can lead to a cancerous tumor. In nutshell we can say cancer results when cells accumulate genetic errors and multiply without control.

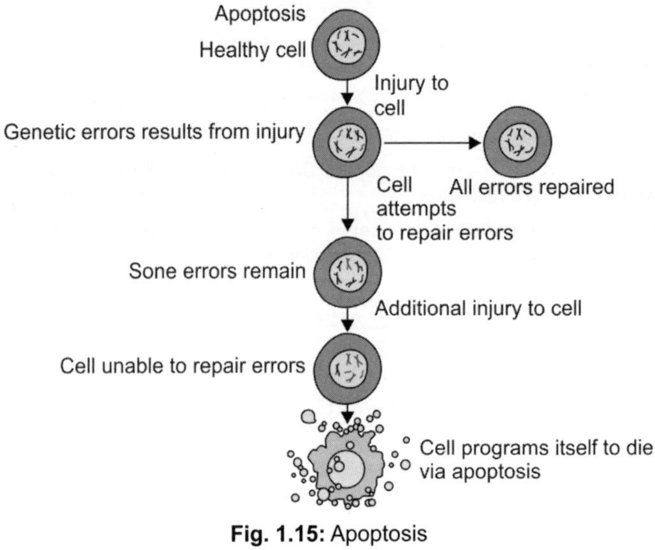

Fig. 1.15: Apoptosis

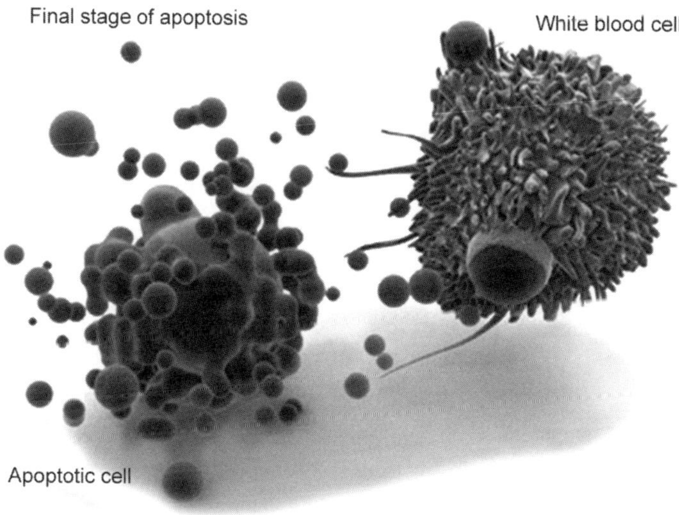

Fig. 1.16: Macrophage activity

CHARACTERISTICS AND STRUCTURE OF GENES

The term gene was introduced by Johanssen in 1909. Prior to him Mendel had used the word factor for a specific, distinct, particular unit of inheritance that takes part in expression of a trait. *Johanssen has defined gene, as an elementary unit of inheritance, which can be assigned to a particular trait.* Morgan's work suggested gene to be the shortest segment of chromosome, which can be separated through crossing over, can be undergo mutation and influence expression of one or more traits.

Presently, *a gene is defined as a unit of inheritance composed of a segment of DNA or chromosome situated at a specific locus (Gene locus), which carries coded information associated with a specific function and can undergo crossing over as well as mutation* (Fig. 1.17). Some of the specific features of genes are:

- A specific portion of the DNA code is called a *gene*, which has genetic information.
- The term gene is often used to refer genetic material on a chromosome that code for a trait. For example, one person has a gene for hair color.
- A unit of genetic material, which is able to replicate.

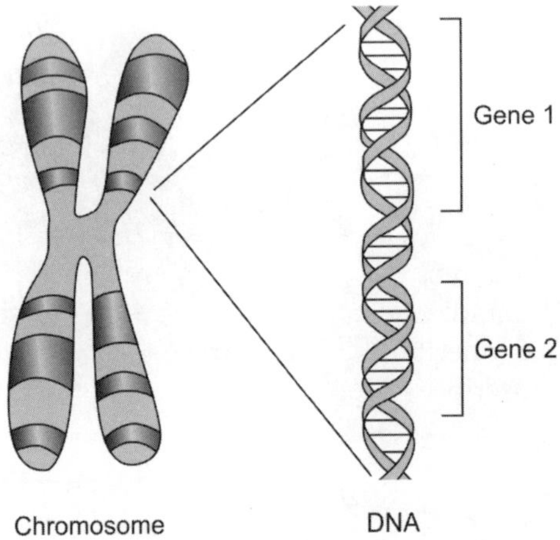

Genes

Fig. 1.17: Structure of gene
(Genes are made-up of DNA. Each chromosome contains many genes.)

- It is a unit of recombination or capable of undergoing crossover.
- A unit of genetic material, which can undergo mutation.
- A unit of heredity connected with somatic structure or function that leads to a phenotype expression.
- *A* gene is the basic physical and functional unit of heredity.
- Genes, which are made-up of DNA, act as RNA instructor to make molecules called proteins.
- In humans, genes vary in size from a few hundred DNA bases to more than 2 million bases. The Human Genome Project has estimated that humans have between 20,000 and 25,000 genes.
- Every person has two copies of each gene, one inherited from each parent. Most genes are the same in all people, but a small number of genes (less than 1 percent of the total) are slightly different between people. Alleles are forms of the same gene with small differences in their sequence of DNA bases. These small differences contribute to each person's unique physical features.
- Genes consists of a long strand of DNA that contain promoter, which control the activity of a gene and coding and non-coding sequence.

- Gene coding sequence determines what will be the produce, while non-coding sequence can regulate the conditions of gene expression.
- When gene is active, the coding and non-coding sequence is copied in a process called transcription, producing an RNA copy of the gene's information. This RNA can then direct the synthesis of protein via genetic code. These RNA or proteins are know as gene products.
- Gene is a locatable region of genomic sequence, corresponding to a unit of inheritance, which is associated with regulatory region, transcribed region and/or other functional sequence regions.
- A gene is a union of genomic sequences encoding a coherent set of potentially overlapping functional products.
- The physical development and phenotype of a person can be thought of as a product of genes interacting with each other and with environment.
- Total set of genes in a person are known as genome.
- Genes is basically an instruction for human body. Each gene has a specific purpose and every single function of the human body is coded in one or more genes.
- A person's unique genetic constitutes called the genotype are made-up of about 30,000 to 40,000 genes.
- A person's phenotype, the observable characteristics of his or her genotype, includes the physical appearance and other biological, physiological and molecular traits.

Types of Genes

- *Constitutive Genes:* Genes which are constantly expressing themselves in a cell because their products are required for the normal cellular activities, e.g. gene for glycolysis, ATP-ase.
- *Non-constitutive genes (Luxury genes):* The genes are not always expressing themselves in a cell. They are switched on or off according to the requirement of cellular activities, e.g. genes for lactose system in *Escherichia coli*. They are further classified as inducible and repressible.
- *Inducible genes:* The genes are switched on in response to the presence of a chemical substance or inducer, which is required for functioning of the product of gene activity.

- *Repressive genes*: They are those genes which continue to express themselves till a chemical inhibits or represses their activity.
- *Multigenes:* It is a group of similar or nearly similar genes for meeting requirements of time and tissue specific products.
- *Repeated genes*: The genes which are present in multiple copies, e.g. histone genes, tRNA genes, rRNA genes, actin genes.
- *Single copy genes:* The genes are present in single copy.
- *Pseudogenes:* Genes, which have homology to sfunctional genes but are unable to produce functional products due to intervening nonsense codons, inactivation of promoter genes, e.g. several snRNA genes.
- *Split genes:* Split genes are those genes, which possess extra or nonessential region interspersed with essential or coding part.
- *Jumping genes (Transposons):* They are segments of DNA that can jump or move from one place in the genome to another.
- *Overlapping genes:* Genes those overlap other genes.
- *Structural genes:* Structural genes are those genes, which have encoded information for the synthesis of chemical substance (polypeptides for synthesis of structural and transport proteins, enzymes, hormones, several other proteins and no translated and noncoding RNAs) required for cellular machinery.
- *Regulatory genes:* Regulatory genes do not transcribe RNAs and, therefore, produce no chemicals. They are meant to controlling the function of structural genes.
- *Mitochondrial genes:* The cell nucleus is not the only site where DNA and genes are present. In human, they are also present in mitochondria. The mitochondria are bodies located in cell cytoplasm that are concerned with energy production and metabolism and are thus known as the 'Power Plant' of the cell. One of the function of the Mitochondrial Oxidative Phosphorylation System (OXPHOS) is to generate adenosine triphosphate (ATP) for cell energy. Cell contains hundreds of mitochondria (mt) and each mitochondrium can contain upon 10 copies of mtDNA meaning that thousands of copies of mtDNA are present in some cells. The amount of DNA present in mitochondria is far less than in the nucleus. The mitochondrial genes are virtually only maternally transmitted, since sperm does not contain mitochondria. It is known that some genetic disorders are result of mtDNA mutation.

Functions of Genes

- Genes are components of genetic material and are thus unit of inheritance.
- They control the morphology or phenotype of individual.
- Replication of genes is essential for cell division.
- Genes carry the hereditary information from one generation to next.
- They control the structure and metabolism of the body.
- Reshuffling of genes at the time of sexual reproduction produce variation.
- Different linkages are produced due to crossing over.
- Genes undergo mutation and change their expression.
- New genes and consequently new traits develop due to reshuffling of different parts of genes.
- Genes change their expression due to position effect.
- Differentiation or formation of different type of cells, tissues and organs in various parts of the body is controlled by expression of certain genes and nonexpression of others.
- Development or production of different stages in the life history is controlled by genes.

Nucleic Acid

Any of a group of complex compounds found in all living cells and viruses, composed of purines, pyrimidines, carbohydrates, and phosphoric acid. Nucleic acids in the form of DNA and RNA control cellular function and heredity.

Deoxyribonucleic acid (DNA): It is a nucleic acid that contains the genetic instructions for the development and function of living things. All known cellular life and some viruses contain DNA. The main role of DNA in the cell is the long-term storage of information. It is often compared to a blueprint, since it contains the instructions to construct other components of the cell, such as proteins and RNA molecules. The DNA segments that carry genetic information are called *genes*, but other DNA sequences have structural purposes, or are involved in regulating the expression of genetic information.

In eukaryotes, such as animals and plants, DNA is stored inside the cell nucleus, while in prokaryotes, such as bacteria, the DNA is in the cell's cytoplasm. Unlike enzymes, DNA does not act directly on other molecules; rather, various enzymes act on DNA and copy its information into either more DNA, in DNA replication, or transcribe it into protein. In chromosomes, chromatin proteins, such as histones compact and organize DNA, as well as help in control of its interactions with other proteins in the nucleus.

DNA is a long polymer of simple units called nucleotides, which are held together by a backbone made of sugars and phosphate groups. This backbone carries four types of molecules called bases and it is the sequence of these four bases that encodes information. The major function of DNA is to encode the sequence of amino acid residues in proteins, using the genetic code. To read the genetic code, cells make a copy of a stretch of DNA in the nucleic acid RNA. These RNA copies can then be used to direct protein synthesis, but they can also be used directly as parts of ribosomes or spliceosomes.

Ribonucleic acid (RNA): It is a nucleic acid polymer consisting of nucleotide monomers. RNA nucleotides contain ribose rings and uracil unlike deoxyribonucleic acid (DNA), which contains deoxyribose and thymine. It is transcribed (synthesized) from DNA by enzymes called RNA polymerases and further processed by other enzymes. RNA serves as the template for translation of genes into proteins, transferring amino acids to the ribosome to form proteins, and also translating the transcript into proteins.

RNA is primarily made-up of four different bases: adenine, guanine, cytosine, and uracil. The first three are the same as those found in DNA, but in RNA thymine is replaced by uracil as the base complementary to adenine. This base is also a pyrimidine and is very similar to thymine. Uracil is energetically less expensive to produce than thymine, which may account for its use in RNA. In DNA, however, uracil is readily produced by chemical degradation of cytosine, so having thymine as the normal base makes detection and repair of such incipient mutations more efficient. Thus, uracil is appropriate for RNA, where quantity is important but lifespan is not, whereas thymine is appropriate for DNA where maintaining sequence with high fidelity is more critical.

There are also numerous modified bases and sugars found in RNA that serve many different roles. Pseudouridine (Ψ) and the DNA nucleoside thymidine are found in various places (most notably in the TΨC loop of every tRNA). Another notable modified base is Inosine (a deaminated Guanine base), which allows a 'wobble codon' sequence in tRNA. There are nearly 100 other naturally occurring modified bases, of which pseudouridine and 2′-O-methylribose are by far the most common. The specific roles of many of these modifications in RNA are not fully understood. However, it is notable that in ribosomal RNA, many of the post-translational modifications occur in highly functional regions, such as the peptidyl transferase center and the subunit interface, inferring that they are important for normal function. Single stranded RNA exhibits a right handed stacking pattern that is stabilized by base stacking.

The most important structural feature of RNA that distinguishes it from DNA is the presence of a hydroxyl group at the 2′-position of the ribose sugar. The presence of this functional group enforces the C3′-endo sugar conformation (as opposed to the C2′-endo conformation of the deoxyribose sugar in DNA) that causes the helix to adopt the A-form geometry rather than the B-form most commonly observed in DNA. This results in a very deep and narrow major groove and a shallow and wide minor groove. A second consequence of the presence of the 2′-hydroxyl group is that in conformationally flexible regions of an RNA molecule (that is, not involved in formation of a double helix), it can chemically attack the adjacent phosphodiester bond to cleave the backbone.

Biological Role of RNA

- *Messenger RNA (mRNA):* Messenger RNA is RNA that carries information from DNA to the ribosome sites of protein synthesis in the cell. Once mRNA has been transcribed from DNA, it is exported from the nucleus into the cytoplasm (in eukaryotes mRNA is 'processed' before being exported), where it is bound to ribosomes and translated into protein. After a certain amount of time the message degrades into its component nucleotides, usually with the assistance of RNA polymerases.
- *Transfer RNA (tRNA):* Transfer RNA is a small RNA chain of about 74–93 nucleotides that transfers a specific amino acid to a growing polypeptide chain at the ribosomal site of protein synthesis during translation. It has sites for amino acid

attachment and an anticodon region for codon recognition that binds to a specific sequence on the messenger RNA chain through hydrogen bonding. It is a type of non-coding RNA.

- *Ribosomal RNA (rRNA):* Ribosomal RNA is a component of the ribosomes, the protein synthetic factories in the cell. Eukaryotic ribosomes contain four different rRNA molecules: 18S, 5.8S, 28S, and 5S rRNA. Three of the rRNA molecules are synthesized in the nucleolus, and one is synthesized elsewhere. rRNA molecules are extremely abundant and make-up at least 80% of the RNA molecules found in a typical eukaryotic cell. In the cytoplasm, ribosomal RNA and protein combine to form a nucleoprotein called a ribosome. The ribosome binds mRNA and carries out protein synthesis. Several ribosomes may be attached to a single mRNA at anytime.
- *Non-coding RNA or RNA genes*: RNA genes (sometimes referred to as non-coding RNA or small RNA) are genes that encode RNA that is not translated into a protein. The most prominent examples of RNA genes are transfer RNA (tRNA) and ribosomal RNA (rRNA), both of which are involved in the process of translation. However, since the late 1990s, many new RNA genes have been found, and thus RNA genes may play a much more significant role than previously thought. In the late 1990s and early 2000, there has been persistent evidence of more complex transcription occurring in mammalian cells (and possibly others). This could point towards a more widespread use of RNA in biology, particularly in gene regulation. A particular class of non-coding RNA, micro RNA, has been found in many metazoans (from *Caenorhabditis elegans* to *Homo sapiens*) and clearly plays an important role in regulating other genes. First proposed in 2004 by Rassoulzadegan and published in Nature 2006, RNA is implicated as being part of the germline. If confirmed, this result would significantly alter the present understanding of genetics and lead to many question on DNA-RNA roles and interactions.
- *Catalytic RNA:* Although RNA contains only four bases, in comparison to the twenty amino acids commonly found in proteins, some RNAs are still able to catalyse chemical reactions. These include cutting and ligating other RNA molecules and also the catalysis of peptide bond formation in the ribosome.

- *Double-stranded RNA*: Double-stranded RNA (or dsRNA) is RNA with two complementary strands, similar to the DNA found in all 'higher' cells. dsRNA forms the genetic material of some viruses. In eukaryotes, it acts as a trigger to initiate the process of RNA interference and is present as an intermediate step in the formation of siRNAs (small interfering RNAs). siRNAs are often confused with miRNAs; siRNAs are double-stranded, whereas miRNAs are single-stranded. Although initially single stranded there are regions of intramolecular association causing hairpin structures in pre-miRNAs; immature miRNAs.

Comparison of RNA and DNA: Unlike DNA, RNA is almost always a single-stranded molecule and has a much shorter chain of nucleotides. RNA contains ribose, rather than the deoxyribose found in DNA (there is a hydroxyl group attached to the pentose ring in the 2′ position whereas RNA has two hydroxyl groups). These hydroxyl groups make RNA less stable than DNA because it is more prone to hydrolysis. Several types of RNA (tRNA, rRNA) contain a great deal of secondary structure, which help promote stability.

Like DNA, most biologically active RNAs including tRNA, rRNA, snRNAs and other non-coding RNAs (such as the SRP RNAs) are extensively base paired to form double stranded helices (Fig. 1.18). Structural analysis of these RNAs have revealed that they are not, 'single-stranded' but rather highly structured. Unlike DNA, this structure is not just limited to long double-stranded helices but rather collections of short helices packed together into structures akin to proteins. In this fashion, RNAs can achieve chemical catalysis, like enzymes. For instance, determination of the structure of the ribosome in 2000 revealed that the active site of this enzyme that catalyzes peptide bond formation is composed entirely of RNA.

Synthesis of RNA: Synthesis of RNA is usually catalyzed by an enzyme - RNA polymerase, using DNA as a template. Initiation of synthesis begins with the binding of the enzyme to a promoter sequence in the DNA (usually found 'upstream' of a gene). The DNA double helix is unwound by the helicase activity of the enzyme. The enzyme then progresses along the template strand in the 3′ → 5′

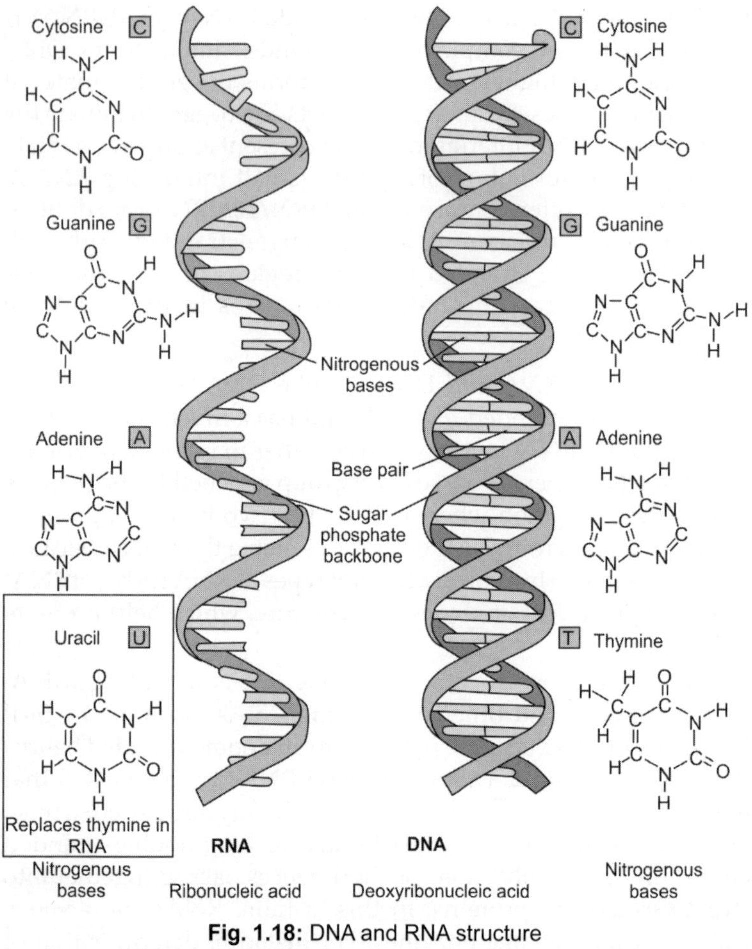

Fig. 1.18: DNA and RNA structure

direction, synthesizing a complementary RNA molecule with elongation occurring in the 5′ → 3′ direction. The DNA sequence also dictates where termination of RNA synthesis will occur.

There are also a number of RNA-dependant RNA polymerases as well that use RNA as their template for synthesis of a new strand of RNA. For instance, a number of RNA viruses (such as poliovirus) use this type of enzyme to replicate their genetic material. Also, it known that RNA-dependent RNA polymerases are required for the RNA interference pathway in many organisms.

DNA Replication

Cell division is essential for an organism to grow, but when a cell divides it must replicate the DNA in its genome so that the two daughter cells have the same genetic information as their parent. The double-stranded structure of DNA provides a simple mechanism for DNA replication. Here, the two strands are separated and then each strand's complementary DNA sequence is recreated by an enzyme called DNA polymerase. This enzyme makes the complementary strand by finding the correct base through complementary base pairing, and bonding it onto the original strand. As DNA polymerases can only extend a DNA strand in a 5′ to 3′ direction, different mechanisms are used to copy the antiparallel strands of the double helix. In this way, the base on the old strand dictates which base appears on the new strand, and the cell ends up with a perfect copy of its DNA.

In following figure 1.19 the double helix (blue) is unwound by a helicase. Next, DNA polymerase III (green) produces the leading strand copy (red). A DNA polymerase I molecule (green) binds to the lagging strand. This enzyme makes discontinuous segments (called Okazaki fragments) before DNA ligase (violet) joins them together.

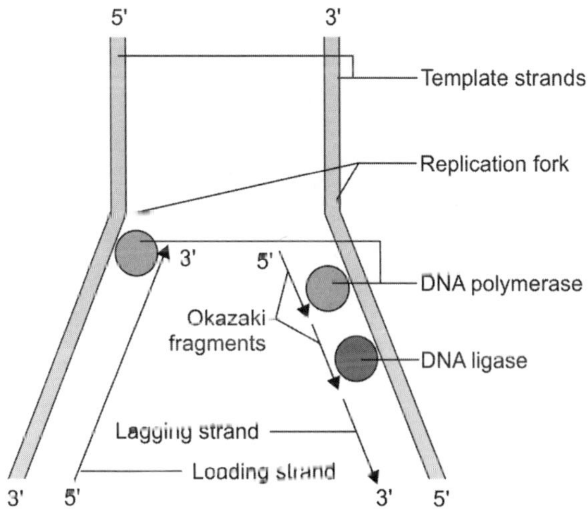

Fig 1.19: DNA replication

PROTEIN BIOSYNTHESIS

Protein biosynthesis (Synthesis) is the process in which cells build proteins. The term is sometimes used to refer only to protein translation but more often it refers to a multi-step process, beginning with amino acid synthesis and transcription which are then used for translation. Protein biosynthesis, although very similar, differs between prokaryotes and eukaryotes (Fig. 1.20).

An overview of protein synthesis: Within the nucleus of the cell (*light blue*), genes (DNA, *dark blue*) are transcribed into RNA. This RNA is then subject to post-transcriptional modification and control, resulting in a mature mRNA (*red*) that is then transported out of the nucleus and into the cytoplasm (*peach*), where it undergoes translation into a protein. mRNA is translated by ribosomes (*purple*) that match the three-base codons of the mRNA to the three-base anti-codons of the appropriate tRNA. Newly synthesized proteins (*black*) are often further modified, such as by binding to an effector molecule (*orange*), to become fully active.)

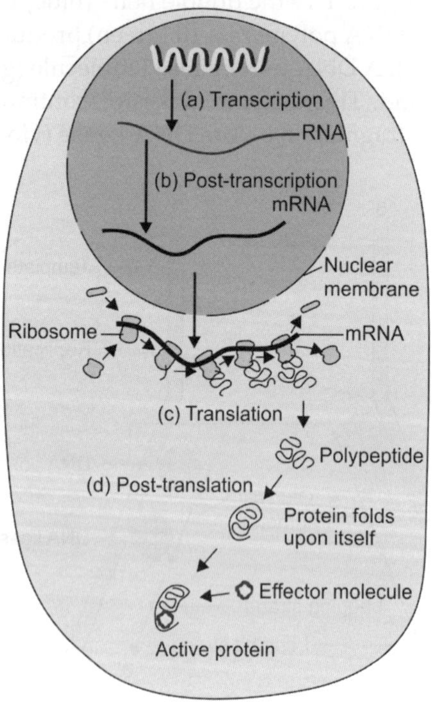

Fig. 1.20: Protien synthesis proess

Steps of the Protien Synthesis

Amino acid synthesis: Amino acids are the monomers which are polymerized to produce proteins. Amino acid synthesis is the set of biochemical processes (metabolic pathways) which build the amino acids from carbon sources like glucose. Not all amino acids may be synthesized by every organism, e.g. adult humans have to obtain 8 of the 20 amino acids from their diet. The amino acids are then loaded onto tRNA molecules for use in the process of translation.

Transcription: Transcription is the process by which an mRNA template, carrying the sequence of the protein, is produced for the translation step from the genome. Transcription makes the template from one strand of the DNA double helix, called the template strand. Transcription takes place in 3 stages.

1. Transcription starts with the process of *initiation*. RNA polymerase, the enzyme which produces RNA from a DNA template, binds to a specific region on DNA that designates the starting point of transcription. This binding region is called the promoter. As the RNA polymerase binds onto the promoter, the DNA strands are begin to unwind.
2. The second process is *elongation*. RNA polymerase travels along the template (non-coding) strand, synthesizing a ribonucleotide polymer. RNA polymerase does not use the coding strand as a template because a copy of any strand produces a base sequence complementary to the strand which is being copied. Therefore DNA from the non-coding strand is used as a template to copy the coding strand.
3. The third stage is *termination*. As the polymerase reaches the termination stage, modifications are required for the newly transcribed mRNA to be able to travel to the other parts of the cell, including cytoplasm and endoplasmic reticulum for translation. A 5′ cap is added to the mRNA to protect it from degradation. In eukaryotes a poly-A tail is added on the 3′ end for protection and as a template for further process. Also in eukaryotes (higher organisms) the vital process of splicing occurs at this stage.

Translation: During translation, mRNA previously transcribed from DNA is decoded by specialized cellular structures called ribosomes to make proteins.

The ribosome has sites, which allow another specialized RNA molecule, known as tRNA, to bind to the mRNA. Binding of the correct tRNA to the mRNA on the ribosome is accomplished by an 'anticodon' that is part of the tRNA. Thus, the correct tRNA, chemically linked to a specific amino acid, is directed to the ribosome to be added to a growing (nascent) polypeptide. The chemical process of connecting two amino acids is shown in (Fig. 1.21).

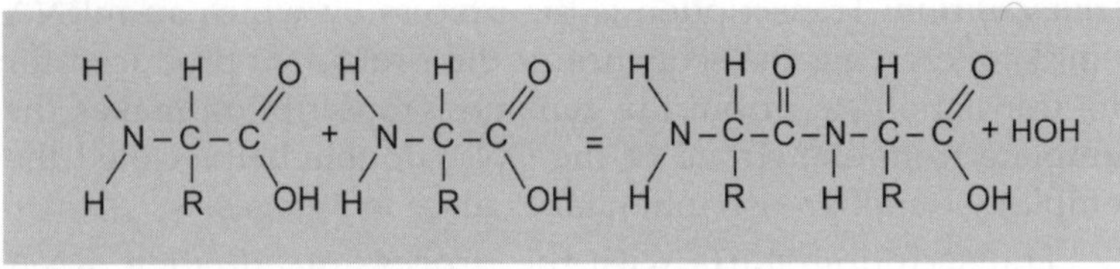

Fig. 1.21: The chemical process of connecting two amino acids resulting in a dipeptide and a water molecule

As the ribosome travels down the mRNA one codon at a time, another tRNA is attached to the mRNA at one of the ribosome sites. The first tRNA is released, but the amino acid that is attached to the first tRNA is now moved to the second tRNA, and binds to its amino acid. This translocation continues on, and a long chain of amino acid (protein), is formed. When the entire unit reaches the stop codon on the mRNA, it falls apart and a newly formed protein is released. This is termination. It is important to know that during this process, many enzymes are used to either assist or facilitate the whole procedure.

The events following biosynthesis (Protein Synthesis) include post-translational modification and protein folding. During and after synthesis, polypeptide chains often fold to assume, so called, native secondary and tertiary structures. This is known as *protein folding*. Many proteins undergo *post-translational modification*. This may include the formation of disulfide bridges or attachment of any of a number of biochemical functional groups, such as acetate, phosphate, various lipids and carbohydrates. Enzymes may also remove one or more amino acids from the leading (amino) end of the polypeptide chain, leaving a protein consisting of two polypeptide chains connected by disulfide bonds.

GENETIC CODE

The *genetic code* is the set of rules by which information encoded in genetic material (DNA or RNA sequences) is translated into proteins (amino acid sequences) by living cells. Specifically, the code defines a mapping between tri-nucleotide sequences called *codons* and amino acids; every triplet of nucleotides in a nucleic acid sequence specifies a single amino acid. Most organisms use a nearly universal code that is referred to as the *standard genetic code* (Fig. 1.22). Even viruses, which are not cellular and do not synthesize proteins themselves, have proteins made using this standard code. For a time, therefore, the code was thought to be universal. However, there are notable exceptions. It is also possible for a single organism to translate different parts of the genome in different ways. For example, in humans, protein synthesis in mitochondria relies on a modified genetic code that varies from the standard one.

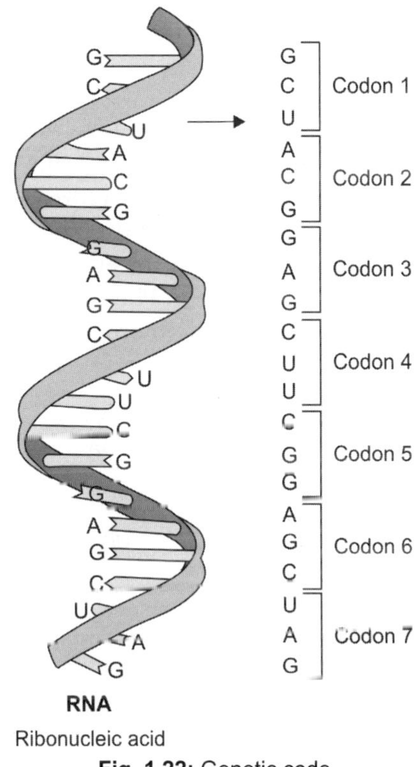

Fig. 1.22: Genetic code

The position or sequence of the bases in DNA ultimately determine the position of the amino acids in the polypeptide chain whose synthesis is directed by the DNA. Therefore, the structure and properties of body proteins are determined by the DNA base sequence of a person's gene. It does this by means of a code. Each amino acid is specified by a sequence of three bases called a codon. There are 20 major amino acid and 64 codons or code words. Sixty-one of the codon specify amino acids and 3 are 'stop' single that terminate the genetic message. One codon that specifies an amino acids usually begins the message. More than one code word may specify a given amino acid, but only one amino acid is specified by any one codon; thus the code is said to be degenerated. For example, the codons that code for the amino acid leucine are UAG, UUG, CUU, CUC, CUA and CUG, but none of these codes for any other amino acid. The relationship between the base sequence in DNA, mRNA, the anticodon in tRNA and the translation into any amino acid is shown in Figure 1.23.

The code is non-overlapping. Therefore, CACUUUAGA is read as CAC, UUU, AGA, and specifies histidine, Phenylalanine, and arginine, respectively. A shorthand way of returning to specific amino acid is to use either specific group of three letters or a single letter to denote specific amino acid. To this system, for example, arginine may be referred to as 'arg' or as simply 'R' while the symbols for phenylalanine are either 'Phe' or 'F'. General genetics referred to in the reference provide more information about the code.

DNA template	3' ... AAA	TGA	CTG ... 5'
mRNA	5' ... UUU	ACU	GAC ... 3'
tRNA	3' ... AAA	UGA	CUG ... 5'
Polypeptide chain	NH_2 ... phe	thr	asp ... COOH

Key: A = Adenine, C = Cytocine, T = Thymine, U = Uracil
phe = Phenylalanine, thr = threonine, asp = aspartic acid

Fig. 1.23: Relationship among the nucleotide base sequence of DNA, mRNA tRNA and amino acids in the polypeptide chain production

NAMING GENES

The HUGO Gene Nomenclature Committee designates an official name and symbol (an abbreviation of the name) for each known human gene. Some official gene names include additional information in parentheses, such as related genetic conditions, subtypes of a condition, or inheritance pattern. The HGNC (Human Genomic Naming Committee) is a non-profit organization funded by the U.K. Medical Research Council and the U.S. National Institutes of Health. The Committee has named more than 13,000 of the estimated 20,000 to 25,000 genes in the human genome. During the research process, genes often acquire several alternate names and symbols. Different researchers investigating the same gene may each give the gene a different name, which can cause confusion. The HGNC assigns a unique name and symbol to each human gene, which allows effective organization of genes in large databanks, aiding the advancement of research. Genetics Home Reference describes genes using the HGNC's official gene names and gene symbols. Genetics Home Reference frequently presents the symbol and name separated with a colon, e.g. Fibroblast growth factor receptor 4 (FGFR4).

CHROMOSOME

In the nucleus of each cell, the DNA molecule is packed into thread-like structures called chromosomes. Each chromosome is made-up of DNA tightly coiled many times around proteins called histones that support its structure. Chromosomes are organized structures of DNA and proteins that are found in cells. A chromosome is a singular piece of DNA, which contains many genes, regulatory elements and other nucleotide sequences. Chromosomes also contain DNA-bound proteins, which serve to package the DNA and control its functions. The word *chromosome* comes from the Greek (*chroma,* color) and (*soma,* body) due to their property of being stained very strongly by some dyes. Chromosomes vary extensively between different organisms. Chromosomes are packaged by proteins into a condensed structure called chromatin.

Chromosomes are not visible in the cell's nucleus not even under a microscope when the cell is not dividing. However, the DNA that makes up chromosomes becomes more tightly packed during cell division and is then visible under a microscope. Most of what researchers know today about chromosomes was learned by observing chromosomes during cell division. Each chromosome has a constriction point called the centromere, which divides the chromosome into two sections, or 'arms.' The short arm of the chromosome is labeled the 'p arm.' The long arm of the chromosome is labeled the 'q arm.' The location of the centromere on each chromosome gives the chromosome its characteristic shape, and can be used to describe the location of specific genes (Fig. 1.24).

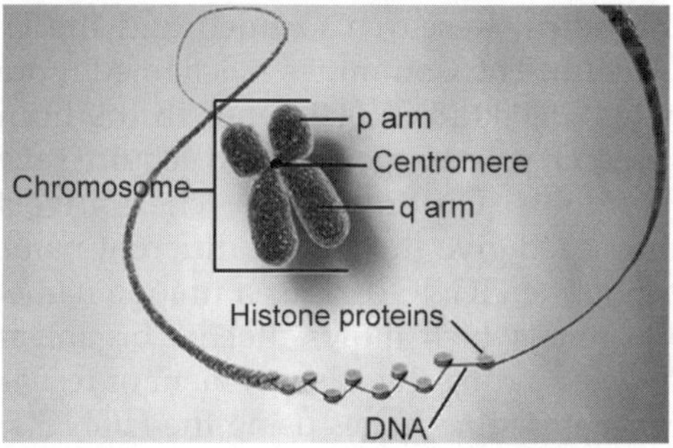

Fig. 1.24: Structure of chromosome

In humans, each cell normally contains 23 pairs of chromosomes, for a total of 46. Twenty-two of these pairs, called autosomes, look the same in both males and females. The 23rd pair, the sex chromosomes, differs between males and females. Females have two copies of the X chromosome while males have one X and one Y chromosome (Fig. 1.25).

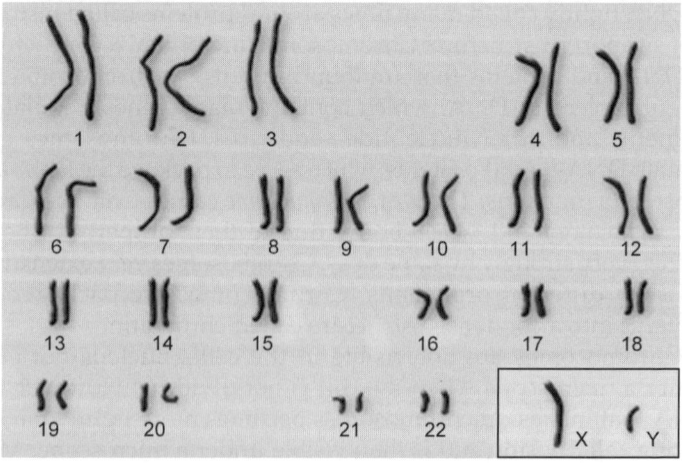

Fig. 1.25: Structure of 23 pairs of human chromosomes

Functions of Chromosome

- Chromosomes contain genes. All the hereditary information is located in the genes
- Chromosomes control the synthesis of structural proteins and thus help in cell division and cell growth
- They control cellular differentiation
- By directing the synthesis of particular enzymes, chromosome control cell metabolism
- Chromosomes can replicate themselves or produce their carbon copies for passage to daughter cells and next generation
- Chromosomes produce nucleoli for synthesis of ribosomes
- Their haploid or diploid number respectively brings about gametophytic and sporophytic characteristics to the individual
- Chromosomes form a link between the offspring and the parents
- Some chromosomes called sex chromosomes (e.g. X and Y) determine the sex of the individual
- Through the process of crossing over, chromosomes introduce variations
- Mutations are produced due to change in gene chemistry.

Chromosomes—Sex Determination

A *sex-determination system* is a biological system that determines the development of sexual characteristics in an organism. Most sexual organisms have two sexes. In many cases, sex determination is genetic: males and females have different alleles or even different genes that specify their sexual morphology. In human being, this is often accompanied by chromosomal differences. In some species of reptiles, including alligators and the tuatara, sex is determined by the temperature at which the egg is incubated or social variables (the size of an organism relative to other members of its population). Sex-determination systems are not yet fully understood in all the species. However it is very clear in human being, which is very well explained by XX/XY chromosomes sex determination theory.

Chromosomal determination of sex: Henking (1891) discovered an X-body in the reproductive cell of firefly. Y-body was discovered by Stevens (1902). Wilson and Stevens (1905) put forward chromosome theory of sex and named the X and Y-bodies on heterogamesis or occurrence of two types of gametes in one of the two sexes. It is of the following type.

- XX-XY Type
- XX-X_0 Type
- ZX-ZZ Type
- ZO-ZZ Type
- Haplodiploidy

However, in human being XX-XY Type of heterogamesis theory is applicable. In human beings the female possess two homomorphic (isomorphic) sex chromosomes, named XX. The males contain two heteromorphic sex chromosome, i.e. XY. The Y-chromosome is often shorter and heterochromatic (made of heterochromatin). Despite of difference in morphology, the XY chromosomes are homologous and syapse during zygotene phase of meiosis. It is because they have two parts, homologous and differential. Homologous region of the two help in pairing. They carry same genes which may have different alleles. Such genes present on both X and Y chromosomes are *XY-linked genes*. They are inherited like autosomal genes, e.g. xeroderma pigmentation, epidermolysis bullosa. The differential region of Y-chromosome carries only Y-linked or holandric genes, e.g. testis determining factor (TDF). It is perhaps the smallest gene occupying only 14 base pairs. Other holandric genes are hypertrichosis (excessive hairness) on pinna, porcupine skin, keratoderma dissipatum (thickening of skin of hands and feet) and webbed toes. Holandric genes are directly inherited by son from his father. Genes present on the differential region of X-chromosome also find expression in male whether they are dominant or recessive, e.g. color blindness, hemophilia. It is because the male are hemizygous for these genes.

Human being have 22 pairs of autosomes and one pair of sex chromosomes. All the ova formed by female are similar in their chromosome type (22 + X). Therefore, female are homogametic. The male gametes or sperms produced by human male are of two type, (22 + X) and (22 + Y). Human males are therefore heterogametic (Male digamety).

Sex of offspring: (Fig. 1.26). Sex of the offspring is determined at the time of fertilization. It cannot be changed later on. It does not depends on any characteristic of the female parent because they are homogametic and produce only one type of eggs (22 + X). The male gametes are of two types, androsperms (22 + Y) and gynosperms (22 + X). They are produced in equal proportion. Fertilization of the egg (22 + X) with gynosperm (22 + X) will produce female child (44 + XX), while fertilization of egg (22 + X) with androsperm (22 +Y) gives rise to male child (44 + XY). As the two types of sperms are produced in equal proportion, there are chances of getting a male or female child in a particular mating. As Y-chromosome determines the male sex of the individual, it is also called androsome.

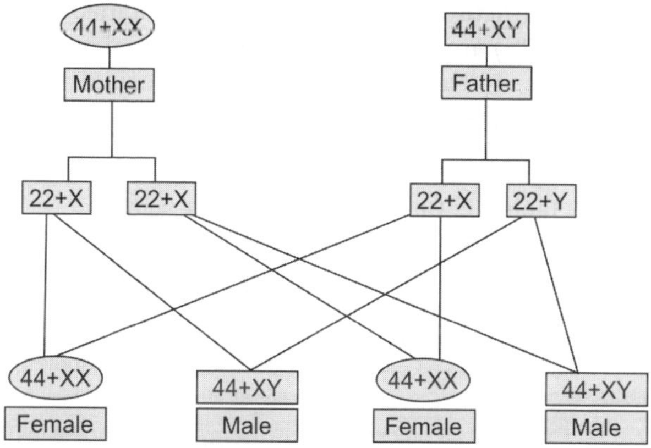

Fig. 1.26: Sex determination schematic presentation

CHROMOSOMAL ABERRATIONS (CHROMOSOMAL MUTATION)

- Chromosomal aberrations are disruptions in the normal chromosomal content of a cell, and are a major cause of genetic conditions in humans, such as Down syndrome.
- In other words, they are changes in the number and or arrangement of genes in the chromosomes.
- Change in number of chromosomes is known as aneuploidy or numerical aberration.
- Change in arrangement of genes in the chromosomes is known as structural aberration.
- Chromosomal aberrations may involve changes in single chromosome, known as intrachromosomal aberrations.
- Chromosomal aberrations may involve changes in two chromosomes, known as interchromosomal aberrations.

- They are also termed as chromosomal abnormalities. Some chromosome abnormalities do not cause disease in carriers, such as translocations, or chromosomal inversions, although they may lead to a higher chance of having a child with a chromosome disorder. Abnormal numbers of chromosomes or chromosome sets, aneuploidy, may be lethal or give rise to genetic disorders.
- Chromosomal abnormalities result in a proportion of congenital anomalies, developmental and intellectual disabilities and behavioral difficulties. The majority of spontaneous abortions (about 50–60%) are the result of chromosomal abnormalities, particularly, if they occur early, numerical changes in chromosomes are summarized in Table 1.2, structural changes are summarized in Table 1.3 and figure 1.27.

Table 1.2: Change in chromosomal number (aneuploidy) (Numerical aberration)

Change	Description	Example
Monosomy	One chromosome is missing	Turner syndrome (Cells in female contain 45 chromosomes with one X chromosome rather than two)
Trisomy	One extra chromosome is present	Trisomy 21 chromosome (Down syndrome) Cells contain 47 chromosome
Tetrasomy	Two extra chromosome are present	Cells contain 48 chromosome (Not compatible with life)
Triploidy	One extra chromosome set of haploid genome is present	Cells contain 69 chromosome (Not compatible with life)
Tetraploidy	Two extra chromosome sets of haploid genome are present	Cells contain 92 chromosome (Not compatible with life)

Table 1.3: Major changes in chromosome structure (Structural aberration)

Change	Description
Deletion (del)	Part of a chromosome is missing with the accompanying DNA, can be at the end (terminal) or in the middle (interstitial). For example, del 5 p, cri-dsi-chat syndrome.

Contd...

Contd...

Change	Description
Duplication (dup)	Part of a chromosome is duplicated along with the accompanying DNA, so that an extra piece of chromosomal material is present. For example, in cat eye syndrome, there is duplication of a certain segment of chromosome 22 resulting in iris coloboma, anal atresia and various congenital malformations.
Inversion (inv)	Alteration in which a portion of the chromosome is rearranged by two breaks occurring 180 degree rotation of the chromosome piece between them and its reinsertion. For example, about 40% are chromosome 9. May or may not result in visible effects.
Ring chromosome (r)	Formed when a segment at the end(s) of one of a pair of chromosome is lost and fuse to form a circular structure. For example, Ring chromosome 14 is associated with psychomotor delay, mental retardation and dysmorphic craniofacial features. It is very rare.
Translocation (t)	Transfer of a chromosome segment to another chromosome after breakage has occurred. In reciprocal translocation two chromosomes exchange piece. A Robertsonism translocation usually involve two acrocentric chromosomes whose long arms fuse. Often small fragments are lost. In a balanced translocation no genetic material added or lost. Balanced reciprocal translocations usually do not cause problems. For example, translocation trisomy 21 or Down syndrome may result from the presence of 46 chromosomes that includes a translocation chromosome, such as t (14 t21) or t (14_q 21_q) so that the genetic material of 47 chromosomes with genetic material of 3 chromosome 21_s is present. There is a normal chromosome, 14, two normal 21 and translocation chromosome consisting of the second chromosome 14 and extra chromosome 21. q

Chromosomal aberrations can lead to a variety of genetic disorders. Human examples include: some of genetic disorder, or genetic disease are:

- ***Cri du chat,*** which is caused by the *deletion* of part of the short arm of chromosome 5. 'Cri du chat' means 'cry of the cat' in French, and the condition was so-named because affected babies make high-pitched cries that sound like a cat. Affected individuals have wide-set eyes, a small head and jaw and are moderately to severely mentally retarded and very short.

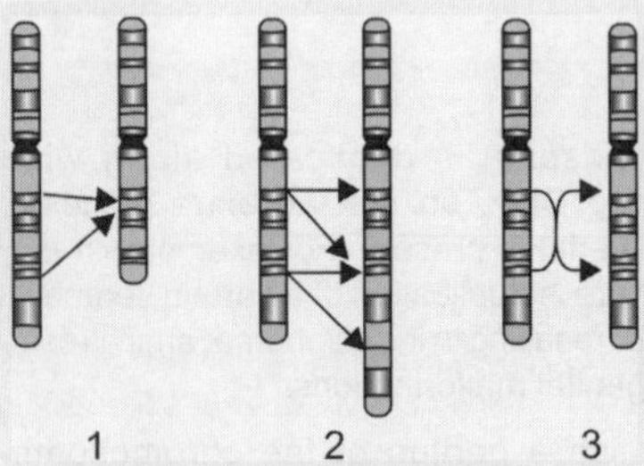

The three major single chromosome mutations: (Intrachromosomal aberration)

- ***Deletion*** (loss of part of a chromosome)
- ***Duplication*** (extra copies of a part of a chromosome)
- ***Inversion*** (reverse the direction of a part of a chromosome)

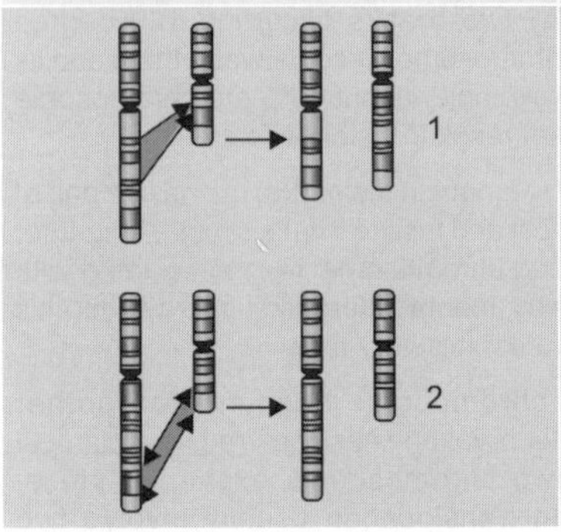

The two major two-chromosome mutations; (Interchromosomal aberration)

- ***Insertion (ring Chromosome) and***
- ***Translocation*** (part of a chromosome breaks off and attaches to another chromosome)

Fig. 1.27: Chromosomal aberrations

- ***Wolf-Hirschhorn syndrome,*** which is caused by partial *deletion* of the short arm of chromosome 4. It is characterized by severe growth retardation and severe to profound mental retardation.
- ***Down's syndrome,*** usually is caused by an extra copy of chromosome 21 (*trisomy 21*). Characteristics include decreased muscle tone, stockier build, asymmetrical skull, slanting eyes and mild to moderate mental retardation.
- ***Edwards syndrome,*** which is the second most common trisomy after Down syndrome. It is a *trisomy of chromosome 18*. Symptoms include mental and motor retardation and numerous congenital anomalies causing serious health problems. Ninety percent die in infancy; however, those who live past their first birthday usually are quite healthy thereafter. They have a characteristic hand appearance with clenched hands and overlapping fingers.
- ***Patau Syndrome,*** also called D-Syndrome or *trisomy-13*. Symptoms are somewhat similar to those of trisomy-18, but they do not have the characteristic hand shape.

- ***Idic15***, abbreviation for Isodicentric 15 on chromosome 15; also called the following names due to various researches, but they all mean the same; IDIC (15), *Inverted duplication 15*, extra Marker, Inv dup 15, *partial tetrasomy 15*.
- ***Jacobsen syndrome***, also called the terminal 11q deletion disorder. This is a very rare disorder. Those affected have normal intelligence or mild mental retardation, with poor expressive language skills. Most have a bleeding disorder called Paris-Trousseau syndrome.
- ***Klinefelter's syndrome*** (XXY). Men with Klinefelter syndrome are usually sterile, and tend to have longer arms and legs and to be taller than their peers. Boys with the syndrome are often shy and quiet, and have a higher incidence of speech delay and dyslexia. During puberty, without testosterone treatment, some of them may develop gynecomastia.
- ***Turner syndrome (X instead of XX or XY)***. In Turner syndrome, female sexual characteristics are present but underdeveloped. People with Turner syndrome often have a short stature, low hairline, abnormal eye features and bone development and a 'caved-in' appearance to the chest.
- ***XYY syndrome***. XYY boys are usually taller than their siblings. Like XXY boys and XXX girls, they are somewhat more likely to have learning difficulties.
- ***Triple-X syndrome (XXX).*** XXX girls tend to be tall and thin. They have a higher incidence of dyslexia.
- ***Small supernumerary marker chromosome.*** This means there is an extra, abnormal chromosome. Features depend on the origin of the extra genetic material. Cat-eye syndrome and isodicentric chromosome 15 syndrome (or Idic15) are both caused by a supernumerary marker chromosome, as is Pallister-Killian syndrome.

Incidence

The incidence of the specific chromosomal abnormalities found is summarized in Table 1.4. Autosomal trisomies account for about 25%, sex chromosome abnormalities for about 35% and structural rearrangement for about 40%. These figure represent only a small fraction of chromosomally abnormal conception. Nature exercises considerable selection, as only small percentage of these abnormal conceptions survive to term. Between 10 and 20% of all recognized conception end in spontaneous abortions. Studies of the products of spontaneous abortion have detectable chromosomal abnormalities. Approximately 95 to 99% of all turner syndrome embryos are spontaneously aborted, as are about 95% of those with available data, it appears that chromosome abnormalities are present in 10 to 20% of all recognized conception. This may eventually be higher as techniques for determining cytogenic causes improve, more than 1000 chromosome abnormalities have been described in live births.

Table 1.4: Incidence of selected chromosomal abnormalities in live born child

Abnormality	Incidence
Autosomal trisomies	
• Trisomy 21 (Down syndrome)	• 1:650–1:1,000*
• Trisomy 13 (Patan syndrome)	• 1:4000–1:10,000*
• Trisomy 18 (Edwars syndrome)	• 1:3,500–1:7,500*
Sex-chromosome disorders	
• 45, X (Turner syndrome)	• 1:2,500–1:8000#
• 47, XXX (triple X)	• 1:850–1:1,250#
• 47, XXY (Klinefelter syndrome)	• 1:500–1:1,000$
Other Sex-chromosome abnormalities	
• Male	• ~1:1,300$
• Female	• ~1:1,300#
Structural abnormalities	
• Rearrangement (e.g. translocation, duplications)	~ 1:440*

* Live births, # live female birth, $ live male birth

MECHANISM OF INHERITANCE

Heredity is the transmission of genetic character from parents to the offspring. Gregor Johann Mendal (1866) proposed that inheritance is controlled by paired germinal units or factors, now called genes (Fig. 1.28). They are present in all cells of the body and are transferred to the next generation through gametes. Factors or genes are thus physical basis of heredity. They represent small segment of chromosomes. Genes are passed from one generation to the next generation or from one cell to its daughter cell as components of chromosome (chromosomal basis of heredity). The genetic material present in chromosomes is DNA. Genes are the segment of DNA called citrons. Therefore, DNA is the chemical basis of heredity.

Inheritance refers to how genetic information is passed down from one generation to next generation. The basic features of mechanism of inheritance are as follows:

- Genes or chromosomes are physical basis of inheritance.
- Person inherits half of the genetic information from each parent.
- Every gene has two copies of genes; and each parent contributes for one copy of gene to their offspring.
- Genes for different traits are inherited separately from one another. For example, the gene for hair color is not linked with the gene for height. A child may have his mothers' hair color but may not her height. For the most part, each trait is inherited separately.

A particular disorder might be described as 'running in a family' if more than one person in the family has the condition. Some disorders that affect multiple family members are caused by gene mutations, which can be inherited (passed down from parent to child). Other conditions that appear to run in families are not inherited. Instead, environmental factors, such as dietary habits or a combination of genetic and environmental factors are responsible for these disorders.

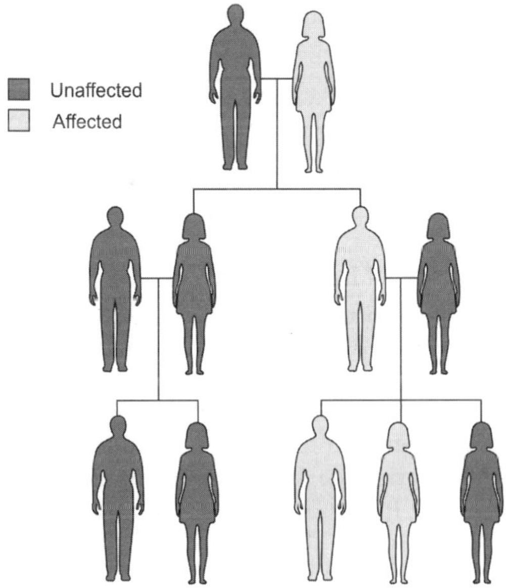

Fig. 1.28: Mechanism of inheritance

Laws of Inheritance

Mendel has given following four laws of inheritance:

- *Law of unit inheritance (paired factors/genes):* A character is represented in an organism or person by at least two factors. The two factors lie on the two homologous chromosomes at the same locus. They may represent the same (homozygous, e.g. TT in case of pure tall, tt in case of dwarf) or alternate expression (heterozygous, e.g. Tt in case of heterozygous tall) of the same character. Factors representing the alternate or same form of a character are called alleles.
- *Law of dominance:* In heterozygous individual, a character is represented by two contrasting factor called alleles. Out of the two alleles, only one is able to express its effect in the individual. It is called dominant allele. The other allele, which does not show its effect in the heterozygous individual is called recessive allele.
- *Law of segregation:* The two factors of a characteristic which remain together in an individual do not get mixed up but keep their identity distinct, separate at the time of gametogenesis or sporogenesis, get randomly distributed to different gametes and then get paired again in different offspring as per the principle of probability.
- *Law of independent assortment:* According to this principle or law the two factors of each character assort or separate independent of the factors of other characters at the time of gamete formation and get randomly re-arranged in the offspring.

Mendelian Theory of Inheritance

Genes provide the information for the growth, development and function of our bodies. When a gene is changed, there is a different message sent to the cells. A gene change that makes the genes faulty is called a *mutation*. A mutated (faulty) gene may cause a problem with the development and functioning of different body systems or organs. However, some faulty genes may be beneficial. Our genes are inherited from our parents, who have inherited theirs from their parents and so on. The great majority of genes come in pairs, the exceptions being the genes on the sex chromosomes (X and Y) of a male. The term *Mendelian inheritance* applies when a characteristic or set of characteristics is due to the information contained in a single gene pair. The characteristic may be 'usual' or it may not: it could be a genetic condition.

Mendelian Inheritance is so called because our understanding of it started with the observations of an Augustinian monk named Gregor Mendel in the 19th century. The inheritance pattern depends on whether the faulty gene is part of one of the numbered chromosomes called an *autosome* or on the X chromosome, which is one of the *sex chromosomes*. It also depends on whether the mutation that makes the gene faulty is 'recessive' or 'dominant'.

When the inheritance pattern is known it is possible to provide families and individuals with information regarding the chance (or risk) that the condition will affect themselves and other family members of future generations. Autosomal recessive inheritance, autosomal dominant inheritance, X-linked recessive inheritance and X-linked dominant inheritance are the some Mendelian patterns of inheritance.

Patterns of Inheritance

Some genetic conditions are caused by mutations in a single gene. These conditions are usually inherited in one of several straightforward patterns, depending on the gene involved. Following are the main patterns of inheritance.

- **Mendelian patterns of inheritance.** This includes:
  - Autosomal dominant
  - Autosomal recessive
  - Sex Linked inheritance
    - *X-linked dominant*
    - *X-linked recessive*
    - *Y- linked (Holandric) inheritance*
- **Non-Mendelian patterns of inheritance**
  - Codominant pattern of inheritance
  - Mitochondrial pattern of inheritance
  - Multifactororial pattern of inheritance

Autosomal Dominant

One mutated copy of the gene in each cell is sufficient for a person to be affected by an autosomal dominant disorder (Table 1.5). Each affected person usually has one affected parent (Fig. 1.29). Autosomal dominant disorders tend to occur in every generation of an affected family.

Table 1.5: Selective genetic disorders showing autosomal dominant inheritance

Disorder	Occurrence	Brief description
Aniridia	1:100,000–1:200,000	Absence of the iris of the eye to varying degree, glaucoma may develop, may be associated with other abnormalities in different syndrome
Achondroplasia	1:10,000–1:12,000	Short limbed type of dwarfism with large hands
Adult polycystic kidney disease	1:250–1:1250	Enlarged kidney, hematuria, proteinuria, renal cysts, abdominal mass, eventually renal failure, may be associated with hypertension hepatic cyst, diverticular, cerebral hemorrhage may occur, cystic kidney seen on X-ray films.
Facioscapulo-humeral muscular dystrophy-IA	1:100,000–3:100,000	Facial weakness, atrophy in face, upper limb and shoulder girdle and pelvic girdle muscles, speech may become indistinct: much variability in progression and age of onset.
Familial hyper cholesterolemia (type-IIA)	1:200–1:500	Low-density lipoprotein receptor mutation resulting in deviated LDL, xanthomas, archs lipoidy, corneal and coronary disease.
Hereditary sphenxytosis	1:4500–1:5000	Red cell membrane defect leading to abnormal shape, impaired survival and hemolytic anemia.
Huntington disease	1:1800–1:25000	Progressive neurological disease due to urinucleotide repeat expansion of CAG, involuntary muscle movements with jerkiness, gait changes, lack of coordination, mental retardation with memory loss, speech problems, personality changes, confusion and deceased mental capacity usually begin in mid-adulthood.
Nail-patella syndrome	1:50,00	Nail abnormalities, hypoplasia or absent patella and iliac horns, elbow dysplasia, renal lesions and disease, iris and other eye abnormalities, glaucoma, gastrointestinal problems.

Contd...

Contd...

Disorder	Occurrence	Brief description
Neurofibromatosis-1	1:3000-1:3,300	Café-an-lait spots, neurofibromas and malignant progression are common, complications include hypertension, variable expression.
Osteogenesis imperfecta type-1	1:30,000	Fragile bones with multiple fractures, mitral valve proleapse, short stature in same cases, progressive hearing loss, and wornian bones.
Polydactyly	1:100–1:300	Extra (supernumeracy) digit on hand and feet.
Tuberous sclerosis-I	About 1:10,000	White leaf shaped macules, seizures, intellectual delay, facial angiofibromas, erythemic nodular rash in butterfly pattern on face, learning and behavioral disorder, shagreen patches may develop retinal pathology and rhebdomyoma of the heart.
Van-der-wonde syndrome	1: 80,000–1:100,000	Cleft lip pits, missing premolars.
Van-willebrand disease	1:1000–30:1000	Deficiency or defect in plasma protein called van willebrand factor, leading to prolonged bleeding time, bleeding from mucous membranes.

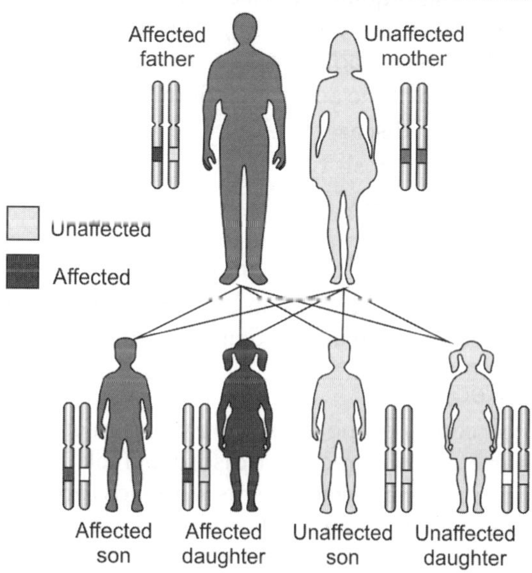

Fig. 1.29: Autosomal dominant pattern of inheritance

Main characteristics of autosomal dominant inheritance and disorders:

- Gene is on autosome
- One copy of the mutant gene is needed for effects
- Males and females are affected in equal number on average
- No sex difference in clinical manifestations
- Vertical family history through several generations may be seen
- There is wide variation in expression
- Penetrance may be incomplete (gene can appear or skip in a generation)
- Increase paternal age effect may be seen
- Fresh gene mutation is frequent
- Later age of onset is frequent
- Male-to-male transmission is possible
- Normal offspring of an affected person will have normal children and grandchildren
- Least negative effect on reproductive fitness
- Structural protein defect is often involved
- In general disorders tends to be less severe than the recessive disorders
- Men and woman equally affected, variable expression, reduced penetrance (in some disorders), and advanced paternal age associated with sporadic cases.

Common examples of the autosomal dominant disorders:

- Huntington disease
- Neurofibromatosis type 1
- Marfan syndrome
- Colon cancer
- Hereditary breast and ovarian cancer

In this example, a man with an autosomal dominant disorder has two affected children and two unaffected children (Fig. 1.29).

Autosomal Recessive

Two mutated copies of the gene are present in each cell when a person has an autosomal recessive disorder (Table 1.6). An affected person usually has unaffected parents who each carry a single copy of the mutated gene (and are referred to as carriers). Autosomal recessive disorders are typically not seen in every generation of an affected family.

Table 1.6: Selective genetic disorders showing autosomal recessive inheritance

Disorder	Occurrence	Brief description
Albinism (tyrosinase negative)	1:15,000–1:40,000 1:85–1:630 (in Americans)	Melanin lacking in skin hair and eyes, nystagmus, photophobia, susceptible to neoplasm, strabismus, impaired vision.
Argininosuccinic aciduria (ASA)	1:60,000–1:70,000	Urea cycle disorder, hyperammonemia, mild mental retardation, vomiting, seizures, coma, abnormal hair shaft.
Cystic-fibrosis	1:2000–1:2500	Pancreatic insufficiency and malabsorption, abnormal exocrine gland, chronic pulmonary disease.
Ellis-van crereld syndrome	Rare	Short-limbed dwarfisms, polydactyly, congenital heart disease, nail anomalies.
Glycogen storage disease-Ia (Von gierke disease)	1:20,000	Glucose-6 phosphatase deficiency, bruising, hypoglycemia, enlarged liver, hyperlipidemia, hypertension, short stature.
Glycogen storage disease-II (pomple disease)	3:100,000– 4.5:100,000	Infant, juvenile and adult form acid maltage deficiency. In infant form cardiac enlargement, cardiomyopathy, hypotonia respiratory insufficiency, developmental delay, macroglossia, death from cardio-respiratory failure by about 2 years of age.
Hemochromatosis	1:3000	Iron storage and tissue damage can result in cirrhosis, diabetes, pancreatitis and other disease, skin pigmentation.
Homocystinuria	1:40,000– 1:1,40,000	Mental retardation, skeletal defects, lens displacement, tall risk for myocardial infraction, caused by cystathionine beta-synthase deficiency.
Metachromatic leukodystrophy	1:40,000	Arylsofatase:A deficiency leading to disintegration of myelin and accumulation of lipids in white matter of brain, psychomotor degeneration, hypotonia, adult, juvonilo and infantile form.
Sickle cell disease	1:400–1:600	Hemoglobinopathy with chronic hemolytic anemia, growth retardation, susceptibility to infection, painful crisis, leg ulcers, dectylitis.

Contd...

Contd...

Disorder	Occurrence	Brief description
Tay-sachs disease	1:3600	Progressive mental and motor retardation with onset at about 6 months, poor muscle tone, deafness, blindness, convulsions, decelerate rigidity, death usually by 3 to 5 years of age.
Usher syndrome	Rare	A group of syndrome characterized by congenital sensorineural deafness, visual loss due to retain-iris pigmentations, vestibular ataxia, occasionally mental retardation, speech problems. Several sub types.
Xeroderma pigmentosa (Complementation group A-G)	1:60,000–1:100,000	Defective DNA repair, sun sensitivity, freckling, atrophic skin lesions, skin cancer develops, photophobia and keratosis, death usually by adulthood.

Main characteristics of autosomal recessive inheritance and disorders:

- Gene is located on autosome
- Horizontal occurrence seen in families
- Two copies of the mutated gene are needed for phenotypic manifestations
- Male and females are affected in equal number on average
- No sex difference in clinical manifestations
- Family history is usually negative especially for vertical transmission (in more than one generation)
- Other affected individual in family in same generation (Horizontal transmission) may be seen
- Consanguinity or relatedness is more often present than in other type of inherited conditions
- Fresh gene mutation is rare
- Age of disease onset is usually early newborn, infancy, early childhood
- Greater negative effect on reproductive fitness
- Associated with particular ethnic groups.

Common examples of the autosomal recessive disorders:

- Cystic fibrosis
- Sickle cell anemia
- Tay-Sachs disease
- Phyenylketonuria
- Thalassemia

In this example, two unaffected parents each carry one copy of a gene mutation for an autosomal recessive disorder. They have one affected child and three unaffected children, two of which carry one copy of the gene mutation (Fig. 1.30).

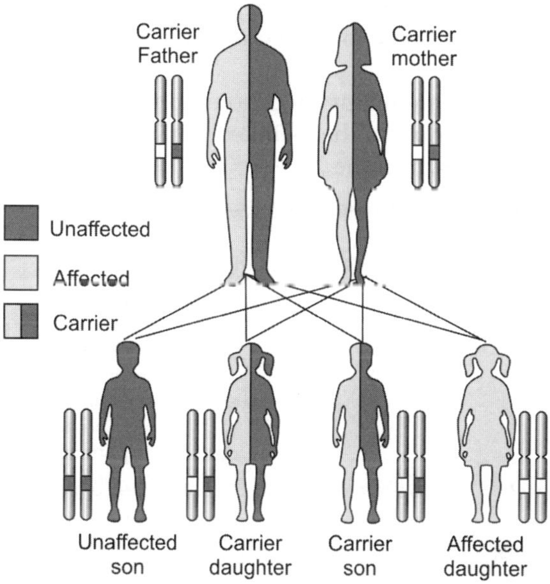

Fig. 1.30: Autosomal recessive pattern of inheritance

Sex-linked Inheritance

- ***X-linked dominant :*** X-linked dominant disorders are caused by mutations in genes on the X chromosome. Females are more frequently affected than males, and the chance of passing on an X-linked dominant disorder differs between men and women. Families with an X-linked dominant disorder often have both affected males and affected females in each generation (Table 1.7). A striking characteristic of X-linked inheritance is that fathers cannot pass X-linked traits to their sons (no male-to-male transmission).

  Major characteristics of X-linked Dominant inheritance and disorders:
  - Mutant gene is located on X-chromosome
  - One copy of the mutant gene is needed for phenotypic manifestations

- X-inactivation modifies the gene effect in females
- Often lethal in males and so many see transmission only in the female line
- Affected families usually show excess of female offspring (2:1)
- Affected male have affected mother (unless new mutation)
- There is no male to male transmission
- There is no carrier state
- Disorders are relatively uncommon.

Common example of the X-linked dominant disorders:
- Fragile X syndrome

Table 1.7: Selective genetic disorders showing X-linked dominant inheritance

Disorder	Occurrence	Brief description
Albright osteodystrophy	Rare	Short stature, delayed dentition, brachy dactyly, hereditary hypocalcemia pseudohypoparathyroidism, many endocrine problem, muscular atrophy, mineralization of skeletone; round faces, possible intellectual disability, hypertension.
Focal dermal hypoplasia	Very rare, exactly unknown	Atrophy, liner pigmentation, papillomas of skin on lips, axilla and umbilicus, digital anomalies, hypoplastic teeth, ocular anomalies (oloboma, microphthalmia) .
Lucontincotia pigmenti	Very rare	Irregular swirling pigmentation of skin lesion, dental anomalies, alopecia, intellectual disability common, seizures, uveitis, retinal abnormalities.
Ornithine transcarbamylase (OTC) deficiency	1:80,000 in Japan, rare among others	Inborn error in urea cycle metabolism, failure to thrive hyperammonemia, vomiting, headache, confusion, rigidity, lethargy, seizure, coma, many males die in neonatal period.
Orofaciodigital syndrome type-I	1:50,000	Cleft palate, tongue, jaw and or lip, facial hypoplasia, intellectual disability, syndactyly, short digits polycystic kidney with renal failure.
X-linked hypophosphatemia or vitamin D resistant	1:25,000	Disorder of tubular phosphate transport, bowed legs, growth deficiency, rickets with ultimate short stature, possible hearing loss.

In this example, a man with an X-linked dominant condition has two affected daughters and two unaffected sons (Fig. 1.31).

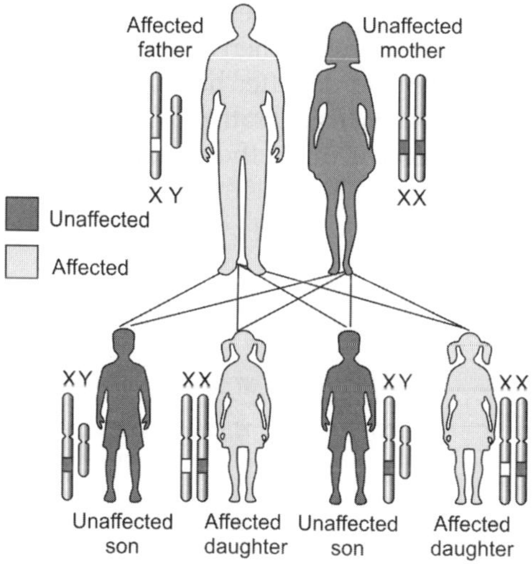

Fig. 1.31: X-linked dominant pattern of inheritance: affected father

In this example, a woman with an X-linked dominant condition has an affected daughter, an affected son, an unaffected daughter, and an unaffected son (Fig. 1.32).

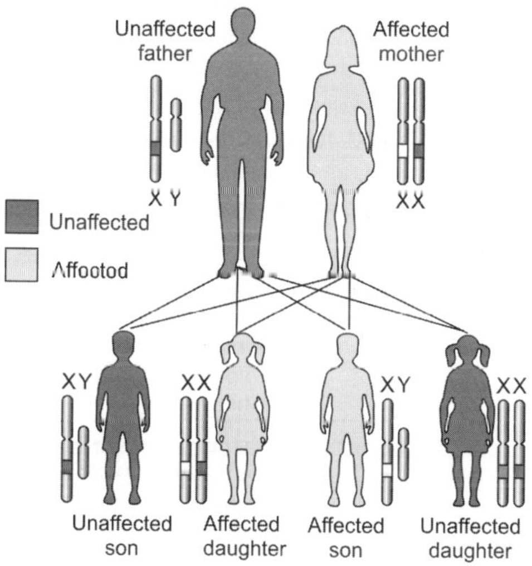

Fig. 1.32: X-linked dominant pattern of inheritance: affected mother

- ***X-linked recessive***: X-linked recessive disorders are also caused by mutations in genes on the X chromosome. Males are more frequently affected than females, and the chance of passing on the disorder differs between men and women. Families with an X-linked recessive disorder often have affected males, but rarely affected females, in each generation. A striking characteristic of X-linked inheritance is that fathers cannot pass X-linked traits to their sons (no male-to-male transmission).

  Major characteristics of X-linked recessive inheritance and disorders (Table 1.8):

Table 1.8: Selective genetic disorders showing X-linked recessive inheritance

Disorder	Occurrence	Brief description
Color blindness (dentan)	8:100	Normal vision actually, defective color vision with green series defect.
Duchenne muscular dystrophy	1:3000–1:5000	Eventual respiratory insufficiency and death
Fabry disease (diffuse angiokeratoma)	1:40,000	Lipid storage disorder ceramide trihexosidase deficiency, α- galactosidase deficiency, on set in adolescence to adulthood, angina, pain attacks, autonomic dysfunction, angiokeratoma.
G_6PD deficiency	1:10–1:50	Enzyme deficiency with subtype shows effect in RBC, usually asymptomatic unless under stress or exposed to certain drugs or infection.
Hemophilia-A	1”250–1:4000	Coagulation disorder due to coagulation factor X deficiency
Hemophilia-B (Christmas disease)	1:4000–1:7000	Coagulation disorder due to coagulation factor X deficiency
Hunter syndrome	1:100,000	Mucopolysaccharide storage disorder with iduronote 2 sulfate deficiency, intellectual disability usual hepatomegaly, spleenomegaly, dwarfing, stiff joints, hearing loss, mild and severe form.
Lesch-Nyban syndrome	Rare	Deficiency of purine metabolism enzyme HPRT; hyperuremia, spasticity, athetosis, self-mutilation, developmental delay.

Contd...

Contd...

Disorder	Occurrence	Brief description
X-linked ichthyosis	1:5000–1:6000	Symptoms usual by 3 months may be born with sheets of scales (collodion babies) dry scaling skin often appears as it unwashed, developmental delay, bone changes, vascular complications, corneal opacities, steroid sulfatase deficiency.
Menkes disease	1:200,000	Copper deficiency caused by defective transportation, short stature, seizure, spasticity, hypothermia, kinky, sparse hair (pili torti); intellectual disability.

- Mutant gene is located on X chromosome
- One copy of the mutant gene is needed for phenotypic effect in male (hemizygous)
- All daughters of affected males will be carriers, if the mother is normal
- All sons of affected males will be normal, if the mother is normal
- Males are more frequently affected than females
- There are some fresh gene mutations
- There is no male to male transmission
- Transmission is often through heterozygous (carrier) females
- Two copies of the mutant gene are usually needed for phenotypic effect in females.
- Unequal X- inactivation can lead to manifesting heterozygotic in female carriers.

Common examples of the X-linked recessive disorders;
- Hemophilia
- Fabry disease
- Duchenne muscular dystrophy
- Protan and deutan form of color blindness
- Hunter syndrome.

In this example, a man with an X-linked recessive condition has two unaffected daughters who each carry one copy of the gene mutation, and two unaffected sons who do not have the mutation. (Fig. 1.33)

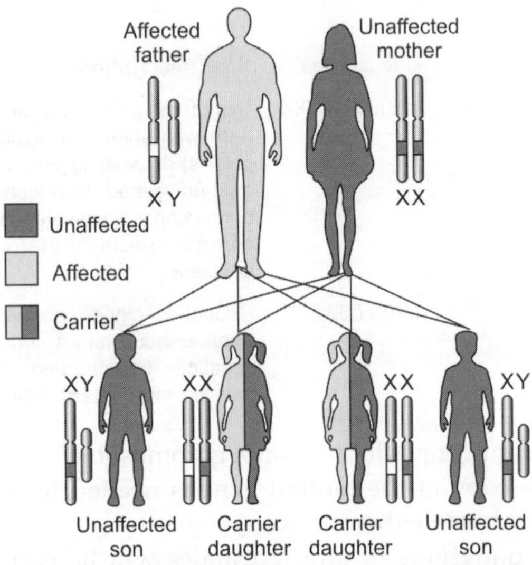

Fig. 1.33: X-linked recessive pattern of inheritance: affected father

In this example, an unaffected woman carries one copy of a gene mutation for an X-linked recessive disorder. She has an affected son, an unaffected daughter who carries one copy of the mutation, and two unaffected children who do not have the mutation. (Fig. 1.34)

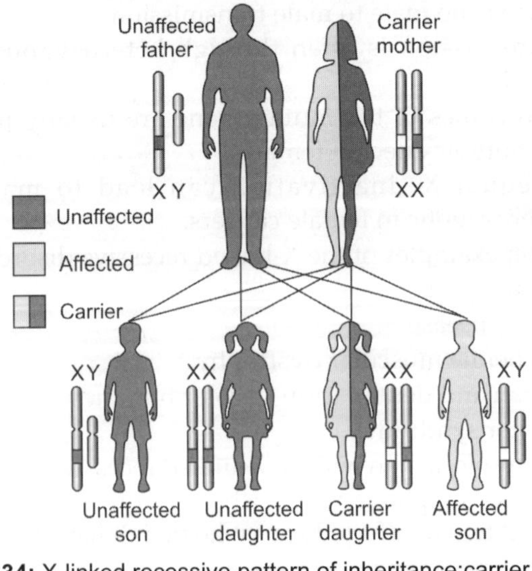

Fig. 1.34: X-linked recessive pattern of inheritance:carrier mother

- **Y-linked (Holandric) inheritance:** Few genes are known to be located on the Y-chromosome and so this type of inheritance has little clinical significance. Most Y-linked genes manifest their effect with one copy and show male-to-male transmission exclusively. All sons of an affected male would eventually develop trait. Although the age at which they develop disorders do varies. None of the affected male's daughter would inherit the trait. It can be hard to distinguish Y-linked inheritance form autosomal dominant disorders that are male sex limited. Some gene on the Y-chromosome are to determine height, male sex determination, such as the 'SRY' gene for the testis determining factor, tooth enamel and size, hairy, ear and finger protein. Male infertility disorder with genetic component can be inherited through this pattern of inheritance.

Codominant Pattern of Inheretance

In codominant inheritance, two different versions (alleles) of a gene can be expressed, and each version makes a slightly different protein (Fig. 1.35). Both alleles influence the genetic trait or determine the characteristics of the genetic condition.

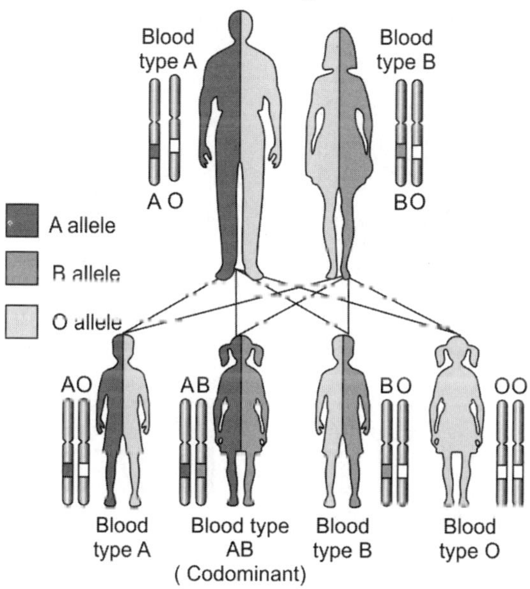

Fig. 1.35: Codominant pattern of inheritance

Example:

- ABO blood group,
- Alpha-1 antitrypsin deficiency

The ABO blood group is a major system for classifying blood types in humans. Blood type AB is inherited in a codominant pattern. In this example, a father with blood type A and a mother with blood type B have four children, each with a different blood type: A, AB, B, and O.

Mitochondrial Pattern of Inheritance

This type of inheritance, also known as maternal inheritance, applies to genes in mitochondrial DNA. Mitochondria, which are structures in each cell that convert molecules into energy, each contain a small amount of DNA. Because only egg cells contribute mitochondria to the developing embryo, only females can pass on mitochondrial conditions to their children (Fig. 1.36). Mitochondrial disorders can appear in every generation of a family and can affect both males and females, but fathers do not pass mitochondrial traits to their children.

Example: Leber's hereditary optic neuropathy (LHON)

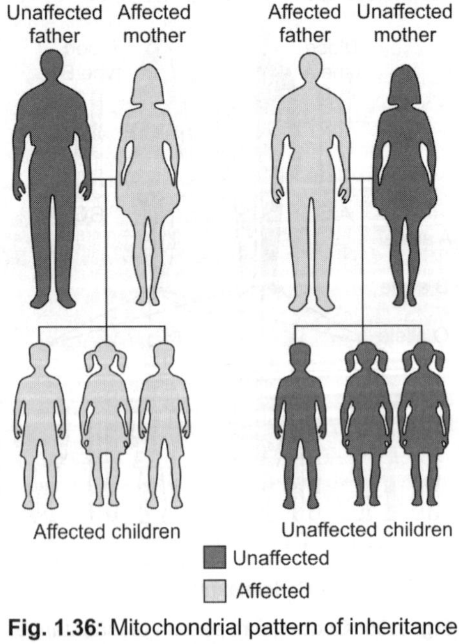

Fig. 1.36: Mitochondrial pattern of inheritance

In one family, a woman with a mitochondrial disorder and her unaffected husband have only affected children. In another family, a man with a mitochondrial condition and his unaffected wife have no affected children.

Multifactorial Pattern of Inheritance

This a common cause of many birth defects as well as common adult onset conditions, such as diabetes, heart disease and cancer. Multifactorial inheritance conditions are believed to be the result of multiple mutations and environmental influence that combine to cause birth defects or disease. Genetic conditions with a multifactorial cause tend to cluster in families but do not follow the characteristic pattern of inheritance seen with single gene disorder. (Fig. 1.37)

Examples:

- Congenital heart disease
- Cleft lip/palate
- Neural tube defect
- Congenital hip dislocation
- Diabetes
- High blood pressure.

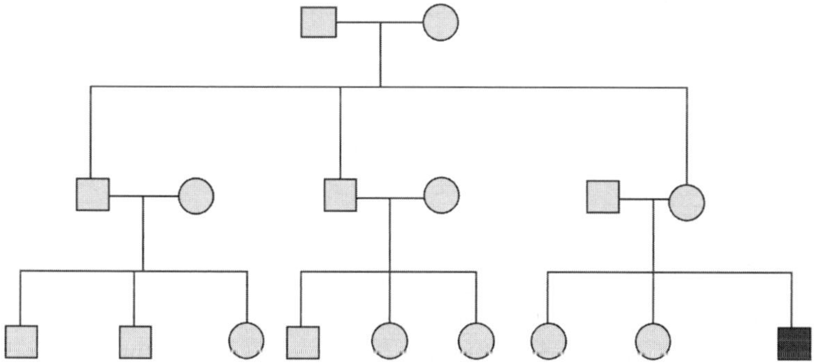

Fig. 1.37: Genetic conditions inherited in a multifactorial manner tend to cluster in families but do not follow the characteristic pattern of inheritance seen with single gene disorders

FACTS ABOUT TRANSMISSION OF GENETIC DISORDERS

When a genetic disorder is diagnosed in a family, family members often want to know the likelihood that they or their children will develop the condition. This can be difficult to predict in some cases because many factors influence a person's chances of developing a genetic condition. One important factor is how the condition is inherited. For example:

- *Autosomal dominant inheritance:* A person affected by an autosomal dominant disorder has a 50 percent chance of passing the mutated gene to each child. The chance that a child will not inherit the mutated gene is also 50 percent.
- *Autosomal recessive inheritance:* Two unaffected people who each carry one copy of the mutated gene for an autosomal recessive disorder (carriers) have a 25 percent chance with each pregnancy of having a child affected by the disorder. The chance with each pregnancy of having an unaffected child who is a carrier of the disorder is 50 percent, and the chance that a child will not have the disorder and will not be a carrier is 25 percent.
- *X-linked dominant inheritance:* The chance of passing on an X-linked dominant condition differs between men and women because men have one X chromosome and one Y chromosome, while women have two X chromosomes. A man passes on his Y chromosome to all of his sons and his X chromosome to all of his daughters. Therefore, the sons of a man with an X-linked dominant disorder will not be affected, but all of his daughters will inherit the condition. A woman passes on one or the other of her X chromosomes to each child. Therefore, a woman with an X-linked dominant disorder has a 50 percent chance of having an affected daughter or son with each pregnancy.
- *X-linked recessive inheritance:* Because of the difference in sex chromosomes, the probability of passing on an X-linked recessive disorder also differs between men and women. The sons of a man with an X-linked recessive disorder will not be affected, and his daughters will carry one copy of the mutated gene. With each pregnancy, a woman who carries an X-linked recessive disorder has a 50 percent chance of having sons who are affected and a 50 percent chance of having daughters who carry one copy of the mutated gene.
- *Codominant inheritance:* In codominant inheritance, each parent contributes a different version of a particular gene, and both versions influence the resulting genetic trait. The chance of

developing a genetic condition with codominant inheritance, and the characteristic features of that condition, depend on which versions of the gene are passed from parents to their child.

- *Mitochondrial inheritance:* Mitochondria, which are the energy-producing centers inside cells, each contain a small amount of DNA. Disorders with mitochondrial inheritance result from mutations in mitochondrial DNA. Although mitochondrial disorders can affect both males and females, only females can pass mutations in mitochondrial DNA to their children. A woman with a disorder caused by changes in mitochondrial DNA will pass the mutation to all of her daughters and sons, but the children of a man with such a disorder will not inherit the mutation .

It is important to note that the chance of passing on a genetic condition applies equally to each pregnancy. For example, if a couple has a child with an autosomal recessive disorder, the chance of having another child with the disorder is still 25 percent (or 1 in 4). Having one child with a disorder does not 'protect' future children from inheriting the condition. Conversely, having a child without the condition does not mean that future children will definitely be affected.

Although the chances of inheriting a genetic condition appear straightforward, factors, such as a person's family history and the results of genetic testing can sometimes modify those chances. In addition, some people with a disease causing mutation never develop any health problems or may experience only mild symptoms of the disorder. If a disease that runs in a family does not have a clear-cut inheritance pattern, predicting the likelihood that a person will develop the condition can be particularly difficult.

Estimating the chance of developing or passing on a genetic disorder can be complex. Genetics professionals can help people understand these chances and help them make informed decisions about their health.

MULTIPLE ALLELES AND BLOOD GROUPS

Multiple Alleles

More than two alternative forms of a gene present on the same locus are called multiple alleles. They are produced due to repeated mutation of the same gene but in different directions. Thus, the wild type of allele for red eye color (w^+ or W) in Drosophila melanogster mutated to form allele for white eye (w), further mutation in both have incomplete intermediate dominance over one another. Some of these alleles are wine (w^w), coral (w^{co}), blood (w^{bl}), cherry (w^c), apricot (w^a), eosine (w^e), buff (w^b), tinged (w^t), honey (w^h), ecru (w^{ec}), pearl (w^p) and ivory (w^i). Despite the presence of several alleles of the same gene in a population, an individual can have only two alleles.

Characteristics includes:

- There are more than two alleles of the same gene, e.g. 15 alleles for eye color in Drosophila, 3 alleles for blood group in human, 4 alleles for coat color in Rabbit.
- All the multiple alleles occur on the same gene locus of the same chromosome or its homologue.
- Chromosome contains only one alleles of the group.
- An individual possesses only two alleles while the gametes carry single allele.
- Multiple alleles express different alternatives of the same character.
- Different alleles show codominance-recessive or intermediate dominance amongst themselves. They however, follow mendelian pattern of inheritance.

Blood Group System

Immunogenetics began in when Lanssteinner discovered the ABO blood group system. At this time 26 such systems, plus 5 collections and 2 series are known in humans, but all did not have clinical significance. A six-digit number is given to every blood group antigen, in which the first three digits represent the system, collection or series and the second three digit represent the antigen. The system that are best characterized and most important are ABO, Rhesus, Kell Lewis, Duffy, MNSs, Lutheran, P, Kidd, Diego, Yt, Xg, Domfrock, childol Rogers and Scianna.

ABO Blood Group System

ABO blood group system in human beings is an example of multiple alleles. Human have four blood groups or blood group phenotypes; A, B, AB, and O. The ABO system is the most clinically important, the major alleles present at the ABO locus chromosomes are A, B, and O. Both A and B alleles are dominant to the O but codominant to each other. The A and B alleles code for certain enzymes and glycosyltransferanses and add sugar to the H substrate precursor to form the A and B glycoprotein antigen. The O allele does not produce an enzyme. These A and B antigens are not confined to the red cell but are widely distributed through the body. There are various subtype of the A, B and O alleles with more polymorphisms being revealed by newer DNA technique, but only A_1 and A_2 appear to have any antigenic importance. The relationship between genotype and blood group is shown in Table 1.9 and example of the inheritance of the ABO blood group are illustrated in Table 1.10 and 1.11.

Persons with blood group O are sometimes said to have a 'null' phenotype. Independent of the ABO system are the H and secretor systems. Person with the genotype HH or Hh produce the H substrate, which is the precursor for the A and B antigen and is modified by the enzymes produced by the A and B allele does not produce a transferase, it exerts no effect on this pathway, the H substrate is unmodifiable and more H antigen remains present. The allele h is a rare silent allele recessive to H. Person with hh who have the A and B allele do not express them due to the absence of the H substrate. The secretor (Se, se) locus determines whether the ABH antigen will be secreted in body fluids, such as saliva, individuals who are nonsecretors (se, se) do not secrete ABH antigens. Approximately 80 percent of the white population is secretors. The secretor gene appears to have a regulatory function on the 'H' gene.

The clinical significance of this relationship is illustrated by the case of women who contacted the genetic counseling center at PGIMER, Chandigarh. She was believed to have blood group O, her husband was A and her child was AB, she had been told by the local health professionals that this was not possible unless her husband was not the child's father. The situation was causing considerable stress in their married relationship. Investigation demonstrated that she in fact had the B allele, but was homozygous for the rare Bombay phenotype known as hh. B antigen production was blocked by the two h alleles, even though she had one B gene. This client had contacted the genetic counseling center on her own.

The health professionals involved in this case had simply accepted what they considered to be the most likely explanation, without further investigation or consultation. Rare cases of other variance are known. This is an example of why it is necessary to recognize the limits of one's own knowledge. Another approach would have been to do DNA testing to establish parentage.

A human being carries two of the three alleles, one from each parent. The maximum number of possible genotype is six for the four phenotypes. The phenotypes are tested by two antisera, anti-A and anti-B.

Table 1.9: Relationship in ABO blood group system

Blood group (Phenotype)	Genotype(s)	Red cell antigen(s)	Antibodies in serum
A	AO, AA	A (+H)	Anti-B
B	BO, BB	B (+H)	Anti-A
AB	AB	A,B (+H)	None
O	OO	H	Anti-A, Anti-B

Table 1.10: Chart showing inheritance of blood groups by children of various parentages

Blood group of mother	**Blood group of father**	**O**		**A**		**B**		**AB**	
	Blood group allele in sperm								
	Blood group allele in ova	*O*	*O*	*A*	*O*	*B*	*O*	*A*	*B*
O	O	*OO* **(O)**	*OO* **(O)**	*AO* **(A)**	*OO* **(O)**	*BO* **(B)**	*OO* **(O)**	*AO* **(A)**	*BO* **(B)**
	O	*OO* **(O)**	*OO* **(O)**	*AO* **(A)**	*OO* **(O)**	*BO* **(B)**	*OO* **(O)**	*AO* **(A)**	*BO* **(B)**
A	*A*	*AO* **(A)**	*AO* **(A)**	*AA* **(A)**	*AO* **(A)**	*AB* **(AB)**	*AO* **(A)**	*AA* **(A)**	*AB* (AB)
	O	*OO* **(O)**	*OO* **(O)**	*AO* **(A)**	*OO* **(O)**	*BO* **(B)**	*OO* **(O)**	*AO* **(A)**	*BO* **(B)**

Contd...

Contd...

Blood group of mother	Blood group of father	O		A		B		AB	
B	*B*	BO (B)	*BO* (B)	*AB* (AB)	*BO* (B)	*BB* (B)	*BO* (B)	*AB* (AB)	*BB* (B)
	O	*OO* (O)	*OO* (O)	*AO* (A)	*OO* (O)	*BO* (B)	*OO* (O)	*AO* (A)	*BO* (B)
AB	*A*	AO (A)	*AO* (A)	AA (A)	AO (A)	AB (AB)	AO (A)	AA (A)	AB (AB)
	B	BO (B)	BO (B)	AB (AB)	BO (B)	BB (B)	BO (B)	AB (AB)	BB (B)

* Every column presents offspring genotype of blood group and letters in parentheses are possible blood group phenotype of offspring

Table 1.11: Example of transmission of blood group genes (ABO system*)

Parents	AO x BO	AB x OO	AA x BB	AA x BO	AB x BB	BB x OO
Offspring genotype	AB, AO, BO, OO	AO, BO	AB	AB, AO	AB, BB	BO
Theoretical proposition of each pregnancy	¼, ¼, ¼, ¼	½, ½	All	½, ½	½, ½	All
Blood group phenotype	AB, A, B, O	A, B	AB	AB, A	AB, B	B

* *Not all possible combinations are shown*

Table 1.12: Example of transmission of blood group genes (Rh system)

Parents	DD x dd	Dd x dd	Dd x Dd
Offspring genotype	DD	Dd, dd	DD, Dd, dd
Theoretical proposition of each pregnancy	All	½, ½	¼, ½ , ¼
Blood group phenotype	Rh (+)	Rh (+), Rh (-)	Rh (+), Rh (+), Rh (-)

The Rhesus (Rh) System

It was not until 1940 that Landsteiner and Wiener discovered the rhesus (Rh) system. This system has become increasingly more complex. Many variants and about 45 antigens are known and various symbols have been used to describe the major components. The most common the one proposed by Fisher, Race and Sanger, reflected the existence of three very closely linked lock C, D or d (ho d) antiserum for the 'd' antigen has been found and those who are RhD negative actually lack the gene; however 'd' is used here for convenience and E or C and E alleles are much less antigenic than D. The D alleles are considered responsible for determining Rh positivity (+) in a dominant relationship to 'd'. This inheritance pattern is illustrated in Table 1.12; the percentage of Rh negative individuals in the white population is approximately 15 percent, few native Americans or Asians are Rh negative. In the black population approximately 7 percent are Rh negative.

GENE MUTATION (ERRORS OF TRANSMISSION)

They are new sudden inheritable discontinuous variations, which are caused by a change in the nucleotide type and sequence of a DNA segment representing a gene. *In other words a gene mutation is a permanent change in the DNA base sequence that makes up a gene. Mutations range in size from a single DNA building block (DNA base) to a large segment of a chromosome.* The first recorded gene mutations are Ancon Sheep (1791) and hornless (polled) cattle (1889). Following are the main features of the gene mutation:

- All genes can mutate. However, mutability differs from gene to gene.
- The direction of gene mutation cannot be predictable. It can occur in any possible direction to any possible degree.
- A mutated gene can mutate back to its permutation state.
- Gene mutation can be lethal. Harmful, neutral or advantageous.
- Most of the mutations are recessive and involve loss of function. A few are dominant ones.
- The gene mutation may occur naturally and automatically due to several reason, termed as spontaneous mutation and others

are produced by external factors or chemicals, they are termed as induced mutations.

- Individuals also possess mutator genes (cause mutations through altering polymerase activity) and antimutator genes (Check alteration in nucleotide through sequence during replication).
- A spontaneous mutation happens through mechanisms of tautomerism (a base change by the repositioning of a hydrogen atom), depurination (loss of purine base- A or G), deamination (change a normal base to an atypical base), transition (a purine change to another purine or a pyrimidine to another pyrimidine) and transversion (a purine become a pyrimidine or vice versa).
- Mutation can occur in somatic or germinal cells.

Gene mutations occur in two ways:

1. ***Germline or inherited mutation:*** Mutations that are passed from parent to child are called inherited mutations or germline mutations (because they are present in the egg and sperm cells, which are also called germ cells). This type of mutation is present throughout a person's life in virtually every cell in the body. Mutations that occur only in an egg or sperm cell, or those that occur just after fertilization, are called new (*de novo*) mutations. *De novo* mutations may explain genetic disorders in which an affected child has a mutation in every cell, but has no family history of the disorder.
2. ***Somatic or acquired mutation:*** Acquired during a person's lifetime. Acquired (or somatic) mutations occur in the DNA of individual cells at some time during a person's life. These changes can be caused by environmental factors, such as ultraviolet radiation from the sun, or can occur if a mistake is made as DNA copies itself during cell division. Acquired mutations in somatic cells (cells other than germ cells) cannot be passed onto the next generation. Mutations may also occur in a single cell within an early embryo. As all the cells divide during growth and development, the individual will have some cells with the mutation and some cells without the genetic change. This situation is called mosaicism.

Some genetic changes are very rare; others are common in the population. Genetic changes that occur in more than 1 percent of the population are called polymorphisms. They are common enough to be considered a normal variation in the DNA. Polymorphisms are responsible for many of the normal differences between people, such as eye color, hair color, and blood type. Although polymorphisms generally have no negative effects on a person's health, some of these variations may influence the risk of developing certain disorders.

Causes of Gene Mutation

Any extracellular physical or chemical factor, which can cause mutation, or increase the frequency of mutation in an individual is called mutagen.

- *Physical factors:* They are two types, temperatures and high-energy radiations.
  a. *Temperature*: Increase in temperature increase the rate of mutations. Rise in temperature breaks the hydrogen bonding between the two strands of DNA and hence denatures the letters.
  b. *High energy radiations*: They include neutrons, *alpha particles, cosmic rays, gamma particles, beta rays, X-rays, ultraviolet rays,* etc. Ultraviolet rays are nonionizing radiations, which affect DNA by forming thymine dimers. It causes bends in DNA duplex that bring about misreplication. Other high-energy radiations are ionizing radiations. They ionize DNA constituents that can react with several biochemicals, X-rays are known to deaminate and dehydroxylation nitrogen bases, from peroxides and oxidize deoxyribose.
- *Chemical factors:* They are of several types. The common ones are nitrogen acid, alkylating agents, base analogs and acridines. Even some of drugs are known to cause gene mutation, like chemotherapeutic drugs for cancer.

Types or Mechanism of Gene Mutation

The smallest part of a gene that undergoes mutation is known as *muton*. It can be as small as a single nucleotide. Most of the gene mutations involvea change in only a single nucleotide or nitrogen base. These gene mutations are called *point mutations*. A mutation involving more than one base pair is termed as *gross mutation*. Gene mutation usually occurs during replication of DNA. It is therefore, also called *copy error mutation*. During gene mutation a gene may undergo several point mutations. This produces multiple alleles. Gene mutations have varying effects on health, depending on where they occur and whether they alter the function of essential proteins. The DNA sequence of a gene can be altered in a number of ways. The main types or methods of gene mutations are as follows:

- *Inversion mutation:* A distortion of DNA by mutagen can change the base sequence of a gene in the reverse order. The process is called inversion. The new sequence will naturally have different codones. *In example, there is reverse order of DNA base after mutation (Fig. 1.38).*

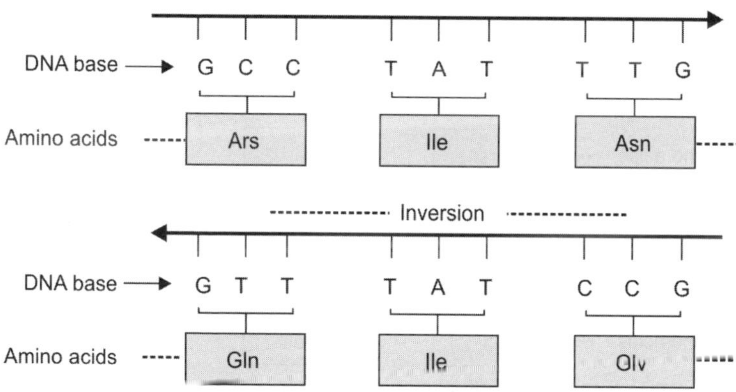

Fig 1.38: Inversion mutation

- *Substitution mutation (replacement):* In substitution a nitrogen base is changed with another. It is of two type, transition and transversion.

    a. *Transition mutation:* A nitrogen base is replaced by another of its type, that is one purine is replaced by another purine (Adenine ↔ guanine), while one pyrimidine by another pyrimidine (cytosine ↔ thymine or uracil). *In example, a purine (guanine) is replaced by another purine (adenine) (Fig. 1.39).*

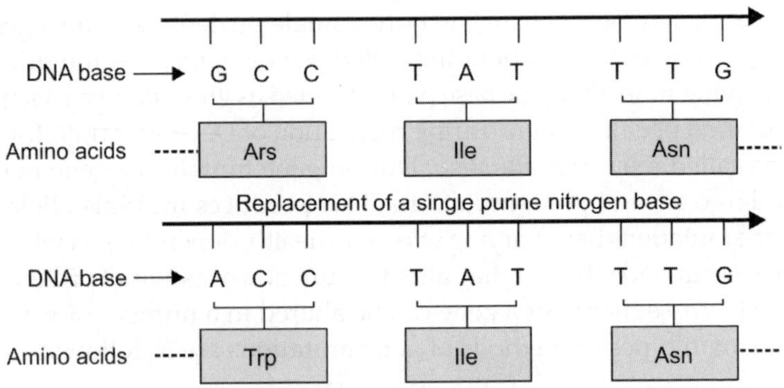

Fig. 1.39: Transition mutation

b. *Transversion mutation:* Hence a purine base is replaced or substituted by a pyrimidine base and vice versa, e.g. Uracil or thymine with adenine and cytosine with guanine *In example, cytosine replaced guanine (Fig. 1.40) and in Fig. 1.41 thymine replaced adenine.*

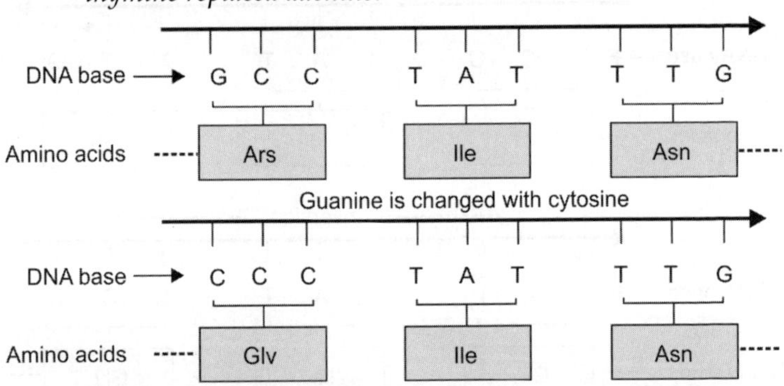

Fig. 1.40: Transversion mutation (cytosine replaces guanine)

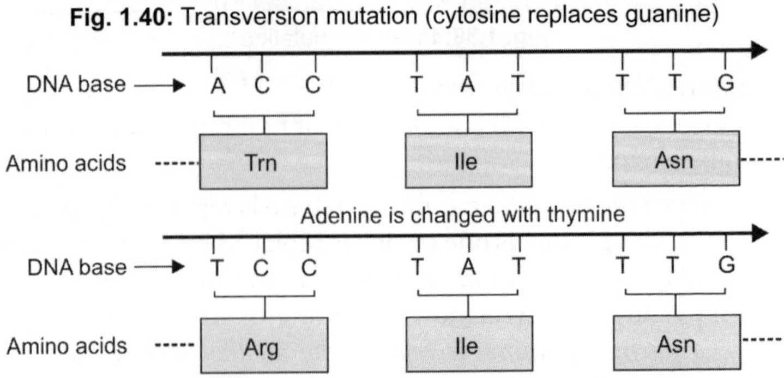

Fig. 1.41: Transversion mutation (Thymine replaces adenine)

- *Frame-shift mutation:* They are those mutations in which the reading of the frame of base sequence shift laterally either in the forward direction due to insertion (addition) of one or more nucleotide or in the backward direction due to deletion of one or more nucleotides. Therefore, frame-shift mutations are of two kinds insertion and deletion. A frameshift mutation changes the amino acid sequence from the site of the mutation.
  - *Insertion mutation:* An insertion changes the number of DNA bases in a gene by adding a piece of DNA. As a result, the protein made by the gene may not function properly. *In this example, one nucleotide (adenine) is added in the DNA code, changing the amino acid sequence that follows (Fig. 1.42).*

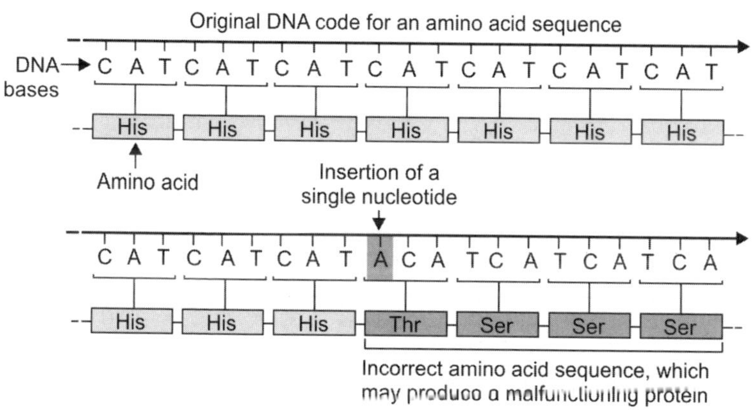

Fig. 1.42: Inserion mutation

  - *Deletion mutation:* A deletion changes the number of DNA bases by removing a piece of DNA. Small deletions may remove one or a few base pairs within a gene, while larger deletions can remove an entire gene or several neighboring genes. The deleted DNA may alter the function of the resulting protein(s). In this example, one nucleotide (adenine) is deleted from the DNA code, changing the amino acid sequence that follows *(Fig. 1.43).*

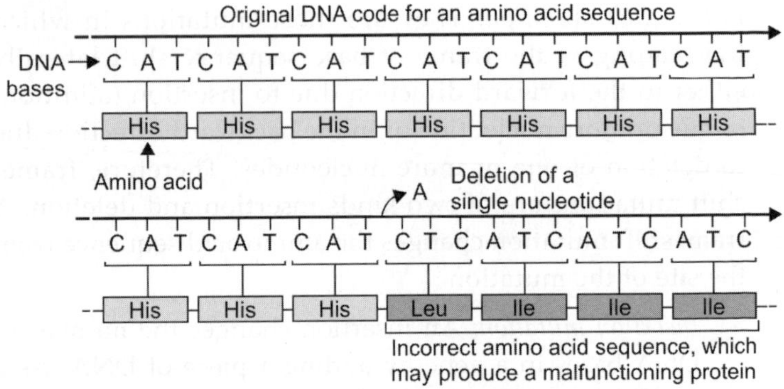

Fig. 1.43: Deletion mutation

- *Missense mutation:* This type of mutation is a change in one DNA base pair that results in the substitution of one amino acid for another in the protein made by a gene. *In this example, the nucleotide adenine is replaced by cytosine in the genetic code, introducing an incorrect amino acid into the protein sequence. (Fig. 1.44)*

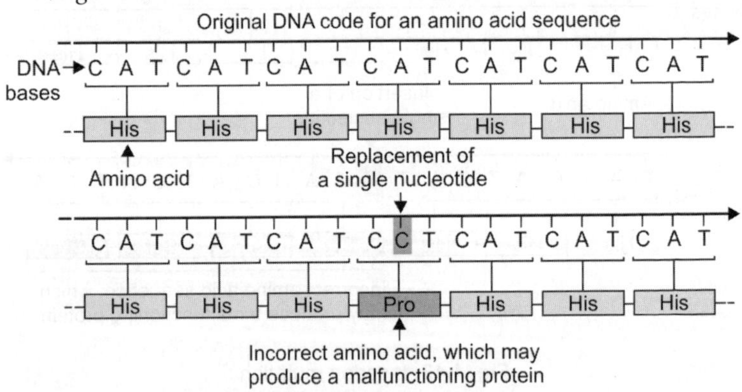

Fig. 1.44: Missense mutation

- *Nonsense mutation:* A nonsense mutation is also a change in one DNA base pair. Instead of substituting one amino acid for another, however, the altered DNA sequence prematurely signals the cell to stop building a protein. This type of mutation results in a shortened protein that may function improperly or not at all. *In this example, the nucleotide cytosine is replaced by thymine in the DNA code, signaling the cell to shorten the protein (Fig. 1.45).*

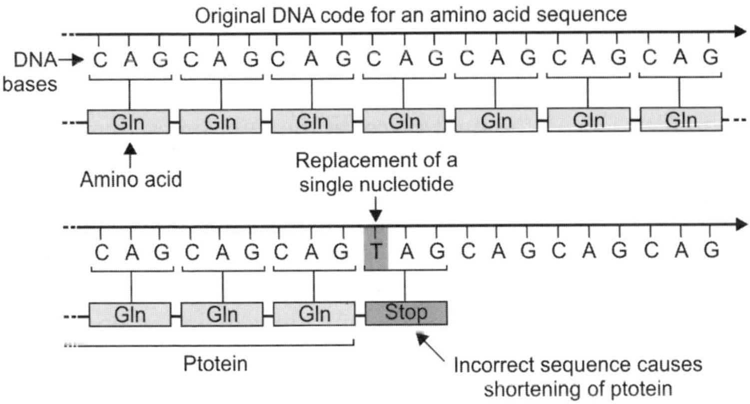

Fig. 1.45: Nonsense mutation

- *Repeat expansion:* Nucleotide repeats are short DNA sequences that are repeated a number of times in a row. For example, a trinucleotide repeat is made-up of 3-base-pair sequences, and a tetranucleotide repeat is made-up of 4-base-pair sequences. A repeat expansion is a mutation that increases the number of times that the short DNA sequence is repeated. This type of mutation can cause the resulting protein to function improperly. In this example, a repeated trinucleotide sequence (CAG) adds a series of the amino acid glutamine to the resulting *protein (Fig. 1.46).*

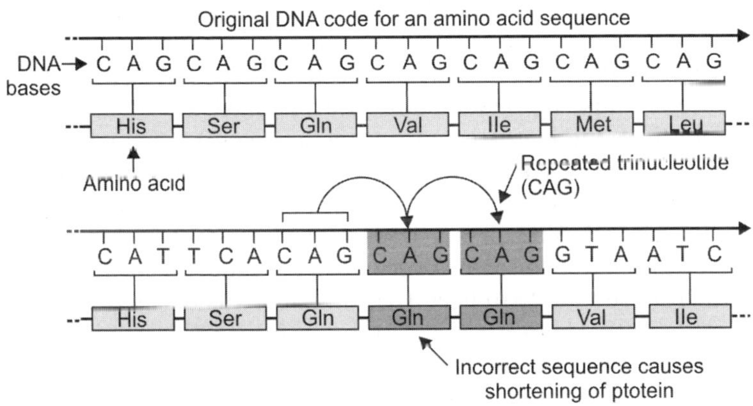

Fig. 1.46: Repeat expansion

EFFECT OF GENE MUTATIONS ON HEALTH AND DEVELOPMENT

To function correctly, each cell depends on thousands of proteins to do their jobs in the right places at the right times. Sometimes, gene mutations prevent one or more of these proteins from working properly. By changing a gene's instructions for making a protein, a mutation can cause the protein to malfunction or to be missing entirely. When a mutation alters a protein that plays a critical role in the body, it can disrupt normal development or cause a medical condition. A condition caused by mutations in one or more genes is called a genetic disorder.

In some cases, gene mutations are so severe that they prevent an embryo from surviving until birth. These changes occur in genes that are essential for development, and often disrupt the development of an embryo in its earliest stages. Because these mutations have very serious effects, they are incompatible with life. It is important to note that genes themselves do not cause disease. Genetic disorders are caused by mutations that make a gene function improperly. For example, when people say that someone has 'the cystic fibrosis gene,' they are usually referring to a mutated version of the CFTR gene, which causes the disease. All people, including those without cystic fibrosis, have a version of the CFTR gene.

Only a small percentage of mutations cause genetic disorders; most have no impact on health or development. For example, some mutations alter a gene's DNA base sequence but do not change the function of the protein made by the gene. Often, gene mutations that could cause a genetic disorder are repaired by certain enzymes before the gene is expressed (makes a protein). Each cell has a number of pathways through which enzymes recognize and repair mistakes in DNA. Because DNA can be damaged or mutated in many ways, DNA repair is an important process by which the body protects itself from disease. A very small percentage of all mutations actually have a positive effect. These mutations lead to new versions of proteins that help an organism and its future generations better adapt to changes in their environment. For example, a beneficial mutation could result in a protein that protects the organism from a new strain of bacteria.

REDUCED PENETRANCE AND VARIABLE EXPRESSIVITY

Reduced penetrance and variable expressivity are factors that influence the effects of particular genetic changes. These factors usually affect disorders that have an autosomal dominant pattern of inheritance, although they are occasionally seen in disorders with an autosomal recessive inheritance pattern.

Reduced penetrance: Penetrance refers to the proportion of people with a particular genetic change (such as a mutation in a specific gene) who exhibit signs and symptoms of a genetic disorder. If some people with the mutation do not develop features of the disorder, the condition is said to have reduced (or incomplete) penetrance. Reduced penetrance often occurs with familial cancer syndromes. For example, many people with a mutation in the BRCA1 or BRCA2 gene will develop cancer during their lifetime, but some people will not. Doctors cannot predict which people with these mutations will develop cancer or when the tumors will develop.

Reduced penetrance probably results from a combination of genetic, environmental, and lifestyle factors, many of which are unknown. This phenomenon can make it challenging for genetics professionals to interpret a person's family medical history and predict the risk of passing a genetic condition to future generations.

Variable expressivity: Although some genetic disorders exhibit little variation, most have signs and symptoms that differ among affected individuals. Variable expressivity refers to the range of signs and symptoms that can occur in different people with the same genetic condition. For example, the features of Marfan syndrome vary widely; some people have only mild symptoms (such as being tall and thin with long, slender fingers), while others also experience life-threatening complications involving the heart and blood vessels. Although the features are highly variable, most people with this disorder have a mutation in the same gene (FBN1). As with reduced penetrance, variable expressivity is probably caused by a combination of genetic, environmental, and lifestyle factors, most of which have not been identified. If a genetic condition has highly variable signs and symptoms, it may be challenging to diagnose.

ANTICIPATION

The signs and symptoms of some genetic conditions tend to become more severe and appears at an earlier age as the disorder is passed from one generation to the next. This phenomenon is called anticipation. Anticipation is most often seen with certain genetic disorders of the nervous system, such as Huntington disease, myotonic dystrophy, and fragile X syndrome. Anticipation typically occurs with disorders that are caused by an unusual type of mutation called a trinucleotide repeat expansion. A trinucleotide repeat is a sequence of three DNA building blocks (nucleotides) that is repeated a number of times in a row. DNA segments with an abnormal number of these repeats are unstable and prone to errors during cell division. The number of repeats can change as the gene is passed from parent to child. If the number of repeats increases, it is known as a trinucleotide repeat expansion. In some cases, the trinucleotide repeat may expand until the gene stops functioning normally. This expansion causes the features of some disorders to become more severe with each successive generation.

Most genetic disorders have signs and symptoms that differ among affected individuals, including affected people in the same family. Not all of these differences can be explained by anticipation. A combination of genetic, environmental, and lifestyle factors is probably responsible for the variability, although many of these factors have not been identified. Researchers study multiple generations of affected family members and consider the genetic cause of a disorder before determining that it shows anticipation.

REVIEW QUESTIONS

Short-note Questions

1. Importance of studying genetics in nursing.
2. Characteristics and structure of genes.
3. Write difference between mitosis and meiosis.
4. Impact of genetic condition on families.
5. Deoxyribonucleic acid (DNA).
6. Mendalian theory of inheritance.
7. Klinefelter's Syndrome.

8. Autosomal dominant pattern of inheritance.
9. Mitosis.
10. Inheritance of Blood groups.
11. Mutation.
12. Allele and haplotype.
13. Blood grouping and cross matching.
14. Sex –linked disorders.
15. Turner's syndrome.
16. Incomplete dominance.
17. Blood groups
18. Define mutation and mention some causes of mutation.
19. Chromosomal aberration.
20. Structural chromosomal abnormalities.
21. Blood group systems.
22. Classify Mendalian disorder, write in detail about autosomal dominant disorder and features of any one type of autosomal disorder.

Short-answer Questions

1. Mention two differences between meiosis and mitosis.
2. Mention two autosomal dominant and two autosomal recessive disorders
3. Define mutation.
4. Define genetics.
5. Nucleotide.
6. Euchromatin.
7. Deletion in chromosomes.
8. Mention two autosomal dominant disorders.
9. Barr body.

Multiple Choice Questions (MCQs)

1. **Observable characters of an organism is called:**
   a. Trait b. Phenotype
   c. Genotype d. Character

2. A segment of DNA that codes for a functional polypeptide or an RNA molecule is called:

a. Allele b. Gene
c. Recon d. Muton

3. The genetic constitution of an organism is called:

a. Genotype b. Trait
c. Phenotype d. Genome

4. The part of the cell that binds to mRNA during protein synthesis is a:

a. Ribosome b. Lysosome
c. Peroxisome d. Centrosome

5. A triplet of bases on mRNA is known as a:

a. Nucleotide b. Anticodon
c. Antinucleotide d. Codon

6. The reproduction of humans requires the genetic process of:

a. Mitosis b. Meiosis
c. Bivalence d. Inheritance

7. In a family, father is having a disease and mother is normal. The disease is inherited to only daughters and not to the sons. What type of disease is this?

a. Sex linked dominant b. Sex linked recessive
c. Autosomal dominant d. Autosomal recessive

8. In man, which of the following genotypes and phenotypes may be the correct result of aneuploidy in sex chromosomes?

a. 22 pairs + Y females b. 22 pairs + XX females
c. 22 pairs + XXY males d. 22 pairs + XXXY females

9. A woman with one gene for hemophilia and one gene for color blindness on one of the X chromosomes marries a normal man. How will the progeny be?

a. Hemophilic and color blind daughters
b. All sons and daughters are hemophilic and color blind
c. 50% hemophilic and color blind sons and 50% normal sons
d. 50% hemophilic color blind sons and 50% color blind daughters

10. Crossing over occurs during which phase of cell division:

a. Pachytene b. Diplotene
c. Diakinesis d. Pachytene

11. Who is regarded as the father of genetics?

a. Bateson b. Morgan
c. Mendel d. Watson

12. The alternate forms of a gene is called:

a. Recessive character b. Dominant character
c. Alleles d. Alternative gene

13. Which of the following is not needed for DNA transcription?

a. Ribosomes b. Nucleotides
c. DNA d. Enzymes

14. A gene showing codominanace:

a. Has one allele dominant to the other
b. Has both alleles independently expressed in the heterozygote
c. Has alleles tightly linked on the same chromosome
d. Has alleles expressed at the same time in development

15. If characteristic requires only one gene to show itself the characteristic is considered:

a. Dominant b. Co-dominant
c. Recessive d. None of these

ANSWER KEY

1. b	2. b	3. a	4. a	5. d	6. b	7. a
8. c	9. c	10. a	11. c	12. c	13. d	14. b
15. a						

FURTHER READING

1. American Society of Human Genetics/American College of Medical Genetics: Points to consider: Ethical, legal, and psychosocial implications of genetic testing in children and adolescents. Am J Hum Genet 1995;57:1223-41.
2. Beauchamp TL, Childress JF: Principles of Biomedical Ethics. New York, Oxford University Press, 1994.

3. Billings PR, Kohn MA, de Cuevas M, et al: Discrimination as a consequence of genetic testing. Am J Hum Genet 1992;50:476-82.
4. Bove C, Fry ST, MacDonald DJ: Presymptomatic and predisposition genetic testing: Ethical and social considerations. Semin Oncol Nurs 1997;13:135-40.
5. Clayton, Julie. (Ed.). 50 Years of DNA, Palgrave MacMillan Press, 2003. ISBN 978-1-40-391479-8.
6. Enkins J: Educational issues related to cancer genetics. Semin Oncol Nurs 1997;13:141-4.
7. Fiers W, et al. Complete nucleotide-sequence of bacteriophage MS2-RNA - primary and secondary structure of replicase gene, Nature, 260, 500-7, 1976.
8. Havens DMH, Kovner R: Genetic testing: How it is transforming the role of health professionals and the implications for pediatric nurse practitioners. Journal of Pediatric Health Care 1997;11:193-7.
9. Holtzman NA, Watson MS: Promoting Safe and Effective Genetic Testing in the United States: Final Report of the Task Force on Genetic Testing. http://www.nhgri.nih.gov /ELSI/TFGT_final. Accessed September, 1997.
10. Judson, Horace Freeland. The Eighth Day of Creation: Makers of the Revolution in Biology, Cold Spring Harbor Laboratory Press, 1996. ISBN 978-0-87-969478.
11. Lippman-Hand A, Fraser FC: Genetic counseling: Provision and reception of information. Am J Hum Genet 1979;3:113-27.
12. Love RR: The accuracy of patient reports of a family history of cancer. Journal of Chronic Disease 1985;38:289-93.
13. MacDonald DJ: The oncology nurse's role in cancer risk assessment and counseling. Semin Oncol Nurs 1997;13:123-8
14. Matloff ET, Peshkin BN: Complexities in cancer genetic counseling: Breast and ovarian cancer. Principles and Practice of Oncology Updates 1998;12:1-11.
15. Michie 5, Bron F, Bobrow M, et al. Nondirectiveness in genetic counseling: An empirical study. Am J Hum Genet 1997;60:40-7.
16. National Society of Genetic Counselors: Position Statements. 1991. National Society of Genetic Counselors: Code of Ethics. 1992.
17. Offit K: Clinical Cancer Genetics: Risk Counseling and Management. New York, WileyLiss, 1998, 249.
18. Olby, Robert. The Path to The Double Helix: Discovery of DNA, first published in October 1974 by MacMillan, with foreword by Francis Crick; ISBN 978-0-48-668117-7; the definitive DNA textbook, revised in 1994, with a 9 page postscript.

19. Peters J, Stopfer J: Role of the genetic counselor in familial cancer. Oncology 1996;10:159-75.
20. Rassoulzadegan M, et al. Nature, doi:10.1038/nature04674 , 2006.
21. Reilly PR, Boshar MF, Holzman SH: Ethical issues in genetic research: Disclosure and informed consent. Nat Genet 1997;15:16-20.
22. Ridley, Matt. Francis Crick: Discoverer of the Genetic Code (Eminent Lives) first published in June 2006 in the USA and then to be in the UK September 2006, by HarperCollins Publishers; 192 pp, ISBN 978-0-06-082333-7.
23. Rieger PT: Overview of cancer and genetics: Implications for nurse practitioners. Nurse Practitioner Forum 1998;9:122-33.
24. Rothenberg K, Fuller B, Rothstein M, et al: Genetic information *an*d the workplace: Legislative approaches and policy changes. Science 1997;275:1755-1757.
25. Rothenberg KH: Genetic discrimination and health insurance: A call for legislative action. J Am Med Womens Assoc 1997;52:43-4.
26. Rothenberg K, Fuller B, Rothstein M, et al. Genetic information and the workplace: Legistative approaches and policy changes. Science 1997;275:1755-7.
27. Rowland LP: Molecular basis of genetic heterogeneity: Role of the clinical neurologist. J Child Neurol 1998;13:122-32.
28. Savage R, Armstrong D. Effect of a general practitioner's consulting style on patients' satisfaction: A controlled study 1990;BMJ 301:968-70.
29. Scanlon C, Fibison W: Managing genetic information: Implications for nursing practice. Washington, DC, American Nurses Association, 1995.
30. Schneider KA: Counseling About Cancer: Strategies for Genetic Counselors. Dennisport, MA, Graphic Illusions, 1994.
31. Shiloh S, Saxe L: Perception of risk in genetic counseling. Psychological Health 1989;3:45 61.
32. Walker AP: Historical perspective and philosophical perspective of genetic counseling. In Emery AEH, Rimoin DL, Connor JM, et al (eds): Principles and Practice of Medical Genetics, ed 3. New York, Churchill-Livingstone, 1996.
33. Wertz DC, Fanos JH, Reilly PR: Genetic testing for children and adolescents. Who decides? JAMA 1994;272:875-81.

Chapter 2

Emerging Paradigm of Genetics in Nursing

Learning Objectives

This chapter is designed to enable the reader to:

- List out the milestones of genetics nursing practices
- Describe the role of nurses in genetics
- Appraise the importance of genetics in nursing curriculum
- Recognize the barriers and approaches for implementation of genetics in nursing
- Discuss the assumptions regarding genetics and health care in future.

Key Terms

- Genetics Nursing
- Genetics Nurses
- Genetics Nursing Network
- Genetics Advanced Practice Nurses
- International Society of Nurses in Genetics
- Genetics Nursing Credentialing Commission

INTRODUCTION

In the last few years, genetic nursing practice has been transformed from a nearly hidden specialty to a recognized specialty practice with formal recognition, publication of scope and standards of practice, and most recently, the availability of credentialing for genetic nurses. All areas of nursing practice have been impacted by recent advances in genetic knowledge and technology. Nearly all diseases are now recognized to have a genetic component.

Nurses now provide education to patients about hereditary risk for developing disease, counsel about the benefits and risks associated with genetic testing, and manage disease risk based on genetic information.

The recent development of commercial testing for susceptibility genes (such as the predisposition genes for breast ovarian cancer syndrome and colon cancer) have had a great impact on nursing's role in the identification and management of individuals at risk for developing many diseases. These developments have led to tremendous changes in genetic nursing practice. Nurses have been involved in managing genetic information since the 1960s, when nurses provided services to children with genetic disorders and their families. Although in some respects the nurse's role today in managing genetic information and caring for individuals and families at risk for or diagnosed with genetic diseases or conditions is similar to this traditional role, the scope of practice is much broader and more encompassing. What has also changed, according to Forsman, is the amount of genetic information available and the population to which this information may be applied. We now know that genetic changes contribute to most, if not all, diseases. Consequently, the scope of genetic knowledge application in nursing is limitless. 'Nursing can ignore genetics no longer. The time for meaningful action is now'.

There is an opportunity for nursing to practice health promotion tailored to highly specific and uniquely personal predispositions; in other words, for individualized health care, nurses can offer care that protects patients and families from the risks associated with genetic information, including addressing family issues. Nurses are also needed to refer patients to genetic specialists and assist patients in making choices as a genetic health care. Every nurse is needed; do not miss the revolution. All nurses have a role in the delivery of genetics services and the management of genetic information. Nurses require genetic knowledge to identify, refer, support, and care for persons affected by or at risk for genetic conditions.

'Genetic nursing is a holistic practice that includes assessing, planning, implementing, and evaluating the physical, spiritual, ethical, and psychosocial aspects of patients and families who have genetic concerns'. Genetics nurses practice in many different environments. Genetic nursing practice includes client and family assessment to identify genetic risk factors and intervention, information, service, and referral needs, take a detailed family history and construct a pedigree, analyze the assessment data, provide genetic education, and develop and carry out a plan of care to address genetic concerns. In addition, nurses in genetics provide genetic counseling, order and interpret genetic tests if within their scope of practice, and provide surveillance and management of persons affected by or at risk for genetic conditions.

In oncology, for example, areas of responsibility begin with risk assessments for cancer in patients and family members. This assessment includes a detailed family history, construction of a pedigree, and assessment of hereditary, environmental and lifestyle cancer risk factors. Once these risk factors are determined, the information is interpreted to the patient. Recommendations for cancer prevention and early detection can be tailored to the specific risks identified. If genetic testing for a cancer susceptibility gene is appropriate, the individual/family should be informed about the risks and benefits associated with the test, and the potential risks and benefits associated with the screening and prevention measures. The nurse also needs to explore possible psychosocial responses to the potential outcomes of a genetic test. This education may be done individually or with several family members. If testing is pursued, results are disclosed in person. At that point, a tailored plan for prevention and early detection is written and given to the family or individual. Long-term follow-up includes assessment of adjustment to the test results and compliance and follow-through with the plan for cancer prevention and early detection.

GENETICS NURSING PRACTICE MILESTONES

Genetics nursing practice has seen several memorable milestones in less than five years. In the past, there has been minimal recognition of the important role that nurses can play in genetics. The International Society of Nurses in Genetics (ISONG) has clearly been the leader in working with nursing leaders to promote genetic nursing practice and develop a credentialing process for genetic nurses. Through these efforts, only five years ago, the American Nurses Association established genetics nursing as an official specialty of nursing practice.

- *1960s:* Nurses published about the nurse's role in genetics and conducting genetics research
- *1984:* Genetics Nursing Network was formed, which later became ISONG
- *1988:* International Society of Nurses in Genetics (ISONG) was incorporated
- *1997:* Genetics Nursing designated an official nursing specialty by American Nurses Association
- *1998:* Statement on the Scope and Standards of Genetics Clinical Nursing Practice published by ISONG and ANA
- *2001:* ISONG approved formation of the Genetic Nursing Credentialing Commission (GNCC)
- *2001:* Credentialing of the first Genetics Advanced Practice Nurses [APNG(c)]
- *2002:* GNCC goes online at [www.geneticnurse.com], develops a logo and becomes incorporated
- *2002:* GCN credential is first offered by GNCC.

ROLES OF NURSES IN GENETICS

Following are the main roles of nurses in the field of genetics:

- Planning, implementing, administering (managing), and evaluating screening and testing programs.
- Monitoring and evaluating clients with genetic disorders in a similar manner to other disorders working with families under stress caused by problems related to a genetic condition.
- Coordinating care and services for individuals or families affected by genetic conditions, managing home care and therapy for persons with genetic disease.
- Following up on positive newborn screening tests, interviewing clients with possible genetically related conditions.
- Assessing needs and interactions in clients and families affected by genetic disease.
- Taking comprehensive and relevant family histories.
- Assessing the client and family's cultural or ethnic health beliefs and practices as they relate to the genetic problem.
- Assessing the client and family's strengths and weaknesses and family functioning.

- Providing health teaching and education related to genetics serving as an advocate for a client and family affected by a genetic disorder.
- Participating in public education about genetics.
- Developing an individualized plan of care, including anticipatory guidance for a person with a genetic condition.
- Explaining the purpose, meaning, and implications of genetic tests and results.
- Reinforcing and interpreting genetic counseling and testing information.
- Supporting families when they undergo counseling and make decisions.
- Recognizing the possibility of a genetic component in a disorder and taking appropriate referral action. Appreciating and ameliorating the social impact of genetic problems on the patient, family, and members of the community.

IMPORTANCE OF GENETICS IN NURSING CURRICULUM

Nursing programs traditionally include certain non-nursing courses, like general biology, microbiology, sociology/anthropology, ethics, pharmacology and genetics depending on the design of the curriculum.

Genetic concepts must be in all courses in the nursing program. They must be included in both didactic teaching and clinical applications. They must include practical and relevant examples with applications. Before making decisions about how and where to include genetic content in the nursing curriculum, it is important first to appraise the content to which students are actively exposed. In a nursing program, sometimes there is more genetic content than is realized. For example, when listing genetic content in a survey, one school did not include discussing cystic fibrosis as genetic under chronic illness for children. The first step is to meet with the instructors of courses both within nursing and outside of nursing and find out what content is already present. If a particular topic is not covered that the nursing program believes is important, they can request that it should be added. If the nursing program believes that a course in molecular biology or human genetics or an interdisciplinary course that focuses on genetics is needed, then they can work directly and collaboratively with the relevant department(s) to design a course that can be added to the basic nursing curriculum. It is also important that the nursing program examines what knowledge students should have retained from prior learning. It may not be necessary to reteach the complete content, such as meiosis, mitosis, and typical patterns of inheritance, etc.

Some other ideas for including genetic content within nursing curricula for both nursing and non-nursing courses are listed later with examples. Graduate programs can use similar ideas by providing more complexity and depth for topics and by incorporating genetic content at a higher level into the specialty courses. The exact nature depends on the area of specialization.

Important knowledge for the basic nursing graduate in regard to genetics includes the following:

- Basic mechanisms of inheritance and transmission of chromosomes and genes, including the concepts of variation and mutation. Nonmendelian mechanisms should be included. A major issue is how much of this should be retaught as it typically is in maternal child health or obstetrics and pediatrics? Should a separate course on molecular biology required for nursing be taught within the university or should all undergraduate students regardless of major have an interdisciplinary course that relates knowledge from biology, anthropology, philosophy, sociology, and other disciplines to genetically related issues?
- Information about the common inherited genetic disorders, for example, cystic fibrosis, Down's syndrome, phenylketonuria, sickle cell anemia, and hemochromatosis. Disorders that are particularly frequent in persons who reside in the geographic location of school should be included.
- An understanding of genetic contributions to human diversity including concepts, such as discrimination and eugenics.
- Ways of thinking about health and disease in relation to genetics, including how genetics and the environment interact and how genes interact with genes. This should lead to new ways of thinking about health promotion and disease prevention.

- Information about genetic contributions to common and complex conditions, such as breast cancer, colorectal cancer, heart disease and hypercholesterolemia, mental illness, certain behavioral traits, and Alzheimer disease.
- Care management of adults with childhood genetic disorders.
- Care management of persons with adult genetic disorders, such as Huntington disease.
- An understanding of genetic approaches to the therapy of genetic and complex diseases.
- Interpretation of genetic risks (i.e. how to explain the meaning of a 1-in-4 risk for having another child with Tay-Sachs disease).
- What constitutes a proper family history specifically, what key information should be obtained and how to construct and read pedigrees.
- Information about genetic risk, genetic testing and screening, and the implications both positive and negative.
- How to interpret the results of genetic tests.
- Awareness of the possibility of an inherited or genetic component for a client's condition and knowledge of cardinal features of familial predisposition, such as early age of disease onset, multiple family members with the same diagnosis, predisposing risk factors.
- An awareness of social, legal, and ethical issues related to genetics, including effects on individuals, groups, and societies, some of which are unique to genetic conditions.
- An understanding of the social and ethical ramifications of possessing a particular genotype or genetic disorder in terms of societal issues, confidentiality, freedom of choice, and risks in terms of insurance and disclosure.
- Application of traditional nursing skills, such as patient education, confidentiality, and counseling to genetic information. The concept of nondirective counseling can be included.
- Ways in which genetic knowledge is used in diagnosis and treatment applications.
- Development of nonjudgmental attitudes about genetics and related disorders.

- Ways to access resources relating to genetics for patient and self-education and the need to keep current.
- Knowledge about referral possibilities knowing not only who should be referred to but also how and to whom it should be done.
- The knowledge that responses to drugs used in therapy are at least in part genetically determined.
- Advanced practice nurses may play direct roles in genetic counseling and in advanced assessment. They also may work within a particular specialty in which genetics plays a role, such as an oncology or cardiology clinic, as well as in long-term management of specific genetic disorders depending on the specialty area in which they are trained. An example of the latter is the nurse who works in a sickle cell clinic. The graduate curriculum should include a higher level of the concepts discussed previously as well as advanced material related specifically to the specialization.

BARRIERS AND APPROACHES FOR IMPLEMENTATION OF GENETICS IN NURSING

Numerous barriers including genetic content in basic nursing education have been identified. The most commonly encountered barrier is lack of time. Knowledge continues to expand but, until recently, nursing programs have continued with essentially the same program length. The intensity of the curriculum has increased and has become more dense at a time when many students have less time to spend on learning or are less qualified than previously. Faculty barriers include perceived lack of knowledge, insecurity in their knowledge, not perceiving genetic content as important, and not recognizing the broad scope of genetics as it influences health care but treating the genetic approach as a collection of rare disorders to be memorized.

Potential approaches to addressing these barriers can include the following:

- *Educating faculty:* As the nursing faculty is aging, education in genetics may have taken place sometime ago and must be refreshed.

- *Instilling confidence in faculty:* Faculty must be confident that they can understand material and are interpreting it correctly. This can be addressed through continuing education and workshops. Faculty must feel secure with content to teach it.
- Providing rewards and incentives for faculty.
- Expanding on what is already in the curriculum after determining what already exists.
- Using genetic examples that may be central or incidental. For example, a person who has a particular genetic condition could be the focus of a surgical case study in which the genetic condition is not central but the genetic information is included.
- Emphasizing a lifespan approach for genetic disorders.
- Emphasizing the relevance of genetic examples and using contemporary examples; for example, cloning or DNA testing as used in the OJ.
- Offering continuing education/workshops for faculty that may include hands on demonstrations.
- Seeking consultation/advice to get started with concrete examples.
- Recognizing need for frequent updating.
- Identifying an advocate or point person in school. This person may be educated to become a resident expert.
- Working with course instructors and the curriculum committee to achieve goals.
- Identifying resources for information about instruction and online information, courses available for faculty updating, core knowledge and curriculum developed for other disciplines and for teaching tools, such as genetic games and deconstructions that are not only informative but also fun. Many scientific supply houses have these products.

ASSUMPTIONS REGARDING GENETICS AND HEALTH CARE IN FUTURE

Some of the guiding principles or basic assumptions in relation to genetics inform that health care must be weighed before considering what core genetic knowledge is needed by the practicing nurses. These assumptions include the following:

- Nurses in all areas of practice will encounter clients with traditional genetic disorders and common disorders with a genetic component.
- Most, if not all, disorders have a genetic basis to a greater or lesser extent, even conditions such as fractures. To a degree, a mutant gene can be thought of as an etiologic agent.
- Traditional genetic disorders are seen across the lifespan. Many inherited biochemical disorders have infant, childhood, and adult forms. Other disorders typically appear or are noticed in adulthood, such as Huntington disease and hemochromatosis.
- The previously existing genetic condition of a particular client influences the choice of care and treatment for any new health problem for which he or she is seeking consultation.
- The so-called common or complex diseases, such as cancer and heart disease have a genetic component evident in origin, diagnosis, treatment, management, and preventive approaches.
- Humans are diverse not only because of cultural and social factors but also because of genetic variation. This is not inherently bad or good but a fact that influences how we all respond to foods, drugs, medications, and chemicals in the environment and profoundly affects how people respond to health care interventions because all people have different degrees of possible health.
- Assessment for genetic risk for specific conditions preceding options of testing followed by counseling will become more prevalent and include persons at risk for common diseases, such as heart disease, various types of cancers, and Alzheimer disease, in addition to those already in common use, such as prenatal diagnosis.
- Technologic advances are such that persons with genetic disorders that appear in infancy or childhood and formerly caused early death are living not only to early adulthood but later. For example, some adults with sickle cell anemia have lived into their eighties. Health care providers must deal with how the genetic disorder impacts the appearance and management of common health problems and aging and vice versa. For example, how will co-illness with type 2 diabetes mellitus influence the course of disease and response in an

adult with cystic fibrosis? How will common conditions such as hypertension be managed against the background of a previously existing genetic disease?

- Ways of thinking about health promotion and disease prevention will change.
- Many diseases will be diagnosed and treated using knowledge from genetics.
- Genetic information that influences health care through the lifespan will be available prenatally.

Genetic knowledge makes it possible to individualize aspects of health care such as prevention and treatment in new ways. In the not-too-distant future, it will be possible to predict the diseases for which a fetus or newborn will have a genetic predisposition, and a fetus or newborn will have a predicted genetic future that may be subject to modulation.

Genetics often has been associated with tertiary health care and rare genetic disorders in the minds of many nurses. Genetics plays and will continue to play a greater role in the common and complex disorders, such as various cancers, infectious diseases, Alzheimer disease, heart disease, and chronic obstructive pulmonary disease, and in relatively common genetic conditions that have significant organ effects, such as hemochromatosis. Clients who see primary care providers such as advanced practice nurses will seek genetically related information and may require assessment for genetic risk at multiple points in the lifespan from prenatal to the older age group. On the basis of such risk assessment, they may choose genetic testing. Studies have demonstrated that a significant percentage of health care professionals misinterpret the results of genetic testing. Often they may not know it is available for a condition relevant to their client or may not recognize that their client is at risk. The curriculum in nursing and other health care professions is deficient in genetic content.

REVIEW QUESTIONS

Short-note Questions

1. Mention genetic nursing practice milestones.
2. What is the role of nurses in genetics?

3. Describe the importance of genetics in nursing curriculum.
4. Discuss the approaches to barriers in implementation of genetics in nursing.
5. Enumerate the assumptions regarding genetics and health care in future.

Short-answer Questions

1. List four recent important genetics nursing practice milestones.
2. List four essential roles of nurses in genetics.
3. List two reasons why genetics should be included in the nursing curriculum.
4. List two barriers of implementation of genetics in nursing.

Multiple Choice Questions (MCQs)

1. **When did the first-time nurses publish about the nurse's role in genetics and conducting genetics research?**
   a. 1970 b. 1960
   c. 1980 d. 1990

2. **In which year was the International Society of Nurses in Genetics incorporated?**
   a. 1977 b. 1988
   c. 1999 d. 2009

3. **Following are the roles of nurses in genetic practices, except:**
   a. Planning and implementing the genetic screening tests.
   b. Monitoring and evaluating the patients with genetics disorders
   c. Conducting the gene therapy on a patient with genetic condition.
   d. Providing genetic counseling services to the patient and family.

4. **Which of the following may be considered as the barrier in the implementation of genetics in nursing?**
   a. Lack of availability of genetics textbook.
   b. Lack of available time in nursing program.
   c. Lack of scope for genetic nurses in health care.
   d. Lack of funds for support of genetics in nursing.

5. **What is the main factor that teaching genetics is essentially important in nursing curriculum?**
   a. There is more scope of jobs for nurses with genetics knowledge.
   b. In all the areas of practices, nurses encounter the patients with genetic conditions.
   c. There is more funding of government on education with genetic knowledge.
   d. Nurses with genetic knowledge will be able to get higher pay.

ANSWER KEY

1. b	2. b	3. c	4. b	5. b		

FURTHER READING

1. Anderson, G, Monsen, RB, Prows, CA, Tinley, S, and Jenkins, J. Preparing the nursing profession for participation in a genetic paradigm in health care. Nursing Outlook. 2000;48(1), 23-7.
2. Anderson, G, Yetter, C, and Monsen, R. Genetics nursing, and public policy: setting an international agenda. Policy, Politics, and Nursing Practice. 2000;1(4), 245-55.
3 Frank, T. Hereditary risk of breast and ovarian carcinoma: the role of the oncologist. The Oncologist. 1998;3, 403-12.
4. Forbes N. The nurse and genetic counseling. Nursing Clinics of North America. 1966;1(4):679-88.
5. Forsman I. Evolution of the nursing role in genetics. Journal of Obstretics, Gynecology and Neonatal Nursing. 1994 July/Aug:481-5.
6. Greco, K. Cancer genetics nursing practice: Impact of the double helix. Oncology Nursing Forum Supplement. 2000;27(9), 29-36.
7. Greco, K. ISONG news. MEDSURG Nursing. 2002;11(3), 152.
8. Greco, K and Anderson, G. Redressing Policy in Cancer Genetics: Moving Toward Transdisciplinary Teams. Policy, Politics, and Nursing Practice. 2002;3(2), 129-39.
9. International Society of Nurses in Genetics and the American Nurses Association. Statement on the scope and standards of genetics clinical nursing practice, Washington DC: American Nurses Association. 1998.
10. Jenkins, JF, Prows, C, Dimond, E, Monsen, R, and Williams, J. Recommendations for educating nurses in genetics. Journal of Professional Nursing 2001. 17(6), 283-90.

11. Lashley, F. Nursing and genetics: the past and the future. In F. Lashley (Ed.), The Genetics Revolution: Implications for Nursing. Washington, DC: American Academy of Nursing. 1997.
12. Lashley, FR. Integrating genetics content in undergraduate nursing programs. Biological Research for Nursing. 1999;1(2), 113-8.
13. Mahon, SM. The role of the nurse in developing cancer-screening programs. Oncology Nursing Forum. 2000;27(9 Suppl), 19-27.
14. National Coalition of Health Professional Education in Genetics (NCHPEG). Retrieved on 01/03/03 from http://www.nchpeg.org
15. National Institutes of Nursing Research (2003b, April). Abstract retrieved on 01/03/03 from http://www.nih.gov/ninr/news-info/geneventposter.pdf
16. National Institutes of Nursing Research. (2003a, June). Retrieved on 01/03/03 from http://www.nih.gov/ninr/research/dir/ogi.html
17. Nussbaum, RL, McInnes, RR, and Huntington, FW. Thompson and Thompson Genetics in Medicine (sixth ed.). Philadelphia: WB Saunders. 2001.
18. University of Iowa, College of Nursing. (n.d.). Retrieved on 01/03/03 from http://www.nursing.uiowa.edu/centers/gnirc/clingenet.htm

Chapter 3

Maternal and Prenatal Genetics

Learning Objectives

This chapter is designed to enable the reader to:

- Explain the dynamics of maternal infections and fetal genetics
- Understand the concept consanguinity and its genetic aspect
- Identify the facts about prenatal nutrition and food allergies in children and role of prenatal nutrition in prevention of genetic disorders
- Recognize the genetic effect of maternal age, maternal drug therapy, and maternal exposure to radiations, drugs and chemicals on fetus
- Describe the invasive and noninvasive prenatal testing and diagnosis
- Enumerate the genetic basis of spontaneous abortion and infertility
- Discuss about neural tube defect and Down syndrome.

Key Terms

- Maternal Infections
- Consanguinity Atopy
- Prenatal Nutrition
- Maternal Genetic Aspect of Advanced Maternal Age
- Maternal Drug Therapy Teratogenicity
- Genetic Effect of Radiation, Drug and Chemicals
- Prenatal Genetic Testing and Diagnosis
- Preimplantation Prenatal Diagnosis
- Infertility
- Spontaneous Abortion
- Neural Tube Defects
- Down Syndrome

INTRODUCTION

The complete sequencing of the human genome in 2003 has opened doors for new approaches to health promotion, maintenance, and treatment. Maternal and prenatal genetics is one of the most important health promotion, maintenance and treatment in the field of the genetics. Genetic research is now leading to a better understanding of the genetic components of common diseases, such as cancer, diabetes, and stroke, and creating new, gene-based technologies for screening, prevention, diagnosis, and treatment of both rare and common diseases. Nurses are on the forefront of care, and therefore will participate fully in genetic-based and genomic-based practice activities, such as collecting family history, obtaining informed consent for genetic testing, and administering gene-based therapies. This new direction in health care calls for all nurses to be able to effectively translate genetic and genomic information to patients with an understanding of associated ethical issues.

GENETICS AND INFECTION

Maternal infections during pregnancy are known to cause deleterious effect on health and development of growing fetus. In case of any infection host response in the form of increased level of cytokines and chemokines. It is observed in various studies that increased level of maternal serum Cytokines interlukin-8 (IL-8) during second trimester can increase the risk of schizophrenia among offspring. *'TORCH'* infections generally refer to a group of maternally acquired communicable diseases that include Toxoplasmosis, Other (varicella, Venezuelan equine encephalitis, mumps, coxsackie, parvovirus, HIV), Rubella, Cytomegalovirus and Herpes. These infections are well known to cause harmful effect on developing fetus.

The following list describes many of the features that can be seen in children who are exposed to TORCH infections during pregnancy.

Table 3.1: Maternal infection, observed effects on effects and preventive measure

Infection	Observed effects	Preventive measures
Cytomegalovirus (CMV)	Birth defects, low birth weight, developmental disorders	Good hygienic practices, such as handwashing

Contd...

Contd...

Infection	Observed effects	Preventive measures
Hepatitis B virus	Low birth weight	Vaccination
Human immuno-deficiency virus (HIV)	Low birth weight, childhood cancer	Practice universal precautions
Human parvovirus B19	Miscarriage	Good hygienic practices, such as handwashing
Rubella (German measles)	Birth defects, low birth weight	Vaccination before pregnancy if no prior immunity
Toxoplasmosis	Miscarriage, birth defects, developmental disorders	Good hygiene practices, such as handwashing
Varicella-zoster virus (chickenpox)	Birth defects, low birth weight	Vaccination before pregnancy if no prior immunity

Following is brief description of selected common maternal infections and their effect on growing fetus.

- *Toxoplasmosis:* Toxoplasmosis is caused by a parasite which is transmitted by raw or uncooked meat, or through infected cat feces. It is also associated with a mononucleosis-like illness. However, unlike CMV, prior infection does confer immunity. Transmission rate to the fetus is 15–20% in the first trimester but rises to 60% in the third trimester. However, sequelae are more severe with first trimester infection and are similar to those seen with CMV infections.

  Diagnosis in a pregnant woman should be made by either rising antibody titers or an IgM specific for toxoplasmosis. Although it is controversial, there is some evidence that treatment with antiparasitical medications can ameliorate the effects in the fetus. Maternal toxoplamosis infection will bring various effects on developing fetus, such as:
  - Central nervous system disorders
  - High-risk of schizophrenia
  - Congenital hepatosplenomegaly
  - Retinitis
  - Brain cyst and mental retardation
  - Risk of epilepsy.

- *Varicella:* Varicella infection during pregnancy is associated with a less than 10% risk for fetal embryopathy. The effects include microcephaly, growth disturbances, ocular abnormalities and limb defects with cicatricial skin scarring in a dermatomal pattern when the mother is infected in the first half of pregnancy. Shingles (or herpes zoster) may be associated with similar findings but in a much smaller percentage of exposed infants.

  Congenitally acquired varicella is associated with overwhelming illness in approximately 25% of babies who are exposed at or near the time of birth. The highest risk is for those infants to develop a rash between 5 and 10 days of age. Varicella Zoster IG antibodies) VZIG may be given to the at-risk newborn. Varicella infection may result in following defects in fetus:
  - Microcephaly
  - Eye defects
  - Limb hypoplesia
  - Risk of spontaneous abortion
  - Neonatal infection
  - Fetal death
- *Mumps:* The data are limited, but suggest an increased rate of pregnancy loss. There is also some evidence for a small risk for endocardial fibroelastosis in the newborn.
- *Measles (rubeola):* Based on a small amount of data, there does not appear to be an increase in the rate of birth defects in exposed fetuses.
- *HIV/AIDS infection:* HIV infection in the mother is currently not felt to be associated with a fetal embryopathy. However, the perinatal transmission rate is approximately 30%. Recent evidence suggests that use of AZT (zidovudine) during pregnancy dramatically reduces the fetal transmission rate.
- *Syphilis:* If syphilis is not treated well, can lead following fetal anomalies:
  - Blindness
  - Mental retardation
  - Hypoplastic nose and limb deformities

- Anemia
- Skin rashes.

- *Rubella:* First described in 1941, this prototype of congenital infections is characterized by congenital heart defects, cataracts, deafness and mental retardation. Maternal infection in the first eight weeks of pregnancy is associated with an 85% risk for congenital rubella syndrome (CRS). The risk decreases to that of the general population by approximately 20 weeks gestation. Despite an active immunization program, it is estimated that 6 to 10% of postpubertal women are seronegative.

  Data collected by the CDC suggests that inadvertent use of rubella vaccination in pregnancy or in the three months prior to pregnancy is not associated with congenital rubella syndrome or any increase in the rate of birth defects. However, theoretical risks dictate that the rubella live-virus vaccine be avoided during pregnancy. It is highly recommended that non-rubella immune new mothers be vaccinated prior to discharge from the hospital. Maternal rubella infection can cause serious central nervous system and heart anomalies in growing fetus, such as:
  - Congenital heart anomalies
  - Mental retardation
  - Deafness
  - Blindness
  - Childhood psychotic disorders.

  Rubella infection brings serious health effect on fetus. Therefore, preconception screening and vaccination need to be provided to all women, and they should avoid pregnancy for at least three months after rubella vaccination.

- *Cytomegalovirus (CMV):* CMV is a member of the herpes virus family and is ubiquitous in the environment. It is associated with a mononucleosis-like illness that may be indistinguishable from other viral illnesses.

  Between 1 and 4% of nonimmune pregnant women have a primary CMV infection during pregnancy. There is forty percent probability that the infection is transmitted to the fetus. The risk for congenital infection appears to be highest when the maternal infection has occurred in the first half of pregnancy.

Of those fetuses that are infected, 10–15% have clinically apparent disease at birth, typically including microcephaly, hepatosplenomegaly and chorioretinitis. The mortality in symptomatic newborns is 20–30%.

Primary infection does not confer total immunity for future pregnancies. However, poor outcome of infected fetuses is substantially less when the infection occurs in a mother who has previously had a CMV infection. Testing for CMV during pregnancy can be difficult. A single high titer does not differentiate between a primary and non-primary infection. Therefore, either two analyses four weeks apart looking for rising titers, or both IgG and IgM titers can be obtained. IgM is often available only at reference laboratories. Due to the difficulties in testing, routine screening of all pregnant women is not recommended.

- *Herpes Simplex Virus (HSV):* The greatest concern for fetal embryopathy (growth, cognitive and ocular abnormalities) is from primary infection in the first half of pregnancy. Although it is very rare, infection of the fetus has also been reported with recurrent maternal infections.

  The more common scenario, accounting for 80% of neonates with HSV, is infection in the intrapartum period which can lead to skin lesions, encephalitis, and disseminated disease involving many organ systems (CNS, lung, liver, adrenals, skin, eye and/or mouth). In addition, because of infection elevated maternal IgG antibodies are known to cause various psychotic mental disorders among offspring. LSCS should be considered if the patient has active genital lesions at the time of delivery. Treatment of the newborn with antiviral medications has been effective.
- *Fifth Disease (erythema infectiosum):* Fifth disease is caused by human parvovirus B19. It produces a mild illness in children and adults consisting of a facial rash (slapped cheek appearance), 'lacy' body rash, malaise, flu-like symptoms and joint pain (especially in adults). It is spread by respiratory droplets. The incubation period is approximately two weeks. Fifty percent of the adult population is immune by virtue of the fact that they had fifth disease in childhood. However, since this is a mild illness in children, previous infection is generally not documented.

Human parvovirus affects red blood cell precursors, causing anemia. In pregnant women, this can lead to non-immune fetal hydrops. The risk for fetal death from hydrops in an infected woman is 5% or less. *In utero* transfusions have been successfully used. However, there have also been several case reports of spontaneous resolution of hydrops with a normal fetal outcome. At this time, there does not appear to be a significant risk for birth defects in the fetus.

Pregnant women can be tested for the presence of IgG and IgM, specific for parvovirus, to determine if they have been infected during the pregnancy. However, testing should be limited to those with significant exposure, an unidentified maternal rash-like illness or fetal hydrops.

- *Bacterial infection:* Listeria a bacterium which causes infection in a pregnant mother may cause selected following fetal abnormalities, such as:
  - Spontaneous abortion
  - Intrauterine fetal death

  Soft cheese, cold deli meats, and raw seafood usually are the cause of this infection; therefore, these foods should be avoided during pregnancy.

Role of Nurses

- Nurse need to assess the mother during antenatal for any possibility of infection.
- Refer for antenatal or prenatal screening to rule out any possibility of maternal infection.
- Obtain an information during preconception counseling that women is immunized with rubella vaccine, and inform them to avoid pregnancy for at least for 3 months after rubella vaccination.
- Inform the mother about possible effects of infections on developing fetus.
- Provide emotional support to mother during periods of the stress due to own illness secondary to infection and fear of possible negative effects of infection on fetus.
- Monitor maternal and fetal well-being during episode of infection.

- Provide medical therapies to treat maternal infections and save the fetus from deleterious effects of maternal infection.

CONSANGUINITY ATOPY

'Consanguinity' comes from two Latin words; *con* meaning shared and *sanguis* that means blood. Consanguinity describes a relationship between two people who share a common ancestor or a 'shared blood' relationship. For example, a relationship between two cousins. The most common form of a consanguineous relationship or marriage is between first cousins and in some societies, can account for a large proportion of relationships. In other words, *Consanguinity is defined as the marriage between close relatives.*

Traditionally, some cultures have practiced and continue to practice marriage between relatives, such as cousins as a means of strengthening family ties and retaining property within the family. The incidence of consanguinity reported in *India* is 5 to 60% and uncle-niece and first cousin are the more commonly occurring relationships in Indian population. In India consanguious marriages are more common among Muslims and south Indian Hindu families. The consanguious marriages are common between first cousins, where preferential patrilateral parallel cousin marriage (where a boy marries his father's brother's daughter or sister's daughter) is often favored.

Genetic Aspect of Consanguinity

- Table 3.2 presents proportion of genes shared between close blood relatives; where it is illustarted that first cousins, share approximately one-eighth (1/8th) of their genes in common.
- Children from a first cousin mating will be genetically identical for one-sixteenth (1/16th) of their genetic material. If any of these identical genetic sites are comprised of recessive disease-causing genes, the child will be affected with that disease.
- In general, unrelated individuals have only a small risk for having children with a recessive genetic disorder. This is because there is only a small chance that each parent would carry the same recessive gene and that both parents would pass this same gene to their child. When individuals are consanguineous (related), they have inherited some of their

genetic information from the same family member. This leads to an increased chance that they would carry the same recessive gene and have a child with a recessive genetic disorder.

- Usually two unrelated people will not carry the same faulty gene copy:
  - Children of unrelated parents are at low risk of inheriting from each of their parents a copy of the same faulty gene that could result in a genetic condition.
  - They have a risk of between 2 and 3% (2 to 3 out of every 100 births) of having a child with a birth defect or disability, many of which will be genetic.
- People who are blood relatives share a greater proportion of the same genes than unrelated people do because they have a common ancestor, such as a grandparent from whom they inherited their genes through their parents.
- The closer the biological relationship between relatives, it is more likely that they will have the same faulty gene in common.
- Children of parents who are blood relatives generally have a small increased risk over that of unrelated parents of inheriting from each of their parents a copy of the same faulty gene that could result in a genetic condition:
  - *For example, if parents are first cousins,* the risk is a little higher (about twice), i.e. 5 to 6% (5 to 6 out of every 100 births).
  - The chances of having a baby with a problem would be higher, and parents more likely to share the same faulty gene copy, if their parents and/or grandparents are also close blood relatives.
- This risk applies only to immediate offspring of related individuals and not to their grandchildren or other family members.
- The increased risk for genetic health problems is related to the possibility of passing on recessive genes.
- Genetic diseases are inherited in several different ways: dominant, recessive and X-linked.
- Children born to a consanguineous couple are primarily at higher risk for a recessive genetic disease.
- A recessive disease is a genetic condition caused by inheriting two copies of a nonworking gene.

- When couples belong to certain ethnic groups in which there is a known increased incidence of a specific genetic disease, it may be possible to screen them for this disease to determine if one or both are carriers. It is not possible to screen for all recessive diseases, however, the increased risk for an affected child cannot ever be removed entirely.

Table 3.2: Proportion of genes shared between close blood relatives

Relationship each other	Relationship type	Proportion of similar genes
Indentical twin (Monozygotic)	--------	All (100%)
Non-identical (dizygotic) twin, brothers and sisters, parents and children	First degree	½ (50%)
Uncles and aunts, nephew and nieces, grandparents and half brothers and half sisters.	Second degree	¼ (25%)
First cousin, half uncles, aunts and half nephews and nieces	Third degree	1/8 (12.5%)

Negative effects of consanguinity: The risk that those marrying a relative are more likely to have offspring with birth defects or a disabling condition is nearly always exaggerated and perceived as being higher than it actually is. All parents who are unrelated carry a risk of between 2 and 3% of having a child with a birth defect or disability, where parents are first cousins and there is no family history of a specific condition, or where there is no other history of parents being related in previous generations, the risk is approximately double that for unrelated parents. So the total risk of having a child with a genetic condition where parents are first cousins is around 5–6%. However, in societies with a tradition of first cousin marriage, and where marriages are usually contracted within the community, many couples are often more closely related than first cousins and consequently their risk may be significantly higher.

Role of Nurses

- A nonjudgmental attitude towards consanguineous couples is essential to foster good working relationships between the

health care provider and communities where consanguineous marriage is prevalent.
- It important to provide premarital genetic counseling to closely related couple that are planning to have marriage.
- Ensure that couples referred for premarital counseling are aware that it is not possible to provide blood tests looking for general 'genetic compatibility', apart from a few basic carrier tests for a limited range of specific conditions.
- Plan to provide genetic counseling for a couples that are close blood relatives and thinking about becoming parents.
- Do not wait to refer for preconception screening a consanguineous couple until a pregnancy is underway, especially if they have a family history of a possible autosomal recessive condition.
- Refer the couple for prenatal testing and counseling for early diagnosis and intervention of genetically abnormal fetus.
- Do not imply that a child's condition is their parents' fault; even if a couple are consanguineous and the child has two identical copies of a mutant gene, no one chooses to pass on an illness and no one is 'to blame'.
- Support the couple and family during prenatal diagnosis and help them to take crucial decisions if needed.
- Implement public awareness programs about negative effects of consanguineous marriages.

PRENATAL NUTRITION AND FOOD ALLERGIES

Role of prenatal nutrition play in causation of food allergy among children is still full of mysteries and controversies (Fig. 3.1). Many researches in the field of prenatal nutrition and food allergy of children had not yielded much significant results. But one thing is clear: Childhood is a crucial turning point. This is when the immune system takes shape, it can go down one of two paths: One leads to allergies, the other leads to tolerance. Experts argue about the best ways to protect baby from allergies during pregnancy.

Prenatal nutrition is an area that needs a lot more research but suggested that pregnant women might want to 'pick foods wisely' because what a pregnant woman eating today may not only nourish her body, but may have an impact on her growing fetus.

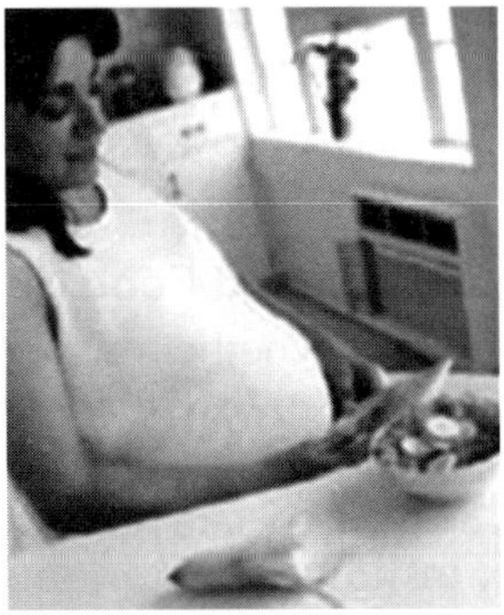

Fig. 3.1: Prenatal nutrition

Recent research suggests that when moms-to-be eat apples during pregnancy, their offspring have lower rates of asthma. And, mothers who consume fish during pregnancy may lower their child's risk of developing the allergic skin condition called eczema. 'There are influences that occur in utero that can have lasting impact,' said Dr. Jennifer Appleyard, chief of allergy and immunology at St. John Hospital and Medical Center in Detroit. 'More and more, we are finding influences for later health develop earlier than we anticipated.'

Dutch researchers recently followed 1,253 children from before birth to age 5. Their mothers completed food questionnaires during their pregnancies, and their children's health was assessed. The children's diets were also assessed. Women who consumed the most apples during pregnancy, more than four a week had children who were 37 percent less likely to have ever wheezed than children of mothers who had the lowest consumption of apples during pregnancy. Additionally, youngsters born to apple-loving moms were 46 percent less likely to have asthma symptoms and 53 percent less likely to have doctor-confirmed asthma than those whose mothers shunned the fruit. The mechanism behind apples' apparent protective effect needs further study, but may have something to do with the flavonoids and other antioxidants contained in apples, said Dr. Devang Doshi, director of pediatric allergy and immunology at Beaumont Hospital in Royal Oak, Mich.

The study, published in the journal *Thorax*, also found that mothers who ate fish more than once a week had children who were 43 percent less likely to have eczema than women who never ate fish. 'This was a good study, but we need a lot more evidence still,' said Doshi, who pointed out that the children in the study generally had well-balanced, nutritious diets, and that may have played a role as well.

Facts of Prenatal Nutrition and Food Allergies in Children

- The verdict is still out on whether nutrition during pregnancy can affect baby's tendency toward food sensitivities or allergies. 'The fairest answer is that we do not really know for sure,' says Scott H. Sicherer, M.D., associate professor of pediatrics at the Jaffe Food Allergy Institute at Mount Sinai School of Medicine in New York. Even so, the American Academy of Pediatrics (AAP) recommends that mothers at high-risk of having an infant with food allergies, who have a family history of food allergy, should consider avoiding peanuts, one of the most highly allergenic of all foods, during the third trimester.
- A family history of allergies is the single most important factor that predisposes a person to develop allergic disease.
- If one parent has allergic disease, the estimated risk of the child to develop allergies is 48%; the child's risk grows to 70% if both parents have allergies.
- Eating peanuts during pregnancy and or while breastfeeding may increase the child's risk for developing a peanut allergy and other food allergies; especially if parents have a family history of allergies. Peanuts are the one food that one might avoid during pregnancy. While other research studies argue that until the parents does not have family history of food allergies, women during pregnant and breastfeeding can enjoy peanut safely, since it is a good source of protein and folic acid, which is essential during pregnancy.
- If one is concerned that consumption of tuna sandwich or milkshake during pregnancy will give baby food allergies, then one can you can relax.
- This genetic tendency, called 'atopy', occurs when allergic individuals' immune systems essentially go into overdrive when they come into contact with an allergen. An allergen refers to any substance, such as pollen, mold or animal dander, which can trigger an allergic response. Food allergies in children can cause a variety of problems that range from eczema to life-threatening allergic reactions.

Prevention of food allergy: Here are some recommendations from the American Academy of Pediatrics (AAP) for prevention of food allergry among childern.

- *Do not eat peanuts during pregnancy*: It has been shown to increase the incidence of peanut allergy in children. Studies are inconclusive regarding other allergens, such as eggs, milk, and fish and given the essential role of these foods in providing balanced prenatal nutrition, no dietary restrictions are currently recommended.
- *Breastfeed exclusively for six months*: By doing so, one reduce infant's exposure to cows' milk and soy, the primary components in most infant formula. Exclusive breastfeeding has been shown to lower rates of infant eczema and good immune system. If it is not possible to breastfeed exclusively, choose hypoallergenic formula brands, such as Enfamil's Nutramigen and Similac's Alimentum.
- *Avoid peanuts while breastfeeding:* Again, studies show lower levels of allergy when nursing mothers avoid peanuts. Research results for other foods are mixed, so the American Academy of Pediatrics suggests that avoidance diets while nursing be determined on a case-by-case basis.
- *Wait to start solid foods*: Allergic eczema has been found to be more common in kids fed solids before 6 months. Wait until child is 6 months old to introduce solid foods. Especially if you have a family history of food allergies, taking steps to prevent early exposure to foods that can cause allergies is a good idea. As a child grows older and the digestive system matures, the body is less likely to absorb food or food components that trigger allergies. Experts believe that waiting to introduce solid foods until your child is 6 months old may help prevent allergies to those foods.
- *Delay introducing allergenic foods*: The American Academy of Pediatrics suggests that children not be fed cows' milk until they are 1 year old. Eggs should be avoided until 2, and tree nuts, peanuts, and fish (e.g. cod, whitefish, and shellfish) until kids are 3 years old.
  - In fact, cutting out foods to protect your child from allergies can have unwanted consequences. A scientific review article published in 2000 in the Cochrane Database of

Systematic Reviews concluded that avoiding cows' milk and eggs during pregnancy does not protect children from developing allergies to foods or to anything else. The only noticeable result was that some women struggled to gain enough weight while pregnant. However it is suggested to introduce cow's milk after one year, which will prevent the chances of developing milk allergy.

- Introduce eggs at age 2. This may help prevent your child from developing an egg allergy.
- Introduce nuts and seafood at age 3. This may help prevent your child from developing an allergy to these foods. (Do not give your child whole nuts until he or she has molars and can chew them well.)

- *Introduce all new foods gradually and one at a time.* Before introducing mixed foods that could cause an allergic reaction, introduce each new food on its own. *Do not mix foods* until you are sure each individual food is tolerated.
- *Give child cooked or homogenized foods.* Many foods are less likely to cause an allergic reaction after they are cooked. (However, be careful. A few foods, such as cod and celery — still contain allergy-causing proteins after cooking.)
- Soft, unpasteurized cheeses like feta, Brie, Camembert, and goat as well as ready-to-eat meats like hot dogs and deli meats may contain Listeria, bacteria that cause mild flu-like symptoms in most adults but can be very dangerous for unborn babies. Listeriosis, the infection caused by the bacteria, in a pregnant mother can cause miscarriage, premature birth, or severe illness or death of a newborn.

Last but not least a question arises that, what a pregnant woman should eat? 'The general consensus is that women should consume a good, well-balanced diet with lots of fruits and vegetables, and not to overindulge in any one food,' in addition peanuts can be avoided.

Role of Prenatal Nutrition in Prevention of Genetic Disorders

Prenatal nutrition plays a major role in prenatal genetics. The discovery that folic acid supplementation to pregnant mother can reduce the risk of neural tube defects is a dramatic success story.

Many of genetic disorders and birth defects are preventable through balanced prenatal and intranatal diet of the mother. Following are some of the examples.

- *Down syndrome:* Down syndrome, also called trisomy 21, is a complex genetic disease that for years was said to be caused by an extra copy of chromosome 21. A recent landmark study indicated that mothers of children with Down syndrome have an imbalance in folate metabolism that may be explained, in part, by a common genetic variation in an enzyme involved in the folic acid pathway. Further studies are expected to see if maternal folic acid supplementation will reduce the incidence of the disorder. If folic acid does prove to reduce incidences of Down syndrome, then this means the chromosome abnormality found in the disorder is a feature associated with the syndrome, but was not the singular cause. Interestingly, before 'bad' genes started getting the sole blame for most birth defects, medical doctors used to think that 'maternal nourishment' was a factor in Down syndrome. Unfortunately somewhere along the line this view fell out of favor. On the mineral front, a number of studies on Down syndrome have linked the syndorme to zinc deficiencies. A 1994 study has shown zinc supplementation had a positive effect on Down syndrome patients.
- *Mitral Valve Prolapse (MVP):* MVP is a common feature of most inherited connective tissue disorders, yet also a common finding among the population on general. Geneticists consider mitral valve prolapse syndrome to be an inherited collagen disorder with overlapping features similar to Marfan syndrome. It is listed in the Marfan nosology as a differential diagnosis to be considered instead of Marfan syndrome. Nutrition oriented research studies, however, show the majority of people with mitral valve prolapse are magnesium deficient and that magnesium supplementation frequently reduces or alleviates MVP symptoms.
- *Wilson's Disease:* People with this inherited disorder have excess copper accumulate in their bodies. Zinc supplementation therapy is used to reduce copper levels and has been successful in treating the disorder.
- *Blue Sclera:* A feature of a wide variety of connective tissue disorders including Ehlers-Danlos syndrome, Osteogenesis

imperfecta and Marfan syndrome. Most cases of blue sclera have been linked to iron deficiency.

- *Cleft Palates:* Reduced significantly through maternal supplementation of folic acid.
- *Spina Bifida:* Reduced significantly through maternal supplementation of multivitamins with folic acid.
- *Cerebral Palsy:* Recent research shows that very low birth weight babies have a lower incidence of cerebral palsy (CP) when their mothers are treated with magnesium sulfate soon before giving birth. The findings come from a study sponsored by the National Institute of Neurological Disorders and Stroke (NINDS) and the California Birth Defects Monitoring Program (CBDMP).

Further understanding of maternal nutrition and birth defects may follow the more typical course of studies of nutrition. Causes of maternal (and hence fetal) nutrient deficiencies include primary deficiencies that arise because of low intake of essential nutrients, a problem that is generally more common in developing as compared industrialized countries, and secondary (conditioned) nutrient deficiencies that arise due to genetic factors, nutrient interactions, toxicants including medications and other chemicals, diseases, and physiological stressors.

MATERNAL AGE

Women are born with all of the eggs, which they will use in their lifetime. The eggs age with the individual and as women get older, their risk increases for having a chromosomally abnormal pregnancy. Once a woman is 35-year-old at the time of delivery, she is considered to be of advanced maternal age.

Chromosomes are the inherited structures in the cells of the body. Normally, there are 46 chromosomes in each cell, arranged into 23 pairs. Chromosomal abnormalities involving an entire missing or extra chromosome are not inherited and are not caused by an exposure during pregnancy. Instead, they are caused by random mistakes in cell division at the time of conception and can occur in anyone's pregnancy. The chance for such an event to occur does increase with a woman's age.

Genetic Aspect of Advanced Maternal Age

Many women today are waiting until later in life to have children. However, an older mother may be at increased risk for miscarriage, birth defects, and pregnancy complications, such as twins, high blood pressure, gestational diabetes, and difficult labors. The risk of having a baby with chromosomal abnormalities increases with maternal age (Table 3.3). Listed below are the risks for having a baby with Down syndrome, one of the most common chromosomal birth defects, as well as the overall risks for having a baby with any type of chromosome abnormality, including Down syndrome:

Table 3.3: Maternal age risks for chromosome abnormalities

Maternal Age	Down syndrome	Any
15 to 24 years	1/1300	1/500
25 to 29 years	1/1100	1/385
35 years	1/350	1/178
40 years	1/100	1/63
45 years	1/25	1/18

It is possible that risks may be higher as many statistics only report live births and do not take into account pregnancies with chromosomal abnormalities that were terminated or ended due to natural pregnancy loss. There are approximately 400 different types of chromosome abnormalities that have been observed in humans, however, many are rare. The risk for Down syndrome makes up almost half of the maternal age risk for chromosome abnormalities.

Common chromosomal abnormality have been seen in children born from mothers with advanced are as follows:

- *Down syndrome (trisomy 21):* The most common chromosomal abnormality in liveborns is Down syndrome (trisomy 21). Down syndrome is caused by an extra chromosome # 21; thus, an affected individual has three rather than two copies of chromosome # 21. It is this extra genetic material that causes the features of Down syndrome, including mental retardation, a characteristic facial appearance, and other health problems.

  In general, for women under the age of 40, after having one child with Down syndrome, the chance of having another baby with Down syndrome is 1 percent. After age 40, the recurrence risk for Down syndrome is based on the age of the mother at delivery. It is important to know that about 75 percent of babies with Down syndrome are born to women under the age of 35. This is because women under the age of 35 have more babies than women over 35. The physician may refer parents to a genetic specialist or genetic counselor who can explain the results of chromosomal tests in detail, including what the recurrence risks may be in another pregnancy and what tests are available to diagnose chromosome problems before a baby is born.

- Some studies have shown a higher chance of miscarriage (early pregnancy loss) in older mothers. When considering all women, about half of first trimester miscarriages occur because of a chromosomal abnormality in the fetus. Because these abnormalities increase with maternal age, miscarriage is also more likely.
- Two other chromosomal abnormalities which are more likely to occur in women of advanced maternal age are trisomy 18 and trisomy 13, resulting from three copies of chromosomes #18 or #13, respectively. Babies with these chromosomal abnormalities have severe mental retardation and serious birth defects. Most infants with these birth defects do not survive their first year of life. Although more severe than Down syndrome, they are also far less common. Other chromosomal abnormalities seen in liveborns occur with the sex chromosomes, the X and the Y. An extra or missing X or Y chromosome may cause mild physical differences, learning disabilities, behavioral and sometimes fertility issues.
- Details of various other genetic disorders seen among children born from parents with advanced are is illustrated in Table 3.4.

Table 3.4: Genetic disorders associated with increased parents age

Disorder	Description	Inheritance mechanism
Achondroplasia	Short limbed type of dwarfism with large hands	AD
Acrodysostomia	Intellectual disability, short limbs with deformities especially in arms and hands growth deficiency, small head, nose and maxilla.	AD

Contd...

Contd...

Disorder	Description	Inheritance mechanism
Apert syndrome	Craniofacial deformities, such as cronio-stenosis skeletal deformities especially 'sock' feet and syndactyly	AD
Basal cell nevus syndrome	Nevi that become malignant, rib and spine anomalies, variable degree of intellectual disabilities, eye abnormalities	AD
Crouzon craniofacial dysostosis	Hypoplasia and abnormalities of skull and face craniosynostosis, premature suture closer, shallow eye orbits	AD
Marfan syndrome	Elongated thin extremities cardiovascular complications, especially of aorta, ocular anomalies, especially lens	AD
Oculodensodigital	Digital anomalies, such as incurved fifth figure or syndactyly, tooth eventual hypoplasia. Other dental abnormalities microphthalmos, glaucoma possible.	AD
Treacher collins syndrome (Mandibulofacial dysostosis)	Molar and mandibular hypoplasia conductive deafness ear malformations, lower eyelid defects, limb abnormalities	AD
Warrdenburg syndrome	Bilateral perception deafness pigment disturbance of hair and eyes (e.g. white lock of hair and uniform light colored irish or heterochromic frises) lateral displacement of inner canthus of eye many have other anomalies	AD
Progeris	Thin skin, alopecia, growth deficiency, atherosclerosis appearance of premature aging	AD
Duchene muscular dystrophy	Progressive muscular disease with weakness	XR
Hemophilia-A	Coagulation disorders with deficiency of factor VIII	XR

AD-Autosomal Dominant, AR-Autosomal Recessive, XR-X-linked Recessive

Role of Nurses

- Nurses need to ensure that any woman pregnant and over the age of 30, should talk with physician about individual health and discuss plans for helping and development of baby to maintain a healthy pregnancy.

- Pregnant mother with age above 35 years should be referred for prenatal testing to diagnose or rule out chromosomal abnormalities and other genetic birth defects. Testing may include blood tests, ultrasound, chorionic villus sampling (testing the tissues around the fetus), or amniocentesis (withdrawing a sample of the amniotic fluid).
- Nurses should provide details about the prenatal testing and support the women during prenatal testing.
- Nurses should help the women and family to take decision about prenatal testing and termination of pregnancy if fetus found to be with chromosomal abnormalities.
- Nurses should plan and implement pre and intra conception counseling about ill effects of advanced parental age.

MATERNAL DRUG THERAPY

The use of drugs in pregnant and lactating women requires a thorough understanding of the unique interactions between the mother, fetus/infant, and the pharmacologic agents that are used in therapy. Any agent that is consumed by a woman may have adverse effects on the fetus/infant. There exists a paucity of data and information for most drugs relative to pregnancy and lactation. Conclusions that can be drawn remain speculative, and the use of any drug during pregnancy and lactation requires extreme caution. Factors involved in fetal drug exposure include the dynamic changes of maternal physiology related to drug absorption, distribution, metabolism, and excretion. Placental transfer of drug occurs with almost all agents, each to varying degrees. The notion that the placenta provides an impervious barrier must be dismissed. The least understood of factors involving potential fetal harm is teratogenicity. The mechanisms and types of teratogenic agents, poorly understood in humans. Most drugs appear in the breast milk and, therefore, carry some degree of potential harm. Minimizing exposure is a goal that can be obtained when taking into account the maternal physiology, basic pharmacokinetic factors, physiochemical interactions between drug and membranes, and the chemical composition of breast milk.

The topic of 'drug safety in pregnancy' embraces the effect of drugs on the pregnancy, fetus or neonate, and the effects of the pregnancy on drug disposition. Almost all drugs cross the placenta to some extent and may pose risk to the developing fetus. A few exceptions exist (e.g. insulin, heparin) which are very large molecules that do not cross biological membranes readily.

The Effects of Pregnancy on Drug Disposition (Pharmacokinetics)

The physiological changes that occur with pregnancy may affect pharmacokinetics. These effects vary with the drug and with the individual, are generally difficult to predict and frequently poorly studied.

- *Oral availability:* Gastrointestinal motility may be reduced during pregnancy and this may result in delayed absorption of orally administered drugs. However, in the vast majority of cases this is unlikely to be of clinical significance, as the total amount of drug that is systemically available will not change appreciably.
- *Distribution:* Maternal water and fat content increases in pregnancy and may increase the volume of distribution of drugs. This should only impact on those drugs that are initiated with a loading dose, when higher doses may be required. Plasma albumin concentrations decrease in pregnancy and may result in reduced protein binding of some drugs. For most drugs these changes should not impact on drug dosing because the unbound (active) concentration should not change. However, problems may arise when drug concentrations are used to tailor drug therapy (e.g. anticonvulsants). Routine measured drug concentrations are usually the total concentrations, i.e. bound plus unbound (free). Total drug concentrations may decline in pregnancy so for drugs, such as phenytoin it is important to measure unbound concentrations just prior to and during pregnancy. Total phenytoin concentrations must not be used to make dosage adjustments in pregnant women. Interpretation of phenytoin concentrations during pregnancy is very complicated and specialist consultation is usually required.
- *Metabolism/elimination:* Maternal drug clearance often increases because of changes that include increased renal and hepatic blood flow and enzyme induction. This generally means that increased maintenance doses of both metabolised and renally

eliminated drugs may be required in pregnancy. For example, drugs that are extensively renally eliminated (e.g. penicillins) will have enhanced clearance in pregnancy because of increased glomerular filtration rates. Increased hepatic metabolism of drugs is variable but can be expected to result in increased dosage requirements in the third trimester for agents such as phenytoin and methadone.

The Effect of Drugs on the Pregnancy, Fetus or Neonate (Teratogenicity)

First-trimester drug exposure has the largest risk of malformations and ideally all drug therapy should be stopped before attempting conception. Accidental drug exposure is a frequent occurrence because approximately half of all pregnancies are unplanned. Major malformations are thought to affect 2 – 4% of all live births. In the majority of cases, the cause of the abnormalities cannot be identified. Exogenous factors, such as drugs are thought to cause only 1 – 5% of all malformations (i.e. affecting < 0.2% of all live births). The percentage of pregnancies affected by drugs is small but largely preventable.

It is difficult to predict which pregnancies exposed to teratogens will result in a malformation. This is because most known teratogens only cause problems in a small percentage of exposed pregnancies. Accurate timing of the exposure can help in assessment of fetal risk as some drugs only cause specific abnormalities at a certain time period in the pregnancy (Table 3.5). For example, folic acid antagonists (e.g. carbamazepine) will not cause neural tube defects if exposure to the drug occurred after the fourth week postconception, by which time neural tube closure has occurred. However, folic acid antagonists may cause other types of malformations beyond this time.

Table 3.5: Stages of fetal development during pregnancy

- *Pre-embryonic (days 0–17 postconception):* Drug exposure during this time is not usually considered to pose risk of malformations. An 'all or nothing response' is said to occur. There is early abortion or no adverse effect on fetal development. However, the half-life of the drug must be considered because many drugs remain in the maternal circulation for a long period after discontinuation.

Contd...

Contd...

- *Embryonic (days 18–56 postconception):* This is the most important time in terms of risk of fetal malformations.
- *Fetal period (days 56–term):* The risk of malformations is lower, but some abnormalities may still occur because development of organs/tissues, such as the central nervous system, teeth and genitalia continues. For example, ethanol exposure may affect central nervous system development, and tetracyclines may adversely discolor deciduous teeth and suppress bone growth.

A number of drugs are suspected of being teratogenic, but only a few have been identified with certainty (Table 3.6). Perhaps the best known of these drugs is thalidomide, which was shown to give rise to a full range of malformations including phocomelia (short flipper like appendages) of all four extremities. Other drugs known to cause fetal abnormalities are the antimetabolites that are used in the treatment of cancer, the anticoagulants drugs (warfarin), several of the anticonvulsant drugs. Some drugs affect a single developing structure, for example, prophylthiouracil can impair thyroid development. More recently vitamin A and its derivative (the retinoids) have been targeted for concern because of their teratogenic potential.

Fetal abnormalities, such as cleft palate, heart defects, retinal and optic nerve abnormalities and CNS malformations were observed in women ingesting therapeutic doses of the drugs during the first trimester of pregnancy. There is also a concern about teratogenic effect of vitamin A, such as those contained in some dietary supplements or vitamin pills. It is currently recommended that doses greater than 10,000 IU should be avoided.

In 1983, the US food and drug Administration established a system for classifying drugs according to possible risk to the fetus. According to the system, drugs are put into five categories A, B, C, D and X. Drugs in category-A are the least dangerous and category B, C and D are increasingly more dangerous. Those in category-X are contraindicated during pregnancy, because of proven teratogenicity (Table 3.7). Because many drugs are suspected of causing fatal abnormalities and even those that were once thought to be safe are now being viewed critically. It is recommended that women in their childbearing years avoid unnecessary use of drugs. This pertains to nonpregnant women as well as pregnant women because many developmental defects occur early in pregnancy. As happened with thalidomide, the damage to the embryo may occur before pregnancy is suspected or confirmed.

Table 3.6: Drugs considered to be human teratogens (not exhaustive)

Teratogenic drugs	
ACE inhibitors	Misoprostil
Androgens	Penicillamine
Antineoplastics (some)	Phenytoin
Carbamazepine	Tetracyclines
Carbimazole	Thalidomide
Danazol	Valproic acid
Diethylstilboestrol	Vitamin A and derivatives, e.g. isotretinoin
Ethanol	Warfari
Lithium	

Table 3.7: Harmful or teratogenic effect selected drugs on fetal

Drugs	Reported effect
ACE inhibitors	• Renal dysfunction, oligohydramnios, intrauterine growth retardation
	Antibiotic
Aminoglycosides	------As streptomycin....
Chloramphenicol	Gray baby syndrome, hypothermia, failure to feed, collapse and death
Streptomycin	Ototoxic to fetal ear, eight cranial nerve damage, other aminoglycosides
Tetracycline	Yellow/blown discoloration of tooth enamel hypoplasia, inhibits bone growth
	Anticancer drugs
Alkylating agent	Chlorambucil has been associated with renal agenesis, busulfan has association with growth retardation, cleft palate, microphthalmia and increased incidence of multiple malformations, all apparently cause a risk of increased spontaneous abortion
Aminopterin	Cranial dystosis, hydrocephalus, hypertelorism, micro-gnathia, limb and hand defects, multiple congenital malformations

Contd...

Contd...

Drugs	Reported effect
Antimetabolites	Cyclophosphamides has been associated with increased incidence of multiple malformations, especially skeletal defects and cleft palate
Methotrexate	Increased incidence of miscellaneous congenital malformations, especially of the central nervous system and limbs
Anticoagulants	
Warfarin	Fetal warfarin syndrome, facial abnormalities, nasal hypoplasia, respiratory difficulties, hypoplastic nails, microcephaly, hemorrhage, ophthalmic abnormalities, bone stippling, developmental delay
Anticonvalescents	
Phenytoin	Fetal hydentoin syndrome, growth retardation, metal deficiency, dysmorphic features, short nasal bridge, mild hypertelorism, cleft lip and palate, cardiac defects, transplacental carcinogenesis (neuroblastomas)
Trimethadione	Apparent syndrome of developmental delay, v-shaped eyebrow and paramethadione, low-set ears, high or cleft palate, irregular teeth, cardiac defects, growth retardation, speech difficulties, increased risk of spontaneous abortion
Valproic acid	Spinal bifida
Antimalarial	
Chloroquine	Slight risk of choriretinitis, may cause otoxicity
Quinine	Deafness, limb anomalies, visceral defects, visual problems, other multiple congenital anomalies
Antithyroid	
Iodides and thlouracils	Depression of fetal thyroid, hypothyroidism, goiter
Carbimazole	Scalp defects, dysmorphic defects, other possible anomalies
Antidepressants	Withdrawal reactions
Antihypertensives	Fetal hypoxia with excessive treatment due to decreased placental perfusion
Corticosteroids	Fetal adrenal suppression
NSAIDs	Premature closure of the ductus arteriosis, renal impairment
Opioids	Withdrawal reactions

Role of Nurses

- Educate mother to remember following basic principles regarding drug therapy during maternity period.
  - Avoid all drugs in pregnancy where possible, especially in the first-trimester.
  - Herbal and other complementary therapies are often perceived by the lay public as 'safe'. Unfortunately, data on many of these products are very limited and insufficient to determine their safety in pregnancy. In general, herbal remedies should be avoided during pregnancy.
  - Consider tapering and discontinuing unnecessary pharmacotherapy prior to attempting conception. Remember that some drugs or their metabolites may have long half-life and persist for some time after stopping therapy.
  - Many conditions are self-limiting and do not require drug treatment. Reassurance or lifestyle measures (e.g. avoidance of migraine triggers) may be sufficient.
  - Where possible, delay treatment until after results of laboratory testing (e.g. swabs), or until after delivery (e.g. for treatment of hypercholesterolemia).
  - If drug therapy is needed, select drugs with the most established safety record. For example, amitriptyline (or nortriptyline) or fluoxetine should be selected over moclobemide or nefazodone for depression.
  - Use the lowest effective dose for the shortest possible time.
  - Poor control of some maternal disease states may carry significant risk to the development of the fetus. In addition, the severity or frequency of some maternal diseases (e.g. migraines) may improve in pregnancy allowing a reduction in the dosage of some drugs, or cessation of treatment.
  - Teach women that over counter products including vitamins, herbs, or iron are considered drugs and should not be taken without discussion with her health care provider.
  - Educate women as to the dangers of self-medication in pregnancy.

  - It is also important to realize that some mothers may be very anxious about the risks that their drug therapy possess to their baby. This may lead to noncompliance with drug therapy, or unnecessary pregnancy terminations.
- Before administering any drug to any women in fertile age does not forget to ask about her pregnancy status.
- Consider every drug unsafe during pregnancy, and try to avoid as far as possible.
- Question any prescription of the doctor, if you find that drug prescribed may be teratogenic.
- Provide preconception or prenatal counseling about harmful effects of drugs on fetus if taken during pregnancy.
- Integrate the previous information into school health programs.
- Provide teaching related to non-pharmacological management to common conditions, such as common cold, can be managed by rest, steam inhalation and plenty of water, anxiety can be managed by relaxation techniques instead of medication.
- Involve the client in decision-making, if drug therapy is being considered, as an informal pattern in her own care.
- Instruct her to keep an accurate list of all medication ingested during pregnancy with the reason for it.
- Maintain a record of all prescription or recommended drugs with the same information. This should be in a handy form for easy reference as part of the patient profile. If drugs therapy is necessary, the lowest effective therapeutic dose of the least toxic agent should be used.
- The risk and benefit should be always be considered and doses should be individualized.
- Question any drug that appears contraindicated in pregnancy because the practitioner prescribing it may not know that the patient is pregnant.

GENETIC EFFECT OF RADIATION, DRUGS AND CHEMICALS

The concept of the fetus as totally protected by placenta barrier was cracked by the association of specific birth defects with rubella infection and shattered by the thalidomide disaster of the early 1960s. Exposures to radiation, (Fig. 3.2) chemicals and drugs during pregnancy can be teratogenic (harmful for embryo or fetus).

The term 'teratogen' is often used to describe those agents acting during pregnancy that cause structural or functional damage to the unborn child, in contrast to 'mutagen' which damage genetic material. Low risk teratogens are defined as agents that produce congenital defect in less than 10 infants among 1000 maternal exposure (Shepard, 2002). Term, such as embryotoxic, fetotoxic or developmental toxicity may also be used. The term 'fetus' as used in this chapter also includes the embryo. The stage of development of the embryo determines the susceptibility to teratogenes. The period during which the embryo is most susceptible to teratogenic agents is when rapid differentiation of tissues are taking place, usually from 15 to 60 days post-conception. In a given exposure during pregnancy a teratogen can have any of the following consequences:

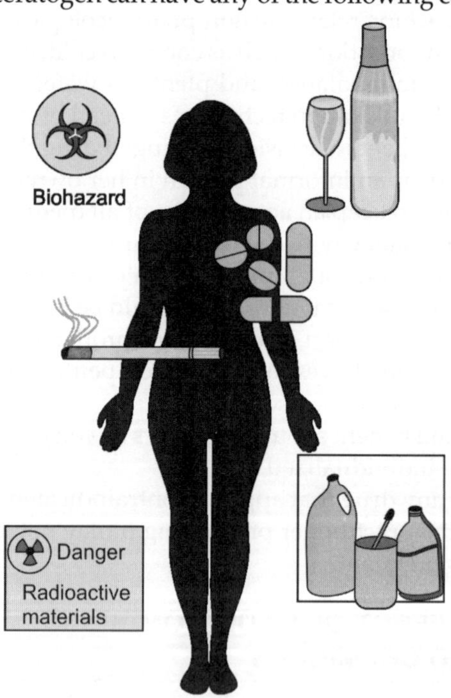

Fig. 3.2: Radiation, drugs and chemicals exposure

- No apparent effect
- Prenatal or perinatal death
- Congenital anomalies

- Altered fetal growth (e.g. growth retardation)
- Postnatal functional and behavioral deficits and aberrations
- Carcinogenesis.

Factors Influence the Effect of the Teratogens

Complex and multifaceted maternal and fetal factors influence the effect of drugs and radiations and chemicals on fetus.

- Agents often act differently in different species and on individuals with same species (e.g. different in genetic constitution, variability in metabolic pathway, etc.) this applies to both the mother and fetus.
- The age of the fetus at the time of exposure, generally when exposed to agents affecting the period from fertilization to implantation the result is either death or regeneration during period of organogenesis. The results is usually gross structural alteration and after oranogenesis in the fetal period the results is usually related to alteration in cell size and number, although the central nervous system and external genitalia remain vulnerable through most of pregnancy (Fig. 3.3).
- The agent access to and disposition within the fetus.
- The chemical, biological and physical properties of the agent (for microorganism type, virulence and number) have varying effects.
- Interactions with other agents and factors (e.g. environment, nutritional, other drugs, etc.) can have negative consequences.
- Level and duration of dosage or exposure influence the agent's effect.
- Maternal biochemical pathway and mechanisms for handling drugs and chemical are altered by pregnancy.
- The degree of interference with maternal system and the extent of modulation that occurs determine the effect on the fetus.
- The genetic constitution of both mother and fetus, dizygotic twins have been born with one having anomalies typical of a drug effect, whereas the other was normal.

Drugs and chemical can cause fetotoxic effect not only by direct fetal interaction but also through interference with maternal system (circulatory, endocrine, excretory, appetite regulatory, etc.)

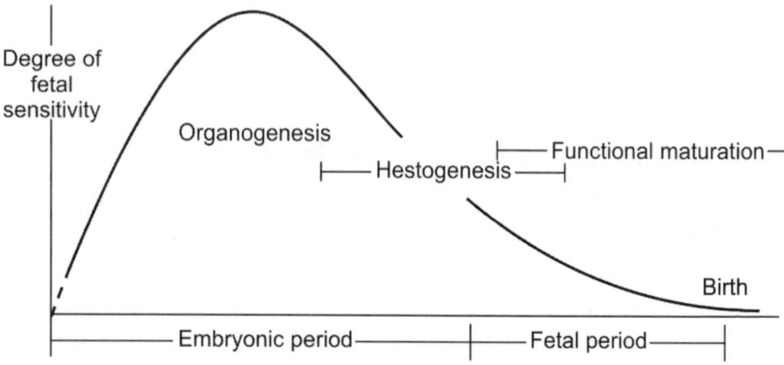

Fig. 3.3: Period of fetal growth and development and susceptibility to deviation

(The highest sensitivity, at least to structure deviation occurs during the period of organogenesis from about days 18 to 20 until about days 55 to 60. The absolute peak of sensitivity may be reached before day 30 postconception. As organogenesis is completed susceptibility to anatomical defects diminished greatly, but probably minor structural deviation is possible until histogenesis is completed late in the fetal period are more likely to involve growth or functional aspects because these are the predominant develop mental features at this time).

Effects of Chemicals and Drugs

Environmental chemicals and drugs can cross the placenta and cause damage to the developing embryo and fetus. Some of the best documented environmental teratogens are the organic mercurials, which cause neurologic deficits and blindness. Sources of exposure to mercury include contaminated food (fish) and water. The precise mechanism by which chemicals and drugs exert their teratogenic effects is largely unknown. They may have cytotoxic (cell killing), antimetabolic or growth-inhibiting properties, often their effects depend on the time of exposure (in terms of embryonic or fetal development) and extend of exposure (dosage).

Drugs including alcohol and illicit drugs, top the list of chemical teratogens, most drugs can cross the placenta and expose the fetus to both the pharmacologic and teratogenic effects. Factors that affect placental drug transfer and drug effect on the fetus includes:

- *The rate at which chemical or drug cross the placenta.* Lipid soluble drugs tend to cross the placenta more rapidly and enter the fetal circulation. The molecular weight of a drug also influences the rate and amount of chemical or drug transferred across the placenta. Drugs with molecular weight less than 500 can cross placenta easily depending on lipid solubility and degree of ionization, those with a molecular weight of 500–1000 cross the placenta with more difficulty and those with molecular weight grater than 1000 cross very poorly.

- The stage of placental and fetal development at the time of chemical or drug exposure.

Illicit use of psychostimulants during pregnancy is an increasing problem in modern society, resulting in increased number of adverse pregnancy outcomes, such a miscarriages, vaginal bleeding, and cognitive effects in newborns (Table 3.8).

Table 3.8: Fetal effect of chemicals and drugs used during pregnancy

Drugs	*Effects on fetus*
Alcohol	Microcephaly, heart defects, mental retardation Fetal Alcohol Syndrome
Tobacco	Miscarriage, premature labor, fetal IUGR (intrauterine growth retardation)
Cocaine and Methamphetamine	Miscarriage, premature labor, fetal IUGR , fetal withdrawal symptoms (tremors, sleeplessness, muscle spasm, and sucking difficulties), learning difficulties.
Heroin and other narcotics	Premature birth, low birth weight babies, hypoglycemia, fetal respiratory distress, intracranial hemorrhage, withdrawal symptoms (irritability, vomiting, diarrhea, joint stiffness)
Marijuana	Premature birth, low birth weight babies
Phencyclidine	Withdrawal symptoms (lethargy, altering tremors)
Organic solvent chemicals inhalants (Paints, glues, etc.)	Varying degree birth as well as microcephaly, heart defects, growth and mental retardation.

- *Alcohol:* The features of fetal alcohol syndrome (FAS) occur in 30–40% of babies born to chronic alcoholics. Another 50–70% of such babies may suffer from fetal alcohol effects (FAE), which is milder than FAS. To be diagnosed with FAS a baby must have the following features:
  - Growth retardation
  - Central nervous system problems

  - Characteristic facial appearance (small head, flat facial profile, thin upper lip)
  - Other major birth defects (heart, gastrointestinal, etc.) are possible
  - Children with FAS have failure to thrive, mild to moderate mental retardation and behavior problems. FAS is the most preventable cause of mental retardation.
- *Thalidomide:* Well known teratogen leading to limb defects in exposed babies. This medication to prevent morning sickness is not used anymore.
- *Cigarette smoking:* Constant exposure to cigarette smoke decreases the amount of oxygen crossing the placenta and can lead to low birth weight and premature babies.
- *Cocaine, street drugs:* Women addicted to street drugs are at increased risk for having babies born addicted to these drugs. The biggest risks to the babies are not from the drugs themselves, but due to poor maternal nutrition and lack of prenatal care. Prenatal cocaine exposure is not associated with a syndrome (a group of seemingly unrelated birth defects found to have a single cause). Studies are still ongoing, looking at long-term effects of exposures in school age children. Cocaine is a vasoconstrictor—causes blood vessels to shrink. There are many prenatal complications due to even one exposure to cocaine:
  - Miscarriage
  - Placental abruption
  - Vascular defects (limb reduction)
  - *In utero* strokes
  - Increased risk for SIDS
  - Infant drug withdrawal
- *Anticonvulsants:* Exposure to antiseizure medications is associated with fetal anticonvulsant syndrome. Approximately 10% of children exposed to Dilantin and other seizure medications will have some growth and mental retardation, digit hypoplasia (shortening), and a characteristic face. Use of valproic acid and carbamazepine in early pregnancy are associated with a 1% risk for spina bifida.
- *Lithium:* Exposure to lithium is associated with an increased risk for congenital heart defects Retinoids.

- *Vitamin A:* Women taking oral vitamin A have a high-risk of having a baby with major birth defects including hydrocephaly (excess fluid in the brain), small head size, mental retardation, malformed ears, facial abnormalities, and heart defects. Topical vitamin A has not proven to increase the risk for birth defects.

Nursing Considerations

- Be proactive, do preconception counseling, which should include, assessment of current alcohol and drug use, environmental exposure and smoking and provide education.
- Females of reproductive age seen in various settings should be taught that medication and social drugs exposure of certain type can affect the fetus, especially in the 1st month or trimester when she may not realize she is pregnant. This should include the danger of medication sharing.
- Encourage the client to tell physician, nurse and other health practitioners involved in her care that she is pregnant.
- Identify those most likely to be users of medications and drugs (including alcohol, caffeine and cigarettes) and inform those who are considering pregnancy or who are already pregnant of the hazards.

Effects of Radiation

Every healthy woman without personal or a family history of reproductive or developmental problems begins her pregnancy with a 3% risk for birth defects and a 15% risk for miscarriage. These are background risks for all healthy pregnant women. Radiation enhances reproductive risk among these women. Heavy doses of ionizing radiation have been shown to cause microcephaly, skeletal malformations, and mental retardations. There is no evidence that diagnostic level of radiation causes congenital abnormalities. However, some of the institution still prefers to ask for pregnancy status of a woman before any radiological investigation. Other institutions may require a pregnancy test before any extensive diagnostic X ray studies.

In routine radiation risk is caused by medical radiation procedures, effect of which is discussed in further discussion of this topic, other sources of radiation which impose the reproductive risk of nonionizing radiation, includes electromagnetic fields emitted from computers, microwave communication systems, microwave ovens, power lines, cellular phones, household appliances, heating pads and warming blankets, airport screening devices for metal objects, and diagnostic levels of ultrasound has been studied extensively. Two national committees of scientists evaluated the risk from these nonionizing radiation sources. Both of the committees published books on the subject. The first came out in 1993 from the Oak Ridge Associated University panel created by the White House while the second was the product of the committee of the National Academy of Sciences. Both of these groups concluded that the reproductive risk of nonionizing radiation is minimal if even existent.

Genetic Aspect of Radiation

This discussion presents facts about effects of radiation in reference to gene damage.

- It is generally believed that radiation is teratogenic. However, Muller's study concluded that no new or unique mutations are produced by radiations, in the range of 25 to 400 R, the frequency of mutation was linear. The majority of radiation-induced mutations were recessive; both parents would have carried the genes for an effect to be observed in the offspring and there was no dose rate or dose frequency effect.
- Epidemiological studies have not demonstrated radiation-induced genetic effects. A largest population study of the atomic bomb survivors and their offspring concluded that blood screening of 27,000 children of atomic survivors for 28 specific disorders that may have been caused by radiation exposure demonstrated only two mutations. However, vivo radiation studies have shown significant teratogenic effect on genes of organisms.
- Principle effects of irradiation on the fetus includes:
  - Prenatal or neonatal death
  - Congenital abnormalities
  - Intrauterine growth retardation
  - Low intelligence (Low IQ)
  - Genetic abnormalities
  - Spontaneous abortion
  - Cancer induction.

- Throughout most of pregnancy, the embryo/fetus is assumed to be at about the same risk for carcinogenic effects as children. Radiation has been shown to increase the risk for leukemia and many types of cancer in adults and children.
- Data on the effect of irradiation *in utero* were obtained by offspring from the atomic bomb survivors; revealed that microcephaly, mental and growth retardation were main abnormalities seen. Abnormalities in eye, genitals and skeletal system occurred less often. Children from Hroshima and Nagasaki who were irradiated *in utero* between 8 and 25 weeks postconception demonstrated lower IQ. Also these children were found with microcephaly.
- Based on the Law of Bergonic and Tribondean (developing embryo is very radiosensitive) and embryo's response to radiation depends on:
  - *Total radiation dose:* Radiation less than 100 mGy is considered safe for fetus. Malformations have a *threshold of 100 to 200 mGy or higher* and are typically associated with central nervous system problems. Fetal doses in excess of 100 mGy can result in some reduction of IQ (intelligence quotient). Fetal doses in the range of 1000 mGy can result in severe mental retardation and microcephaly, particularly during 8 to 15 weeks and to a lesser extent at 16 to 25 weeks
  - *Rate or frequency radiation:* Fatal doses of 100 mGy are not reached even with 3 pelvic CT scans or 20 conventional diagnostic X-ray examinations.
  - *Quality of radiation.*

  Stage of fetal development: During 8 to 25 weeks postconception the CNS is particularly sensitive to radiation (Fig. 3.4).

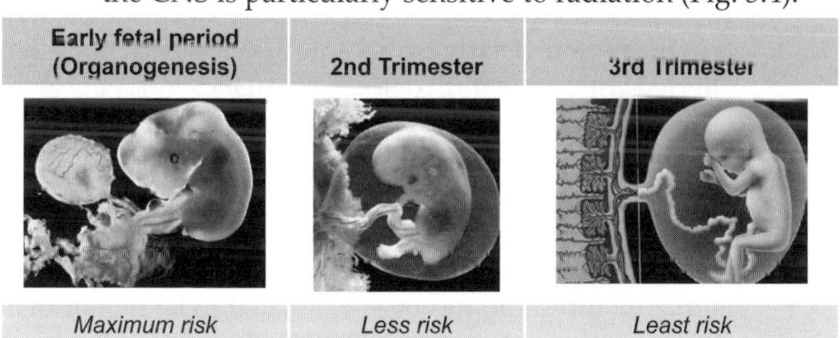

Fig. 3.4: Radiation risk during different stages of fetal developments

Effect of Medical Radiation Procedures

- Ionizing radiation is the kind of electromagnetic radiation produced by X-ray machines, radioactive isotopes (radionuclides), and radiation therapy machines. There is potential for the embryo or fetus to be exposed during the diagnostic or therapeutic procedures for women who are pregnant and have X-rays, fluoroscopy, radiation therapy, or are administered liquid radioactive materials.
- Most diagnostic procedures expose the embryo to less than 5 rad or 50 mSv. This level of radiation exposure will not increase reproductive risks (either birth defects or miscarriage). According to published information, the reported dose of radiation result in an increase incidence of birth defects or miscarriage is above 20 rad or 200 mSv.
- A pregnant medical worker may work in a radiation environment as long as there is reasonable assurance that the fetal dose be kept below 1 mGy during pregnancy. 1 mGy is approximately the dose that all person receive annually from penetrating natural background.
- Another important consideration is the stage of pregnancy in which the radiation exposure occurred:
  - *In the first two weeks postconception* or the second two weeks from the last menstrual period, the embryo is very resistant to the malforming effects of X-rays. The embryo is, however, sensitive to the lethal effects of X-rays although doses much higher than 5 rad or 50 mSv is necessary to cause a miscarriage.
  - From the third to the eighth week of pregnancy, the embryo is in the period of early embryonic development but is not affected with either birth defects, pregnancy loss, or growth retardation unless the exposure is substantially above the 20 rad (200 mSv) exposure.
  - *From the eighth to the fifteenth week of pregnancy*, the embryo or fetus is sensitive to the effects of radiation on the central nervous system. But here again, the exposure has to be very high. The threshold has been estimated to be higher than 30 rad (300 mSv) before an effect can be seen on the IQ of the developing embryo. General diagnostic studies do not

reach these levels and, therefore, these effects are rarely of concern for patients.

- *Beyond the 20th week of pregnancy* when the fetus is completely developed, it has become more resistant to the developmental effects of radiation. In fact, the fetus is probably no more vulnerable to many of the effects of radiation than the mother in the latter part of pregnancy. But the most important thing is that practically none of the diagnostic radiological procedures will affect an embryo at this late stage of pregnancy and certainly there is no risk for birth defects or miscarriage from the range of exposures that occur from diagnostic studies.

Minimizing risk of medical radiation procedures: Health care providers need to follow following principles to minimize the harmful effects of radiation on growing fetus.

- All medical radiation practices (occupational and patient-related) should be justified before performing (more benefit than risk).
- Medical radiation exposures should be justified for each patient before they are performed.
- After it is decided to do a medical radiation procedure, the fetal radiation dose should be reduced while still obtaining the required diagnostic information.
- Radiation therapy and interventional fluoroscopically-guided procedures may give fetal doses in the range of 10 to 100 mGy or more depending on the specifics of the procedure, which is considered safe during pregnancy
- After higher dose medical procedures have been performed on pregnant patients, fetal dose and potential fetal risk should be estimated by a knowledgeable person.
- Most nuclear medicine diagnostic procedures are done with short-lived radionuclides (such as technetium-99^m) that do not cause large fatal doses
- Often, fetal dose can be reduced through maternal hydration and encouraging voiding of urine.
- Some radionuclides do cross the placenta and can pose fetal risks (such as iodine-131). Therefore, use of such radionuclides should be discouraged.

- The fetal thyroid accumulates iodine after about 10 weeks gestational age. High fetal thyroid doses from radioiodine can result in permanent hypothyroidism
- If pregnancy is discovered within 12 h of radioiodine administration, prompt oral administration of stable potassium iodine (60–130 mg) to the mother can reduce fetal thyroid dose. This may need to be repeated several times.
- A number of radionuclides are excreted in breast milk. It is recommended that breastfeeding is suspended as follows:
  - Completely after ^{131}I therapy
  - 3 weeks after ^{131}I, 125_{I}, ^{67}Ga, ^{22}Na, and ^{201}Tl therapy.
  - 12 h after ^{131}I hippurate and all ^{99m}Tc compounds except 4 h after ^{99m}Tc red cells, DTPA, and phosphonates.

Radiation Exposure and Termination of Pregnancy

- High fetal doses (100–1000 mGy) during *late pregnancy* are not likely to result in malformations or birth defects since all the organs have been formed.
- A fetal dose of 100 mGy has a small individual risk of radiation-induced cancer. There is over a 99% chance that the exposed fetus will *NOT* develop childhood cancer or leukemia.
- Termination of pregnancy at fetal doses of less than 100 mGy is *NOT* justified based upon radiation risk.
- At fetal doses in excess of 500 mGy, there can be significant fetal damage, the magnitude and type which is a function of dose and stage of pregnancy.
- At fetal doses between 100 and 500 mGy, decisions should be based upon individual circumstances.

Role of Nurses

- Nurses should be proactive in assessment of a women regarding pregnancy before conducting any radiodiagnostic or radiotherapeutic interventions.
- Estimate risk-benefit ratio for any radiological intervention.
- Take an informed consent from patient after discussing the potential expected risk of medical radiation on fetus before any medical radiation procedure.

- Provide radiation protective devices to pregnant women during radiodiagnostic procedures, like lad jackets during X-ray studies.
- Provide antenatal education to women about reproductive risk of exposure to radiation.
- Conduct several school health programs to enhance awareness of children about reproductive risk of exposure to radiation sources in pre-pregnant age (potential effect of radiation on ova and sperms).

PRENATAL GENETIC TESTING AND DIAGNOSIS

Prenatal genetic testing generally refers to tests that are done during pregnancy to either screen for or diagnose a birth defect. The main goal of prenatal genetic testing is to provide families with information to make informed choices about pregnancy and reproduction, and to assist the health care providers in providing the best care and management of women during pregnancy.

Some prenatal genetic tests are screening tests. They cannot diagnose a birth defect, but only determine if the fetus has a high or low risk for a particular problem. One example is maternal serum screening. Maternal serum screening test for Alfa Fetoprotein (AFP) is conducted to identify pregnancies at increased risk for open neural tube defects, Down syndrome, and trisomy 18, etc. These screening tests do not always give a definitive prenatal diagnosis and may just show the probability of a problem with the fetus. In most cases, further diagnostic tests are required to confirm and diagnose the fetal abnormality.

Other prenatal tests are diagnostic and can diagnose certain fetal problems with a high degree of accuracy. Amniocentesis is an example of a prenatal diagnostic test performed on amniotic fluid (fluid surrounding the developing baby during pregnancy). As the fetus grows and sheds cells, those cells can be found in the amniotic fluid and can be used to study the chromosomes. This test identifies fetal chromosome abnormalities. If, for example, an extra chromosome 21 is seen, a diagnosis of Down syndrome is made.

Purposes of Prenatal Diagnosis

- To enable timely medical or surgical treatment of a condition before or after birth

- To give the parents the chance to abort a fetus with the diagnosed condition
- To give parents the chance to 'prepare' for a baby with a health problem or disability, or for the likelihood of a stillbirth.

Having this information in advance of the birth means that health care staff can better prepare themselves and parents for the delivery of a child with a health problem.

Indications for Prenatal Testing and Diagnosis

In general, genetic testing is offered to couples or individuals identified as being at risk for a particular genetic problem. Some of the risk factors that health care providers consider in deciding who should be offered testing include family history, medical history, and ethnicity. Prenatal diagnosis is therefore offered to all pregnant women if they have positive antenatal screening results. However, some women may be offered definitive prenatal diagnosis from the outset without any preceding screening tests, for example:

- Family history of an inherited condition, mental retardation or birth defects
- History of previous pregnancy with fetal abnormality
- Mother has been exposed to viral illness, such as toxoplasmosis or rubella during the pregnancy
- Mother has been exposed to teratogens, such as certain drugs or radiation, during the pregnancy
- Woman has type 1 diabetes mellitus, epilepsy or myotonic dystrophy.
- Women 35 or older who are pregnant or are planning to become pregnant
- Abnormal ultrasound findings
- Couples who are close blood relatives, such as first cousins
- Ethnicity, e.g. Asians have higher risk of sickle cell anemia
- Unexplained or multiple miscarriages
- Positive maternal serum screening, such as AFP Tetra.

The primary aim of a prenatal diagnosis is to provide an accurate diagnosis that will allow the widest possible range of informed choice to those at increased risk of having children with genetic disorders or with congenital abnormalities.

Prenatal Screening

The following antenatal screening tests are offered:

- *Screening for potential for neonatal infection:* Testing for hepatitis B, HIV, syphilis is offered to all women at antenatal visit. This means that effective postnatal intervention can be offered to infected women to decrease the risk of mother-to-child-transmission.
- *Screening for hemolytic disease of the newborn:* Maternal blood group and RhD status are checked at antenatal visit. Assessment for atypical red cell alloantibodies is also carried out at visit and again at 28 weeks to screen for the possibility of the development of hemolytic disease of the newborn. All nonsensitized pregnant women who are RhD negative are offered routine antenatal anti-D prophylaxis.
- *Screening for sickle cell and thalassemia:* Maternal blood testing for disease and carrier status is carried out and, if necessary, paternal blood testing is undertaken so that the probability of the fetus being affected can be assessed.
- *Downs Syndrome screening:* All pregnant women should be offered this screening. This is done using nuchal transluncency, serum screening or both combined, depending on the gestation of pregnancy.
- *Fetal anomaly screening*: An ultrasound scan is performed between 18 and 20 weeks to screen for structural anomalies including skeletal, genitourinary, gastrointestinal, central nervous system and other organ defects. There is no evidence that ultrasound causes harm to the fetus or the mother.
- *Abdominal palpation and measurement of symphysis-fundal distance:* This is a screening test to help detect babies that are small- or large-for-gestational-age and to help detect poly or oligohydramnios which may suggest an underlying problem with the fetus that requires further investigation and definitive prenatal diagnosis.

Types of Prenatal Testing and Diagnosis

Prenatal testing and diagnosis is offered to a women whose prenatal screening test come to be positive or indicate high-risk. Women who have had a previous fetal abnormality or who have a family history of an inherited condition may be offered these diagnostic tests from the outset. The tests that are carried out include:

Noninvasive Tests

Ultrasound: Ultrasound has become the standard in fetal evaluation because it is safe and noninvasive (Fig. 3.5). It can confirm pregnancy, determine fetal age, growth, and development, identify placental implantation site, determine fetal viability or death, confirm multiple gestation, identify masses associated with pregnancy, assess amniotic fluid volume and placental calcification, and facilitate the use of more invasive studies, diagnostics, and treatment. When assessing for specific congenital anomalies or abnormalities in early pregnancy, the uterus and bladder must be differentiated. To facilitate this, clients are instructed to consume approximately 32 to 48 oz of fluid 1 to 2 hours before the procedure and are encouraged not to void until the procedure is completed. Some discomfort due to the pressure exerted by the transducer over a full bladder is expected. A full bladder is typically not necessary for clients in the late stages of pregnancy.

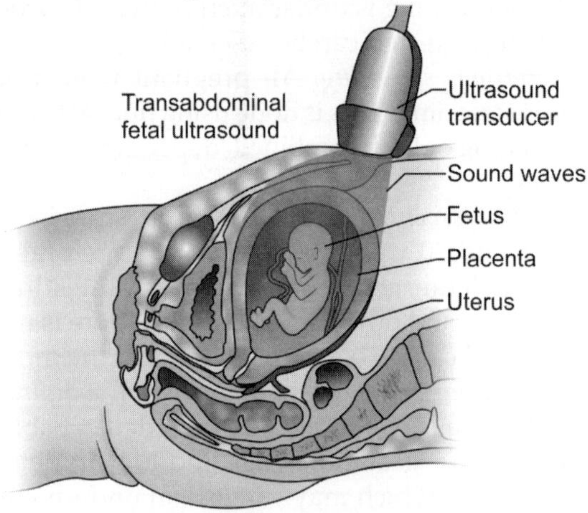

Fig. 3.5: Fetal ultrasonography

Fetal Echocardiography: This is performed through the maternal abdomen when there is suspicion of a congenital cardiac defect (Fig. 3.6). This procedure provides information regarding blood flow velocity and direction, size, position, valves, and chambers of the heart. No specific patient preparation is necessary and no discomfort is involved in the procedure. Client preparation and counseling regarding expected and actual study findings and emotional support to assuage any anxiety about the procedure are necessary.

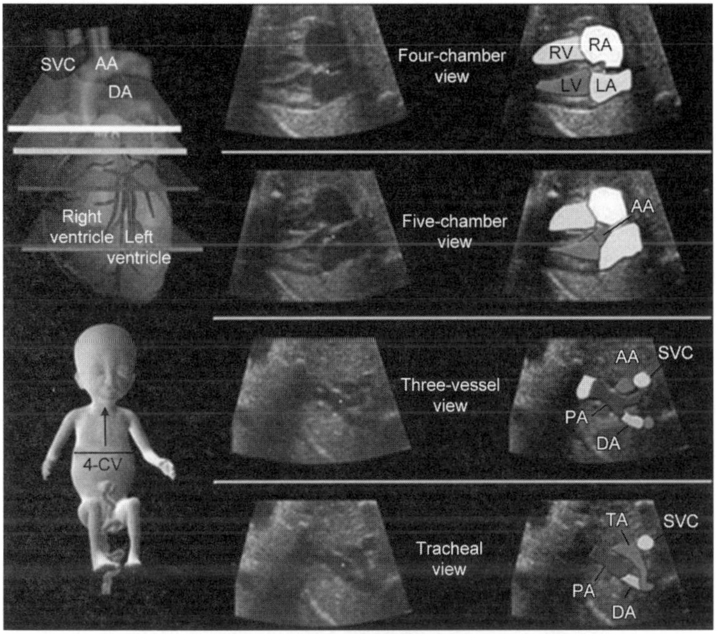

Fig. 3.6: Fetal Echocardiography

Source: Matthews RJ, Fetal echocardiography. Definition: Cardiology. http://www.rjmatthewsmd.com/Definitions/fetal_echocardiography.html retrieved 12/12/2010

Fetal Radiology: In suspected skeletal dysplasia, X-rays can be taken around the same time as the routine anomaly ultrasound scan. Prenatal MRI is also used to assess fetuses with spina bifida, look for associated malformations, and along with ultrasound scanning help to predict neurological deficit and ambulatory potential. Fetal echocardiography can also be carried out if cardiac defects are suspected, for example if there is a family history or in maternal diseases with an increased risk of fetal heart defects, such as diabetes. CT and MR imaging can be used during pregnancy. Concern has been raised as to the long-term side effects, particularly with MR imaging due to the high noise level transferred to the fetus. Risks of the technology and the lack of a long history of its use must be weighed against the benefits of determining a problem *in utero*.

Invasive Tests

Amniocentesis: Amniocentesis is the sampling of amniotic fluid during pregnancy (Fig. 3.7). Amniocentesis involves the insertion of a needle through the maternal abdominal and uterine walls and into the amniotic space. Approximately 10 to 20 ml of amniotic fluid is aspirated. The procedure is performed under ultrasound guidance at approximately 16 to 20 weeks' gestation. Fetal cells are retrieved for analysis. It can be done:

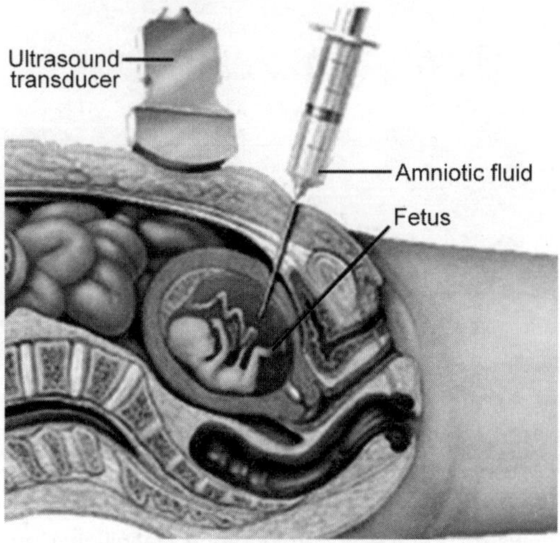

Fig. 3.7: Amniocentesis

- Early in pregnancy (early amniocentesis between 12 and 14 weeks gestation).
- Later in pregnancy (midtrimester amniocentesis between 16 and 18 weeks gestation).

The fluid extracted contains cells from the amnion and fetal skin, lungs and urinary tract. These fetal cells are grown in culture media allowing analysis for:

- *Cytogenetic analysis:* Analysis for chromosomal abnormalities, such as Downs Syndrome can be carried out using cell culture and karyotyping. More recently, rapid aneuploidy techniques using PCR have been used to detect Downs Syndrome which provide results much more quickly than karyotype analysis from cultured cells which usually takes 13–14 days.

- *Molecular genetic tests:* If a disease-causing mutation has been identified in a family, molecular genetic tests can be performed to detect genetic diseases such as cystic fibrosis.
- *Biochemical analysis:* Enzyme levels can be assayed to detect inborn errors of metabolism. Alpha-fetoprotein and acetylcholinesterase levels can be measured to help identify and distinguish between neural tube defects, anencephaly and ventral wall defects, such as gastroschisis and omphalocoele, that may have been suspected during anomaly scanning. Hormone levels can be assessed to diagnose adrenogenital syndrome.

Indications for amniocentesis

- Advanced maternal age (> 35 years) - the most common indication
- Previous child with:
  - Neural tube defect (1 in 20 subsequent pregnancies affected)
  - Chromosomal abnormalities
  - A birth defect
- Positive antenatal screening tests, including for example:
  - Fetal ultrasound findings
  - Raised maternal serum alpha-fetoprotein (ultrasound now also used in neural tube defect screening)
- History of:
  - Parent carrying a balanced chromosomal translocation (1 in 4–10 chance fetus affected)
  - Risk of recessively inherited metabolic disorder
  - Mother carrying X-linked disorder (to determine fetal sex)
  - Mother exposed to certain drugs or infections (which can cause fetal malformations)
- Analysis to detect specific conditions from:
  - DNA (for example fragile X, sickle cell disease, cystic fibrosis)
  - Enzymatic activity in amniocytes (for example Tay-Sachs disease)
  - Fluid biochemistry (for example in congenital adrenal hyperplasia- 17-OH- progesterone).

Procedure of amniocentesis

- Technique:
  - Rhesus immunoprophylaxis should be given where appropriate (fetomaternal transfusion is a risk in amniocentesis and chorionic villus sampling)
  - Preferably performed under ultrasound guidance
  - 22G spinal needle is inserted through maternal abdominal and uterine walls into pocket of amniotic fluid within the amniotic sac
  - 10–20 ml of fluid is aspirated (or approximately 1ml per week of gestation)
  - A cell filtration system may be used
  - Smaller volumes may be aspirated where advanced laboratory techniques require less material
- Midtrimester amiocentesis:
  - Normally performed in second trimester from 14–16 weeks gestation
  - There is relatively more amniotic fluid (enough amniotic fluid for reliable cell culture- about 20 ml)
  - There is still time to terminate the pregnancy (if results indicate this to be advisable)
- Early amniocentesis:
  - This has been conducted at weeks 9–14
  - Less fluid is removed and ultrasound guidance is essential
  - Carries higher risk of loss of pregnancy (around 7%) and talipes equinovarus
  - Preferred over chorionic villus sampling (CVS) where CVS unreliable (in twin pregnancies).

Diagnostic testing of amniotic fluid

The following tests can be performed on aspirated amniotic fluid:

- On the amniotic fluid:
  - AFP and acetylcholinesterase levels (for neural tube defects)
  - Bilirubin levels (for gestational assessment and to detect isoimmune hemolysis)
  - Tests of lung maturity (various but lecithin to sphingomyelin ratio for example)

- Enzyme analysis (many and varied including for inborn errors of metabolism)

- On fetal cells extracted from amniotic fluid testing for genetic and chromosomal disorders:
  - Direct metaphase visualization of chromosomes (e.g. for Prader-Willi syndrome)
  - Direct DNA analysis techniques (e.g. for Tay-Sachs disease, phenylketonuria, Duchenne muscular dystrophy and cystic fibrosis)
  - Indirect DNA analysis (used, e.g. to detect linkage disorders when the exact gene is not known).

Risks and complications of amniocentesis

- Uterine cramping
- Uterine bleeding (about 2%)
- Amniotic fluid leakage (about 3%)
- There is a risk of maternal rhesus sensitization in susceptible pregnancies
- Amnionitis (only about 0.1%)
- Increased risk of miscarriage
- Failure of cell culture from 1% up to 5% if performed under 12 weeks' gestation
- Anxiety for parents caused by delay in diagnosis (may make choices for termination of pregnancy difficult).

Chorionic Villus Sampling (CVS)

Chorionic villus sampling (CVS) or chorionic villus biopsy (CVB), diagnostic procedure in which a sample of chorionic villi from the developing placenta is removed from the uterus of a pregnant woman, using a fine needle inserted through the abdomen (A-approach in Fig. 3.8) or a thin plastic catheter inserted into the vagina and through the cervix (B-approach in Fig. 3.8). Chorionic villi are fingerlike projections of a membrane (the chorion) that surrounds the fetus. The villi develop from the fertilized ovum, or egg, and have a genetic composition similar to that of the fetus. Cells in the sample are grown in the laboratory and studied to detect the presence in the fetus of such genetic birth defects as Tay-Sachs disease and Down syndrome since it allows the examination of the fetal karyotype and/or genotype. The sex of the child can also be ascertained.

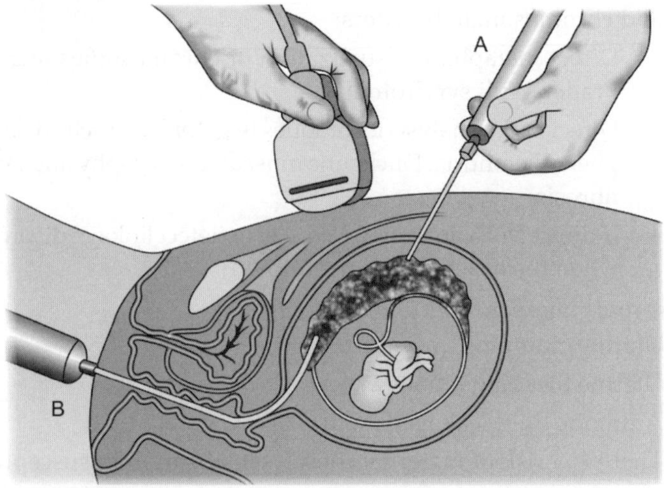

Fig. 3.8: Chorionic Villus Sampling (CVS):
A . Transabdominal needle, and B. Transcervical cannula

Indications of CVS

Aim of procedure: Prenatal diagnosis of chromosomal/single-gene abnormalities.

Most likely to be used in the following situations

- Advanced maternal age
- Past history of genetic/chromosomal abnormality
- Familial chromosomal rearrangement
- Biochemical/molecular diagnosis of a familial genetic disorder.

CVS cannot be used to screen for structural problems, such as neural tube defects, which have no known metabolic or molecular basis (unlike amniocentesis). Women should have serum alpha-fetoprotein and other diagnostic tests to detect this condition.

Contraindications of CVS

- Previous or suspected neural tube defects (as not the appropriate test)
- Active bleeding

- Infection
- Transcervical route of sampling: cervical polyps, fibroids, fundal placenta, retroverted uterus with posterior placement of placenta.

Procedure and Practical Points of CVS

- Procedure is usually performed at 10–13 weeks.
- Written consent should be obtained.
- Sample obtained either by ultrasound-guided transabdominal needle, or transcervical cannula aspiration/biopsy forceps.
- Results are obtained within 7–14 days (direct preparation 1 week, long-term culture 2 weeks).
- Thus CVS allows earlier diagnosis than with amniocentesis (which may only be safely conducted in the second trimester) and earlier opportunity to consider termination of pregnancy in the event of a fetal abnormality.
- Use of biopsy forceps rather than cannula aspiration for transcervical route seems to make the procedure technically easier, and to be preferred by patients and operators alike.
- Diagnostic accuracy 97.5–99.6%, depending on abnormality being screened for. It is slightly less accurate than amniocentesis because of placental mosaicism (the placenta can have populations of cells with different karyotype/genotype in about 0.8–1.6% of cases). If results from direct preparation are inconclusive then amniocytes need to be cultured.

Risk and Complications with CVS

- Repeat procedures are required in 1 to 10% of cases due to laboratory failure, mosaicism, ambiguous results, insufficient sample or maternal cell contamination. The latter occurs more frequently in transcervical CVS.
- In a low risk population, background pregnancy loss is about 2%, and second trimester amniocentesis increases this risk by a further 1%.
- Miscarriage rates following CVS is higher than after second trimester amniocentesis. However, there is some evidence to suggest this continues to improve overtime probably relating to improvements in technique.

- The increase in risk is significantly higher for transcervical CVS in terms of pregnancy loss and miscarriage.
- Transcervical CVS is more technically demanding than transabdominal route and more likely to lead to sample failures and multiple insertions.
- On the whole, second trimester amniocentesis is safer than transcervical sampling or early amniocentesis.
- Where early diagnosis is needed, transabdominal CVS is preferred to early amniocentesis/transcervical CVS.
- Where transabdominal CVS is not technically possible then transcervical CVS or second trimester amniocentesis should be used.
- Amniotic fluid leakage.
- Vaginal bleeding (higher for transcervical vs transabdominal route)
- Sepsis (rare)
- CVS at 8–9 weeks was reported to be associated with an increased incidence in limb deficiencies (oromandibular limb hypoplasia and isolated limb disruption) in the fetus and so procedure no longer performed this early.

Fetal Blood Sampling (FBS)

This technique uses ultrasound guidance to obtain fetal blood cells from the umbilical cord. It enables karyotyping/chromosome analysis as well as being used for the assessment and treatment of rhesus isoimmunization. Intrauterine blood transfusions may be performed using this technique. Fetal viral infection can be confirmed by immunoglobulin assessment of fetal blood and some hematological and metabolic abnormalities can be detected. The fetal loss rate is 1 to 3%. In the past, fetal blood sampling was used only during labor through the mother's open cervix to test blood from the fetal scalp for oxygenation. Today, in many perinatal care centers, fetal blood sampling is performed by specially trained perinatologists as part of diagnosis, treatment, and monitoring fetal problems at various times during pregnancy. Fetal blood sampling is known by several names depending on the sampling site used to collect the specimen including cordocentesis, funicentesis, or percutaneous umbilical blood sampling, or PUBS.

Indications of FBS

FBS is used presently for the following indications:

- *Diagnosis of genetic disorders:* Particularly those that need fetal DNA sample that cannot be diagnosed by other prenatal diagnostic methods, these may include hemoglobinopathies (although DNA analysis of amniotic fluid cells or CVS largely replaced FBS), certain immunologic deficiencies and disorders and certain coagulation disorders.
- *Diagnosis of chromosomal abnormalities:* For the purpose of rapid chromosome analysis (in 24 hours) particularly if ambiguous results, mosaicism, or culture failure results from amniocentesis or CVS.
- *To diagnose and treat severe fetal anemia or other blood problems,* such as Rh disease.
- *Diagnosis of fetal infection,* such as toxoplasmosis, cytomegalovirus, rubella (usually done after 22 weeks).
- *Evaluation of nonimmune hydrops fetalis.*
- *To perform certain fetal blood biochemistry testes,* such as acid-base status of fetus.
- *Evaluation of twin to twin transfusion syndrome.*
- *To give certain medications to the fetus.*
- *To check for fetal oxygen levels in later pregnancy.*

Procedure of Blood Sampling

There are several ways blood can be obtained from the fetus. After cleansing the mother's abdomen with antiseptic, a long, thin needle is inserted into the mother's uterus guided by ultrasound. Blood may be taken from the following sources:

- Blood vessels of the umbilical cord (also called cordocentesis, funicentesis, or percutaneous umbilical blood sampling, or PUBS)
- A fetal blood vessel, usually in the liver or heart

Fetal blood transfusions are performed using a similar technique. The fetus either receives blood or has unhealthy blood exchanged for healthy blood to treat some problems. In this case, it may be necessary to give a sedative medication to keep the baby from moving. After a fetal blood sampling procedure, mothers will need rest in the hospital and have the fetal heart rate monitoring for a few hours.

Risks and Complications with Fetal Blood Sampling

Fetal blood sampling is a very complex procedure that must be performed by a specially trained physician (Table 3.9). It is used when other tests or procedures are not possible or not effective.

Table 3.9: Risk and benefits of fetal blood sampling

Risks	Benefits
• Bleeding from the fetal blood sampling site • Changes in the fetal heart rate • Infection • Leaking of amniotic fluid • Fetal death	• Specialized information about the health of the fetus can often be obtained • Fetuses with severe blood damaging diseases can be treated before birth

Maternal Blood Tests

Maternal serum alpha-fetoprotein levels can be measured to aid the diagnosis of neural tube defects between 15 and 22 weeks. They are also raised in abdominal wall defects but amniotic fluid analysis of acetylcholinesterase can help to differentiate between these conditions. AFP screening involves obtaining a venous sample of maternal blood. Screenings are usually performed between 15 and 22 weeks' gestation. Elevated AFP levels may be indicative of neural tube defect, multiple gestation, Rh incompatibility or isoimmunization, low gestational age, or other congenital anomalies, such as congenital nephrosis, duodenal atresia, esophageal atresia, tetrology of Fallot, or hydrocephaly. Low AFP levels may be indicative of trisomy 13, 18, or 21.

The determination of AFP levels is also done in conjunction with triple marker screening. This consists of testing for AFP, human chorionic gonadotropin, and serum estriol levels. Triple marker screening is especially useful in testing for trisomies. Depending on the results of either of these studies, other studies may be recommended. Sensitive counseling, education, and support by nurses specially trained in this field can help clients make informed decisions regarding the tests, their outcomes, and any additional steps that may be needed.

The triple screen is a blood test typically performed between 15 and 20 weeks of pregnancy to detect women whose pregnancies may be at higher risk for three types of problems: open neural tube defects; Down syndrome and trisomy 18 (chromosome abnormalities).

The triple screen measures the levels of three chemicals in the mother's blood; two are hormones produced by the placenta, and the other is alpha fetoprotein (AFP), a protein made in the baby's liver and secreted into the amniotic fluid surrounding the baby. All three chemicals cross the placenta and enter the mother's bloodstream, where they can be measured (Table 3.10). Openings along the baby's body, such as along the spine or in the abdominal wall, allow more than normal amounts of AFP to leak from the baby and enter the amniotic fluid, increasing the level of AFP in the mother's bloodstream.

Table 3.10: Key points of maternal blood tests

- This test is routinely done to assess Neural Tube Defect
- AFP screening involves obtaining a venous sample of maternal blood
- Test is usually performed between 15–22 weeks
- Elevated AFP level may be indicative of:
  - *Neural Tube Defect*
  - *Multiple gestation*
  - *Rh incompatibility/isoimmunization*
  - *Low gestation age*
  - *Fetal abdominal wall problems (e.g. omphalocele, gastroschisis)*
  - *Fetal kidney disease*
  - *Placental problems*
  - *Other congenital anomalies, such as (nephrosis, duodenal atresia, esophageal atresia, tetrology of fallot, and hydrocephaly)*
- Low level of AFP may be indicative of:
  - *Trisomy 13, 18 or 21*
- Triple marker screening includes AFP, Human Chorionic Gonadotrophin (HCG) and serum estriol level estimation in maternal venous sample
- Triple marker screening is done to detect trisomies.

Fetal Tissue Sampling

Another invasive type of testing involves fetal tissue sampling (Table 3.11). This can also be carried out for skin, muscle, liver and other fetal organ analysis. Fetal tissue sampling is indicated for disorders that are not diagnosable through amniocentesis or CVS and are at increased risk for congenital anomalies. The procedure may be performed at 16 to 22 weeks' gestation, and fetal skin, liver, or muscle tissue may be sampled. Skin specimens approximately 2 mm in diameter typically are taken from the buttocks, back, thorax, and occasionally the scalp. In cases in which potential liver enzyme abnormalities may exist and are not diagnosable by other means, liver biopsy is indicated; however, few have been performed. A muscle biopsy might be indicated when DNA analysis is inconclusive or carrier status cannot be ascertained and there is a risk for such conditions as the X-linked recessive Duchenne muscular dystrophy, Beck muscular dystrophy, or mitochondrial myopathies; few have been performed to date.

Fetal tissue sampling is performed under the guidance of ultrasound with the client mildly sedated in order to decrease fetal movement. Procedural risks include spontaneous abortion, amniotic fluid leakage, maternal or fetal infection or injuries, preterm labor or delivery, hemorrhage due to anterior abdominal wall, uterine, or placental injuries, and cosmetic or functional injuries.

Table 3.11: Key points of fetal tissue sampling

• This is an invasive type of testing, involves fetal tissue sampling.
• Sample may be taken from skin, liver or muscle tissue.
• This is performed for disorders that are not diagnosable through amniocentesis or CVS and are at risk for congenital anomalies.
• The procedure may be performed at 16–22 weeks gestation.
• Skin specimens approximately 2 mm in diameter typically taken from the buttocks, back, thorax and occasionally the scalp.
• In case where potential liver enzyme abnormailites may exist and are not diagnosable by other means liver biopsy is indicated.
• A muscle biopsy might be indicated when DNA analysis is inconclusive or carrier status cannot be ascertained and there is a risk for such conditions as the X-linked recessive Duchene muscular dystrophy, Beck muscular dystrophy or mitochondrial myopathies.
• Fetal tissue sampling is performed under the guidance of ultrasound with client is mildly sedated in order to decrease fetal movement.
• Potential risk involved are; spontaneous abortions, amniotic fluid leakage, maternal or fetal infection or injury, preterm labor, hemorrhage, cosmatic or functional injury, etc.

Fetoscopy

This allows visualization of the fetus using endoscopic techniques. It is usually carried out between 18 and 20 weeks gestation. It allows fetal inspection for structural abnormalities, fetal blood sampling to detect, and possibly allow intervention in, conditions, such as hemophilias, thalassemia and sickle cell disease, as well as fetal skin and liver biopsy. The development of a thin gauge embryofetoscopic technique (TGEF) for endoscopy in the first trimester, with advances in optical system, may revitalized prenatal diagnosis by direct visualization when that in needed. The transabdominal approach is most common, as transvaginal approaches are associated with high fetal losses. This method may also used for access to the embryo for blood and tissue sampling for fetal therapy.

PREIMPLANTATION PRENATAL DIAGNOSIS

Preimplantation genetic diagnosis (PGD) (or also known as Embryo Screening) refers to procedures that are performed on embryos prior to implantation, sometimes even on oocytes prior to fertilization. PGD is considered an alternative to prenatal diagnosis. Its main advantage is that it avoids selective pregnancy termination as the method makes it highly likely that the baby will be free of the disease under consideration. PGD thus is an adjunct to assisted reproductive technology, and requires *in vitro* fertilization (IVF) to obtain oocytes or embryos for evaluation.

Indications of PGD

Currently, there are mainly two groups of patients for which PGD is indicated.

1. The first group consists of couples with a high-risk of transmitting an inherited condition. This can be a monogenic disorder, meaning the condition is due to a single gene only, (autosomal recessive, utosomal dominant or X-linked disorders) or a chromosomal structural aberration (such as a balanced translocation). PGD helps these couples identify embryos carrying a genetic disease or a chromosome abnormality, thus avoiding the difficult choice of abortion. In addition, there are infertile couples who carry an inherited condition and who opt for PGD as it can be easily combined with their IVF treatment.

2. The second group consists of couples who undergo IVF treatment and whose embryos are screened for chromosome aneuploidies. The technique is not used to obtaining a specific prenatal diagnosis but rather for screening, properly referred to as preimplantation genetic screening (PGS), to increase the chances of an ongoing pregnancy. The main indications for PGS are an advanced maternal age, a history of recurrent miscarriages or repeated unsuccessful implantation. It has also been proposed for patients with obstructive and non-obstructive azoospermia.

Genetic Analysis Techniques of PGD

Fluorescent *in situ* hybridization (FISH) and Polymerase chain reaction (PCR) are the two most commonly used technologies in PGD, although other approaches have been proposed or are currently in development (such as whole genome amplification and comparative genomic hybridization). PCR is generally used to diagnose monogenic disorders and FISH is used for the detection of chromosomal abnormalities (for instance, aneuploidy screening or chromosomal translocations). Recently a method was developed allowing to fix metaphase plates from single blastomeres. This technique in conjunction with FISH, m-FISH can produce more reliable results, since analysis is done on whole metaphase plates.

Ethical Issues of Prenatal Testing

- The option to continuing or aborting a pregnancy is the primary choice after most prenatal testing. Rarely, fetal intervention corrective procedures are possible.
- Are the risks of prenatal diagnosis, such as amniocentesis worth the potential benefit?
- Some fear that this may lead to being able to pick and choose what children parents would like to have. This could lead to choice in sex, physical characteristics, and personality in children. Some feel this type of eugenic abortion is already underway (sex-selective, etc.)
- Knowing about certain birth defects, such as spina bifida and teratoma before birth may give the option of fetal surgery during pregnancy, or assure that the appropriate treatment and/or surgery be provided immediately after birth.

- Questions of the value of mentally or physically disabled people in society.
- How to ensure that information about testing options is given in a nondirective and supportive way.
- That parents are well informed if they have to consider abortion vs continuing a pregnancy.

Role of Nurses

Nurses' role in prenatal genetic testing will be different in invasive and noninvasive prenatal testing based on the nature of the test. However, some of the general responsibilities are as follows:

- Provide detailed information about the test, including purposes, risk-benefit ratio, procedure of test, expected results, cost of test, expected risks, total time needed in getting results, etc.
- Help the patient to manage preprocedure anxiety.
- Take an informed written consent from patient.
- For early pregnancy ultrasonography advise the patient to consume 900 to 1200 ml water 1 to 2 hours before procedure.
- Administer Rho (D) immunoglobulin to Rh negative mothers before every invasive test, which incolve risk of fetal blood comes in contact with mother.
- Administer prophylactic antibiotic in invasive tests as per institution's policy.
- In fetal tissue sampling sedate the patient by administering 5–10 mg diazepam as per order.
- Consult the patient and family about expected results of the test.
- Provide relaxing and comforting environment to reduce anxiety.
- Provide emotional support before, during and after the procedure.
- Offer counseling services as per need of the patient and family.
- Inform about follow-up and test result availability contacts, etc.

INFERTILITY

Infertility primarily refers to the biological inability of a man or a woman to contribute to conception. Infertility may also refer to the state of a woman who is unable to carry a pregnancy to full term.

There are many biological causes of infertility, some which may be bypassed with medical intervention. Generally, worldwide it is estimated that one in seven couples have problems conceiving, with the incidence similar in most countries independent of the level of the country's development.

There are strict definitions of infertility used by many doctors. However, there are also similar terms, e.g. subfertility for a more benign condition and fecundity for the natural improbability to conceive. Infertility in a couple can be due to either the woman or the man, not necessarily both.

Reproductive endocrinologists, the doctors specializing in infertility, consider a couple to be infertile if:

- The couple has not conceived after 12 months of contraceptive free intercourse if the female is under the age of 34
- The couple has not conceived after 6 months of contraceptive free intercourse if the female is over the age of 35
- The female is incapable of carrying a pregnancy to term.

Subfertility

A couple that has tried unsuccessfully to have a child for a year or more is said to be *subfertile* meaning less fertile than a typical couple. The couple's fecundability rate is approximately 3 to 5%. Many of its causes are the same as those of infertility. Such causes could be endometriosis, or polycystic ovarian syndrome.

Primary vs Secondary Infertility

Couples with *primary infertility* have never been able to conceive, while, on the other hand, *secondary infertility* is difficulty conceiving after already having conceived and carried a normal pregnancy. Technically, secondary infertility is not present if there has been a change of partners.

Causes: Common causes of infertility are:

- Ovulation problems
- Tubal blockage
- Male associated infertility
- Age-related factors
- Uterine problems
- Previous tubal ligation

- Previous vasectomy
- Unexplained infertility

Factors that can cause male as well as female infertility are:

Genetic factors
  - A Robertsonian translocation in either partner may cause recurrent spontaneous abortions or complete infertility.
- *General factors*
  - Diabetes mellitus, thyroid disorders, adrenal disease
- *Hypothalamic-pituitary factors*
  - Kallmann syndrome
  - Hyperprolactinemia
  - Hypopituitarism
- *Environmental factors*
  - Toxins, such as glues, volatile organic solvents or silicones, physical agents, chemical dusts, and pesticides.

Genetic Basis of Infertility

Fertility, similar to other bodily functions, is the concerted action of numerous processes that result in normal quality sperm. As molecular genetics has advanced, so has our knowledge about the genetics of male infertility. Most recently, it has become obvious that more men may have a genetic basis for infertility than was previously thought. Genetics may contribute to infertility by acting at a variety of physiologic levels including hormonal balance, sperm production and sperm motility. An understanding of the genetic basis for reproductive failure is essential to treat and counsel infertility patients. Although treatments of genetically caused infertility are limited. Because of this, it is important to be conversant in genetic issues to better inform patients (a) about their conditions and (b) about the risks of possible transmission to their offspring.

The **Y chromosome** is a small, but intensely studied chromosome that is known to carry the genes that determine both testis development and spermatogenesis. It has 60 million base pairs and consists of a long arm (Yq) and a short arm (Yp). On the short arm can be found the gene for **Testis Determining Factor (TDF)** and on the long arm, one or more genes that may control spermatogenesis, termed **AZF genes (Azoospermia factor)**.

The long arm (Yq) of the Y chromosome has recently become the focus of renewed interest as it is now recognized that 7% of oligospermic and 15% of azoospermic men may harbor a small gene deletion on this arm. An exact relationship between the gene, its protein product and spermatogenesis is still unclear.

Genetic Diseases Resulting in Infertility

This complex topic will be discussed by dividing the reproductive tract into 3 components, pretesticular, testicular and post-testicular, and examining specific genetic abnormalities that affect each portion of the tract.

Genetic Conditions with Pretesticular Effects

Pretesticular effects are generally hormonal in nature, because spermatogenesis is largely controlled by hypothalamic pituitary axis. Several syndromes are known to affect the hypothalamus and pituitary gland. Most of these result from single gene deletions.

- *Kallman's Syndrome* causes male hypogonadism because of a deficiency in hypothalamic gonadotropin-releasing hormone (**GnRH**). It occurs in 1/50,000 persons and is most commonly an X-linked recessive disease. The clinical features include anosmia, facial asymmetry, color blindness, renal anomalies and cryptorchidism. The hallmark of the syndrome is a delay in pubertal development. Patient's have severely atrophic testes (< 2 cm) with biopsies showing germ cell arrest and Leydig cell hypoplasia. Hormone evaluation reveals a low testosterone, low LH and low FSH. These men can be fertile when given FSH and LH.
- *Prader-Willi Syndrome* is another very rare condition (1/20,000) characterized by obesity, retardation, small hands and feet and hypogonadism. Again, a deficiency of **GnRH** is the problem. The single gene deletion associated with this condition is on chromosome 15. Similar to Kallman's Syndrome, spermatogenesis can be induced with exogenous FSH and LH.
- *Bardet-Biedl Syndrome* is another rare form of hypogonadotropic hypogonadism that results from GnRH deficiency. It is characterized by retinitis pigmentosa, polydactyly hypogonadism. It presents similar to Kallman's Syndrome except the patient has genetic obesity. The hypogonadism can be treated with FSH and LH.

- *Sickle Cell Anemia* is associated with the inheritance of **B S-globin** genes and is found in 1/600 Afro-americans. Men with sickle cell anemia have decreased testosterone and either increased or decreased LH and FSH. Although high or low levels of gonadotropins would appear to implicate very different diseases, it may be that pituitary and testicular microinfarcts from sickle disease account for these two disparate presentations of hypogonadism.
- *b-Thalassemia* patients have mutations in the b**-globin** gene that leads to an imbalance in the alpha and beta globin composition hemoglobin. The trait is present in 3 to 5% of Mediterranean and African peoples. Clinical features range from mild anemia (trait) to iron overload (major thalassemia). Infertility may result from the deposition of iron in the pituitary gland and testis.
- *Cerebellar Ataxia* can be associated with hypogonadotropic hypogonadism. This is a rare condition which can result from consanguinous unions. Cerebellar involvement includes abnormalities of speech and gait. These patients are eunichoid-looking with atrophic testis. Hypothalamic-pituitary dysfunction is thought to cause infertility; the basis for the dysfunction may be from pathological changes in cerebral white matter.

Genetic Conditions with Testicular Effects

Conditions that directly affect the testicle tend to result from structural or numerical chromosomal abnormalities. Unlike with pretesticular conditions that are treatable with hormone replacement, the testicular effects are, at present, largely untreatable. Assisted reproductive technology, however, can provide biological children for men with these conditions, but it virtually ensure that the genetic disease will be transmitted.

- *Klinefelter's Syndrome* is the most common genetic reason for azoospermia. accounting for 14% of cases. It has a classic triad: small, firm testes, gynecomastia, and azoospermia. In this abnormality of chromosomal number, 90% of men carry an extra X chromosome (47 XXY) and 10% of men are mosaic with a combination of XXY/XY. Paternity with this syndrome is rare, but more likely in the mosaic form of the disease. Testes biopsies show sclerosis and hyalinization. Hormones usually demonstrate a decreased testosterone and frankly elevated LH and FSH. This syndrome may present with increased height, decreased intelligence, varicosities, obesity, diabetes, leukemia, increased likelihood of extragonadal germ cell tumors and breast cancer.

- *XYY Syndrome* is another abnormality of chromosomal number that can result in infertility. Typically, men with 47, XYY are tall and 2% exhibit aggressive, often criminal behavior. Hormone evaluation reveals an elevated FSH and normal testosterone and LH. Semen analyses show either severe oligospermia or azoospermia. Testis biopsies demonstrate maturation arrest or Sertoli cell-only syndrome.
- *XX Male Syndrome* presents as a male with azoospermia. Typically, there are normal male external and internal genitalia. Patients usually present with gynecomastia at puberty. Hormone evaluation shows elevated FSH and LH and low or normal testosterone. Testis biopsy reveals an absence of spermatogenesis with hyalinization, fibrosis and Leydig cell clumping. The most obvious explanation is that the SRY or Testis Determining Region is translocated from the Y to the X chromosome so that testis differentiation is present. However, the Azoospermia gene (AZF) is not similarly translocated, resulting in azoospermia.
- *Noonan's Syndrome* presents phenotypically as a male Turner's syndrome (45, X0). However, the karyotype is normal 46, XY and the chromosomal abnormality not yet identified. Typically, these men have dysmorphic features like webbed neck, short stature, low set ears and wide set eyes. At birth, 75% will have cryptorchidism that limits fertility in adulthood. If testis are fully descended, then fertility is possible and likely.
- *Immotile Cilia Syndrome* is a heterogeneous group of disorders in which sperm motility is reduced or absent. The sperm defects are from abnormalities in the motor apparatus or axoneme of sperm and other ciliated cells. Various defects in the dynein arms cause deficits in ciliary and sperm activity. Kartagener's Syndrome is a subset of this disorder that presents with the triad of chronic sinusitis, bronchiectasis and situs inversus. Most immotile cilia cases are diagnosed in childhood due to

respiratory and sinus difficulties. Cilia present in the retina and ear may also be defective and lead to retinitis pigmentosa and deafness in Usher's Syndrome. Men with immotile cilia characteristically have necrospermia or completely nonmotile but viable sperms in normal numbers. Depending on the ciliary defect, there can be some sperm motility and forward progression. Sperm nuclear material is thought to be unaffected. Serum hormones are normal as is the testis biopsy. The Hypo-osmotic Sperm Swelling Test can determine whether nonmotile sperms are viable and may help these men to conceive.

- *The Azoospermia Gene:* It has recently been discovered that approximately 10 to 15% of men with azoospermia will have structural changes in the Y chromosome. This idea was originally postulated in 1976 based on small structural changes in the Y chromosome seen on karyotyping. This led to the concept that an 'azospermic factor (AZF)' existed and its absence or mutation accounted for the azoospermia. Since then, an explosion in molecular genetics technology has allowed far more sophisticated analysis of the Y chromosome. Presently, the DAZ (Deleted in Azoospermia) region is the most likely candidate gene and is the subject of intense study at UCSF by Dr Renee Reijo. The exact function of these genes in spermatogenesis is not clear, as the gene products are only beginning to be recognized. It is expected, however, that men who acquire or inherit these gene deletions will certainly pass them onto offspring if assisted reproductive technology is used to achieve biologic pregnancies.

Genetic Conditions with Post-Testicular Effects

The post-testicular portion of the reproductive tract includes the epididymis, vas deferens, seminal vesicles and associated ejaculatory apparatus. Genetic conditions in these organs are mainly of polygenic or multifactorial nature. This discussion will exclude conditions that present with ambiguous genitalia or intersex.

- *Cystic Fibrosis* is the most common, fatal autosomal recessive disorder in the US. It is associated with more than 600 possible genomic mutations. The disease is associated with fluid and electrolyte abnormalities (abnormal chloride-sweat test) and presents with chronic lung obstruction and infections, pancreatic insufficiency and infertility. Interestingly, 98% of men with cystic fibrosis (CF) have wolffian duct abnormalities: the body and tail of the epididymis, vas deferens, seminal vesicles and ejaculatory ducts are atrophic, fibrotic or completely absent. Serum hormones and spermatogenesis are usually normal. Most afflicted patients die in their twenties of pneumonia or related problems. Gene therapy is being actively applied to this disease. A blood test for CF genetic mutations is available.

- *Congenital Absence of the Vas Deferens (CAVD)* accounts for 1 to 2% of all cases of infertility and up to 5% of azoospermic men. On physical examination, no palpable vas deferens is observed on one or both sides. Similar to CF, the rest of the wolffian duct system may also be abnormal and unreconstructable. Recently, this disease has been demonstrated to be a *forme fruste* of CF. However, the vast majority of these men fail to demonstrate any symptoms of CF. In cases of bilateral vasal absence, 65% of patients will harbor a detectable CF mutation. In addition, 15% of these men will have renal malformations, most commonly unilateral renal agenesis. In patients with unilateral CAVD, the incidence of detectable CF mutations is generally lower, and that of renal agenesis approaches 40%. Serum hormones are normal as is spermatogenesis. Epididymal sperm aspiration is very effective in procurring sperm from these men for use with IVF since virtually all of these men will have an intact caput epididymis.
- *Young's Syndrome* presents with the clinical triad of chronic sinusitis, bronchiectasis and obstructive azoospermia. The obstruction is located in the epididymis, usually near the junction the caput and corpus. Since obstruction may not occur until after puberty, fertility is possible in some patients. The pathophysiology of the condition is unclear but may involve abnormal ciliary function or abnormal mucus quality and slugding within the epididymis. Serum testosterone, FSH and LH are normal, as are the testis biopsies. Reconstructive surgery can be attempted but usually meets with lower success rates than observed with other obstructed conditions.

- *Idiopathic Epididymal Obstruction* is a relatively uncommon, but well-recognized condition found in otherwise healthy azoospermic men. It is successfully treated with epididymovasostomy. There is recent evidence linking this condition with CF: in one series, 37% of men so obstructed were seen to harbor a CF gene mutation. This implies that up to one-half of patients with idiopathic obstruction at the level of the epididymis may in fact have a genetic predisposition or reason for the problem.
- *Myotonic Dystrophy* is the most common reason for adult-onset muscular dystrophy. This usually presents with cataracts, muscle atrophy, and various endocrinopathies. Most men with this condition are noted to have testis atrophy but fertility has been reported. Infertile men may have elevated FSH and LH with low or normal testosterone and testis biopsies show seminiferous tubule damage in 75% of cases.
- *Adult Polycystic Kidney Disease* is an autosomal dominant disorder associated with numerous cysts of the kidney, liver, spleen, pancreas, epididymis seminal vesicle and testis. Disease onset usually occurs in the 3rd or 4th decade with symptoms of abdominal pain, hypertension and renal failure. Ten to fourty percent of patients will also have cerebral berry aneurysms. Infertility with this disease is usually secondary to obstructing cysts in the epididymis or seminal vesicles. Serum hormones are normal and spermatogenesis is undisturbed.

Diagnosis of Infertility

- *Detailed fertility history* including frequency and timing of sexual intercourse, duration of infertility and any previous fertility events, childhood illness and any problems of development, any serious illness (diabetes, respiratory infection, cancer, previous surgeries), sexual history including STDs, any exposure to toxins, such as chemicals or radiation, history of any medications and allergies, any family history of reproductive problems.
- *Physical examination:* Testicular or reproductive examination.
- Postejaculatory urine sample
- Semen analysis
- *Blood test for* gondola hormonal level or infection.

- *Postcoital tests (Cervical penetration test) to;* evaluate the effect of a women's cervical mucus on man's sperms.
- Sperm antibody test
- Testicular biopsy
- Ultrasound
- *Fertilization tests, including* the hamster test, the human zona penetration test, and acrosome reaction test.
- *Genetic testing including* preimplantation genetic diagnosis (PGD), that examines all the chromosomes in a human embryo and detect defective genes, such as those for cystic fibrosis, at the very earliest stages. Genetic analysis to determine DNA fragmentation in the sperm may be a better way of predicting outcome of pregnancy.

Medical Management of Infertility

- Provide higher antioxidant vitamin C and vitamin A diet
- Hormonal monitoring and ovulation period intercourse
- Provide stress management advices and interventions
- *Advise for lifestyle changes:* Man who wants to achieve higher sperm counts need some of the following lifestyle modification, like:
  - Avoid smoking, drugs and increase intake of coffee.
  - Get sufficient rest and exercise, and avoid excessive exercises.
  - Manage stress with yoga, meditation, and spiritual interventions.
  - Prevent overheating of testis.
- Assisted Reproductive Technologies (ART) management: It refers methods used to achieve pregnancy by artificial or partially artificial means. Which includes:
  - *Artificial Insemination (AI)* in when sperm is placed into a female's uterus (intrauterine) or cervix (intracervical) using artificial means rather than by natural copulation.
  - *In vitro fertilization (IVF): In vitro* fertilization (IVF) is the technique of letting fertilization of the male and female gametes (sperm and egg) occur outside the female body (Fig. 3.9).
  - *Intracytoplasmic sperm injection (ICSI)* is beneficial in the case of male factor infertility where sperm counts are very low or

failed fertilization occurred with previous IVF attempt(s). The ICSI procedure involves a single sperm carefully injected into the center of an egg using a microneedle.

- *Gamete intrafallopian transfer (GIFT):* In this a mixture of sperms and eggs is placed directly into a woman's fallopian tubes using laparoscopy following a transvaginal ovum retrieval.
- *Zygote intrafallopian transfer (ZIFT)* In this egg cells are removed from the woman's ovaries and fertilized in the laboratory; the resulting zygote is then placed into the fallopian tube.

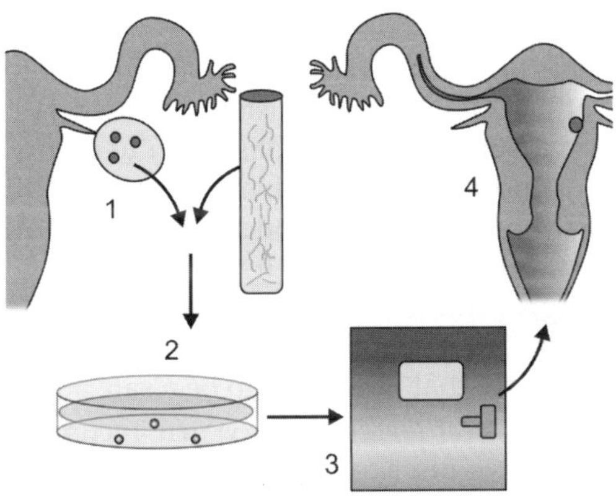

Fig. 3.9: *In vitro* fertilization

- Other techniques:
  - *In vitro maturation:* In this process follicles are harvested a few days before ovulation. These maturing follicles are removed and healthy embryo in produced. This allows the fertilization without the use of fertility drugs.
  - *Blastocyte transfer:* In this instead of implanting the standard 2 to 3 days embryo in the uterus, the procedure implants bastocyte, which are more complex 5 days old embryo.
  - *Ooplastic transfer:* This one of contraversial and experiemental procedure that use the womens's own egg and a female

donor's egg and the male's sperm for fertilization. Genetic material from the donor's egg plus the sperm are added to the women's own egg. This has been successful in a few cases and long-term effects are unknown.

- *Complementary and alternative treatments:* Three complementary or alternative female infertility treatments have been scientifically tested, with results published in peer-reviewed medical journals.
    a. *Group psychological intervention:* A 2000 Harvard Medical School study examined the effects of group psychological intervention on infertile women. The two intervention groups; a support group and a cognitive behavior group had statistically significant higher pregnancy rates than the control group.
    b. *Acupuncture:* Acupuncture performed 25 minutes before and after IVF embryo transfer increased IVF pregnancy rates in a German study published in 2002. In a 2006 similar study conducted by The University of South Australia, the acupuncture group's odds (although not statistically significant) were 1.5 higher than the control group. Although definitive results of the effects of acupuncture on embryo transfer remain a topic of discussion, study authors state that it appears to be a safe adjunct to IVF.
    c. *Manual physical therapy:* The Wurn Technique, a manual manipulative physical therapy treatment, was shown in peer reviewed publications to improve natural and IVF pregnancy rates in infertile women in a 2004 study, and to open and return function to blocked fallopian tubes in a 2008 study. The therapy was designed to address adhesions restricting function and mobility of the reproductive organs.

Role of Nurses

- Infertility has significant psychological and social impact; therefore, nurses need to provide psychological support during throughout diagnosis and treatment of infertility.
- Provide information about causes of infertility including genetic causes, and possible treatment modalities. For example, Artificial Reproductive Technique (ART), etc.

- Take written consent for diagnostic and therapeutic interventions.
- Assist the physical in diagnostic and therapeutic interventions.
- Provide discharge teaching and follow-up information.
- Teach about healthy lifestyle modification and effective stress management strategies.

SPONTANEOUS ABORTIONS

Spontaneous abortions refers to a clinical condition describing the loss of the intrauterine product prior to the viability of the fetus, conventionally accepted as 20 weeks of intrauterine life, or 500 grams of fetal body weight.

In other words *spontaneous abortions or miscarriage* is the natural or spontaneous end of a pregnancy at a stage where the embryo or fetus is incapable of surviving, generally defined in humans at prior to 20 weeks of gestation. Miscarriage is the most common complication of early pregnancy. The medical term 'spontaneous abortion' is used in reference to miscarriages because the medical term 'abortion' refers to any terminated pregnancy, deliberately induced or spontaneous, although in common it refers specifically to active termination of pregnancy.

Determining the prevalence of miscarriage is difficult. Many miscarriages happen very early in the pregnancy, before a woman may know she is pregnant. Treatment of women with miscarriage at home means medical statistics on miscarriage miss many cases. Prospective studies using very sensitive early pregnancy tests have found that 25% of pregnancies are miscarried by the sixth week LMP (Last Menstrual Period). Clinical miscarriages (those occurring after the sixth week LMP) occur in 8% of pregnancies.

Types of Spontaneous Abortions

- *Early pregnancy loss*: Very early miscarriage; those which occur before the sixth week LMP (Last Menstrual Period) are medically termed as *early pregnancy loss* or *chemical pregnancy*.
- *Clinical spontaneous abortion:* Miscarriages that occur after the sixth week LMP are medically termed as *clinical spontaneous abortion*.

Alternatively the following terms are used to describe pregnancies that do not continue:

- *An empty sac* is a condition where the gestational sac develops normally, while the embryonic part of the pregnancy is either absent or stops growing very early. Other terms for this condition are *blighted ovum* and *an embryonic pregnancy*.
- An *inevitable abortion* describes where the fetal heart beat is shown to have stopped and the cervix has already dilated open, but the fetus has yet to be expelled. This usually will progress to a complete abortion.
- A *complete abortion* is when all products of conception have been expelled. *Products of conception* may include the trophoblast, chorionic villi, gestational sac, yolk sac, and fetal pole (embryo); or later in pregnancy the fetus, umbilical cord, placenta, amniotic fluid, and amniotic membrane.
- An *incomplete abortion* occurs when tissue has been passed, but some remains *in utero*.
- A *missed abortion* is when the embryo or fetus has died, but a miscarriage has not yet occurred. It is also referred to as *delayed miscarriage*.

The following two terms consider wider complications or implications of a miscarriage:

- A *septic abortion* occurs when the tissue from a missed or incomplete abortion becomes infected. The infection of the womb carries risk of spreading infection (septicemia) and is a grave risk to the life of the woman.
- *Recurrent pregnancy loss* (RPL) or *recurrent miscarriage* (medically termed *habitual abortion*) is the occurrence of three consecutive miscarriages. If the proportion of pregnancies ending in miscarriage is 15%, then the probability of two consecutive miscarriages is 2.25% and the probability of three consecutive miscarriages is 0.34%. The occurrence of recurrent pregnancy loss is 1%. A large majority (85%) of women who have had two miscarriages will conceive and carry normally afterwards.

Etiology

There are many reasons for pregnancy loss. It is important to realize that in many cases, no cause for past miscarriage(s) is identified.

Most causes of miscarriage are not under our control. It is important to remember that women who have a miscarriage(s) still have a good chance for a successful future pregnancy.

Genetic Causes

- *Fetal chromosomal abnormalities:* Approximately 50% of first trimester miscarriages are due to a chromosome abnormality in the fetus. Chromosomes are the inherited structures in the cells of our bodies. There are 46 chromosomes in each cell, arranged into 23 pairs. A baby has two copies of every chromosome – one inherited from the mother in the egg, and the other inherited from the father in the sperm. Each chromosome holds hundreds to thousands of genes, which are responsible for growth and development. An extra chromosome or a missing chromosome can cause miscarriage, usually in the first or second trimester of pregnancy, or can lead to a child with learning difficulties or mental retardation and birth defects. Chromosome abnormalities involving a missing or extra chromosome are not inherited or caused by an exposure during pregnancy. Instead, they result from a chance mistake in cell division at the time of conception. This error is a random event that can occur in anyone's pregnancy. Once a couple has had a pregnancy affected by a chromosome abnormality, there is a slightly greater chance for their future pregnancies to be affected with chromosome abnormalities. In some cases prenatal diagnosis, such as chorionic villus sampling (CVS) or amniocentesis, are offered in future pregnancies.
- *Inherited chromosomal rearrangements:* An inherited problem with the chromosomes can also cause miscarriage. A parent can have a rearrangement (a 'translocation') of his or her chromosomes, in which the chromosomes are structured differently. The parent should have no health problems because, although his or her chromosomes are rearranged, they are balanced – that is, there are no missing or extra pieces of the chromosomes. However, because of the way the chromosomes are passed from parent to child, the baby may inherit extra or missing pieces of a chromosome. Extra and missing genetic material leads to 'chromosomal imbalance' and can cause mental retardation and birth defects in a liveborn or cause a miscarriage. For couples

who have had multiple miscarriages, the chance that one of the parents has a chromosomal rearrangement is approximately 2 to 4%. While parents who carry chromosomal rearrangements are at increased risk to have further miscarriages or babies born with health problems, they can also produce healthy children. Chromosome studies can be performed on parents' blood to see if either parent is a carrier of a chromosomal rearrangement.

- *Gene Mutation:* Another genetic cause of miscarriage is a change (mutation) in a single gene (or several genes) on the chromosomes. This can cause specific genetic diseases or birth defects. Mutations can occur spontaneously in pregnancies or can be inherited from parents who themselves are healthy. Birth defects associated with these conditions can sometimes be detected during pregnancy by a sonogram. If there is a history of a specific disorder in a parent or family member, single gene disorders can be tested for prenatally in some cases.

Maternal Health Issues

Other reasons for pregnancy loss are related to maternal health. An abnormally shaped uterus can lead to pregnancy loss. Health problems, such as hormonal imbalance, poorly controlled diabetes, lupus and other immune system abnormalities, kidney and heart disease, and hypertension can create difficulties in carrying a pregnancy to term. These causes of miscarriage can be evaluated by blood tests and an ultrasound examination (sonogram) of the uterus. Your doctor can evaluate you for these problems.

Environment

Another cause of pregnancy loss is an environmental exposure during pregnancy. For example, exposure to drugs, alcohol, or high levels of radiation can lead to miscarriage. Infections can cause miscarriage. The risk of miscarriage may be greater in women who smoke.

Clinical Manifestations

- Vaginal bleeding
- Pain does not strongly correlate with miscarriage
- Blood clots with embryotic tissue passes
- Early abrupt disappearance of early signs of pregnancy.

Diagnosis of Spontaneous Abortion

- Hstory of pervaginal bleeding during pregnancy
- Ultrasound exam
- Serial human chorionic gonadotropin (HCG) testing
- Genetic testing for aborted fetal tissue.

Management of Spontaneous Abortion

- No treatment is necessary for a diagnosed complete abortion (as long as ectopic pregnancy is ruled out). However, in cases of an incomplete abortion, empty sac, or missed abortion, there are three treatment options:
  a. *With no treatment (watchful waiting),* most of these cases (65–80%) will pass naturally within two to six weeks. This path avoids the side effects and complications possible from medications and surgery.
  b. *Medical management* usually consists of using misoprostol (a prostaglandin, brand name Cytotec) to encourage completion of the miscarriage. About 95% of cases treated with misoprostol will complete within a few days.
  c. *Surgical treatment* (most commonly vacuum aspiration, sometimes referred to as a D & C or D & E) is the fastest way to complete the miscarriage. It also shortens the duration and heaviness of bleeding, and is the best treatment for physical pain associated with the miscarriage. In cases of repeated miscarriage or later-term pregnancy loss, D & C is also the best way to obtain tissue samples for pathology examination.
- Genetic counseling for the couple and family, if there is genetic cause involved in causation of abortion.

Role of Nurses

- Spontaneous abortion has significant psychological and social impact; therefore, nurses need to provide psychological support during diagnosis and treatment of infertility.
- Provide information about causes of spontaneous abortion including genetic causes, and possible treatment modalities.
- Take written consent for diagnostic and therapeutic interventions.

- Assist the physician in diagnostic and therapeutic interventions.
- Provide discharge teaching and follow-up information.
- Teach about healthy lifestyle modification and effective stress management strategies.

NEURAL TUBE DEFECTS (NTDs)

Complete fusion of the neural tube usually occurs between days 18 and 26 after ovulation. Neural tube defects are malformations of the neuroectoderm and are associated with abnormalities of surrounding mesodermal structures. In other words, NTD is an opening in the spinal cord or brain that occurs very early in human development. The early spinal cord of the embryo begins as a flat region, which rolls into a tube (the neural tube) 28 days after the baby is conceived. When the neural tube does not close completely, an NTD develops (Fig. 3.10). NTDs develop before most women know they are even pregnant.

There are two types of NTDs: Neural tube defects can be classified as:

1. *Open NTDs:* Open NTDs are more common type. Open NTDs occur when the brain and/or spinal cord are exposed at birth through a defect in the skull or vertebrae (back bones). Examples of open NTDs are spina bifida (myelomeningocele), anencephaly, and encephalocele.
2. *Closed NTDs*: Closed NTDs occur when the spinal defect is covered by skin. Common examples of closed NTDs are lipomyelomeningocele, lipomeningocele, and tethered cord. Lastly, spina bifida occulta (SBO) is potentially another form of an NTD in which there is a typically benign (or non-symptom-causing) bony change in one or more vertebrae, but not involving the nerves within the spinal column. The incidence of SBO is not well defined; however, it is more common than the NTDs described above. The cause and potential similarities, or, link to NTDs, has not been established.

Epidemiology

- Incidence has declined significantly in the last 30 years and now occurs in approximately 0.8/1000 total births.
- Anencephaly and spina bifida account for up to 95% of all neural tube defects with equal prevalence.

Cranial presentation	Spinal presentations
• Anencephaly • Encephalocele (meningocele or meningomyelocele) • Congenital dermal sinus	• Spina bifida • Spina bifida occulta • Myelomeningocele • Meningocele • Congenital dermal sinus • Caudal agenesis

Risk Factors

Neural tube defects are considered a complex disorder because they are caused by a combination of multiple genes and multiple environmental factors. Known risk factors include:

- Family history: One type of malformation puts other family members at risk of all types of defect. Studies of twins with NTDs have shown both identical twins have NTDs more than both fraternal twins. Studies of families show that the chance of having a second family member born with an NTD after one child is born with an NTD increases.
- May occur as part of a number of different syndromes and chromosomal disorders. NTDs are a feature (or symptom) of known genetic syndromes, such as trisomy 13, trisomy 18, certain chromosome rearrangements, and Meckel-Gruber syndrome (Fig. 3.10).
- Diet low in folic acid.
- Maternal drug therapy with sodium valproate and folic acid antagonists, e.g. some antiepileptics, trimethoprim.
- Dysraphism is used to describe situations where there is continuity between the posterior neuroectoderm and cutaneous ectoderm.

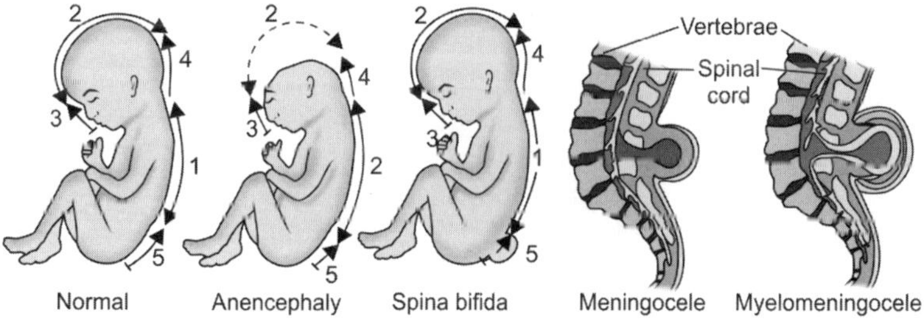

Fig. 3.10: Neural tube defects

Flow Chart 3.1: Genetic and environmental etiology of neural tube defect

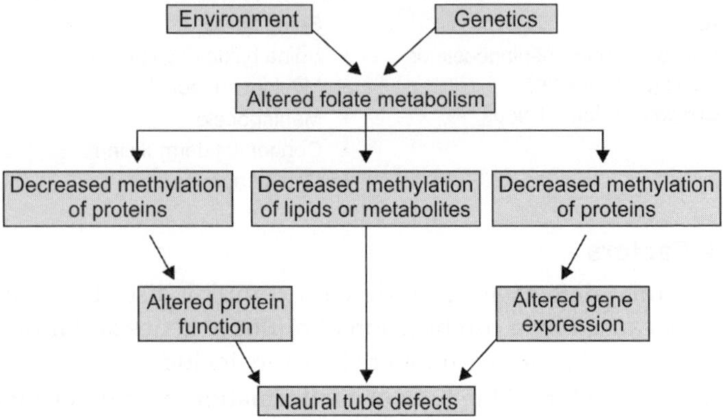

Presentation and Management

Cranial Dysraphism

- *Anencephaly:* Cranial vault is absent (Fig. 3.11)
  - Most cases are now terminated following prenatal diagnosis.
  - In live born babies, initial neurological examination may appear normal if brainstem structures are relatively intact and may have seizures.
  - Infants usually die within hours or days.

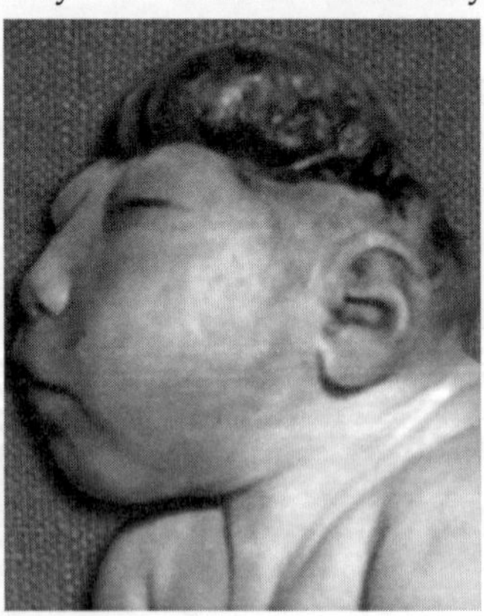

Fig. 3.11: Anencephaly

Source: Anencephaly. Discover and save creative ideas. https://www.pinterest.com/anencephalyx/anencephaly/ retrieved on 15/02/2016

- *Cephaloceles:*
  - Brain matter herniates through a defect in skull. A cranial meningocele contains only meninges, encephalocele contains brain tissue; a ventriculocele contains part of the ventricle within the herniated part of the brain.
  - These are rarer than anencephaly or spina bifida, with an incidence of 1-3/10,000 live births.
  - Associated with other brain abnormalities, e.g. agenesis or corpus callosum or abnormal gyration and may be part of a recognized syndrome.
  - Posterior cephaloceles are commonest in western countries with most being occipital encephaloceles of variable size occurring above or below the tentorium. If below, then they are associated with severe cerebellar defects, e.g. Chiari III malformation.
  - Depending on size, site and associated abnormalities, there may be visual, sensorimotor disturbance, intellectual impairment and seizures.
  - In some parts of Asia, anterior cephaloceles are more common and may protrude into the nose, ethmoid or orbit. Often include olfactory tissue and frontal lobe tissue.

Spinal Dysraphism

Spina bifida includes spina bifida occulta and spina bifida cystica, which may be either a meningocele without neural tissue or a myelomeningocele where the spinal cord forms part of the cyst wall (Fig. 3.12).

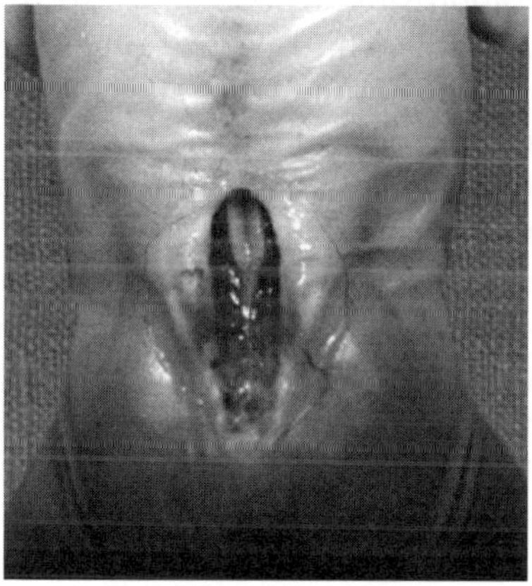

Fig. 3.12: Spina bifida

- *Meningocele:*
  - Protrusion of the meninges outside the spinal canal accounts for 5% of cases of spina bifida cystica.
  - No associated hydrocephalus, and neural examination is often normal.
- *Myelomeningocele:*
  - Occurs in 80–90% of spina bifida cystica cases.
  - 80% are lumbosacral consisting of a sac covered with a thin membrane that may leak CSF.
  - Level of lesion is best assessed by determining upper limit of sensory loss but at all levels there is disturbance of bladder and bowel control.
  - Higher lesions are associated with bladder outlet obstruction with consequent dilatation of the upper urinary tract and chronic pyelonephritis.
  - Hydrocephalus occurs in approximately 90% of cases at birth even with normal head circumference.
  - Usually associated with Chiari II malformation but may also be due to aqueduct stenosis or have no clear cause.
  - Usually detected by ultrasound.
  - If signs of progressive ventricular dilatation or rising intracranial pressure, usually needs insertion of a ventriculoperitoneal shunt.
- *Chiari II malformation*:
  - Occurs in approximately 70% of cases of myelomeningocele.
  - Consists of downward protrusion of the medulla below the foramen magnum overlap the spinal cord.
  - This causes the medulla to be kinked and the cerebellar vermis to be indented, fourth ventricle elongated and midbrain distorted.
  - Problems include palsies and central apnea.
  - Treatment by closure of the defect remains controversial and is not always performed.
- *Spina bifida occulta:*
  - Defect of the posterior arch of one or more lumbar or sacral vertebra (often L5 and S1).
  - Often found incidentally on X-ray in children admitted to hospital; may be considered as a normal variant.

  - However, if examination reveals a naevus, hairy patch, dimple, sinus or subcutaneous mass, then MRI of the spinal cord is recommended even if no associated problems with sphincter or limb control.
  - Can cause asymmetrical lower motor neurone weakness associated with wasting, deformity and diminished reflexes.
  - May also be progressive gait disturbance with spasticity and impaired bladder control.
- *Dorsal dermal sinuses:*
  - Often found in the occipital and lumbosacral areas and can connect the skin surface to the dura or to an intradural dermoid cyst.
  - If open can produce recurrent meningitis so should be explored and removed if possible, before infection occurs.
- *Lipomyelomeningocele:*
  - Seen as a bulge in the lumbosacral region normally lateral to the mid-line.
  - This is a lipoma or lipofibroma attached to the spinal cord which is low-lying.
  - Are often associated with meningocele.
- *Diastematomyelia:*
  - Sagittal cleft dividing the spinal cord in the two halves each surrounded by its pia mater.
  - The cord may be transfixed by a bony or cartilaginous spur.
  - Usually occurs in low thoracic or lumbar regions.
  - Overlying skin abnormality is present in 75% of cases and X-rays show abnormalities in most cases including abnormal segmentation of vertebrae, spina bifida and scoliosis.
  - Neurosurgery is normally indicated if abnormality involves cord or nerve roots with the objective of reducing pressure over spinal cord for normal growth and prevent further damage

Prenatal Screening

- Alpha-fetoprotein in maternal serum: Best detected at 16 to 18 weeks of pregnancy but may not detect closed defects and is less sensitive if a woman is taking valproate.

- Ultrasound: Recommended for all at-risk women (positive serum alpha-fetoprotein, previously affected child) can detect anencephaly from 12th week and spina bifida from 16 to 20 weeks (may occasionally be missed especially in L5 to S2 region).
- Amniocentesis: Only used when unable to obtain adequate ultrasound images; used to measure alpha-fetoprotein and neuronal acetylcholinesterase.

Investigations

- MRI is the study of choice for imaging neural tissue and for identifying contents of the defect in the newborn
- CT scan allows direct visualization of the bony defect and anatomy
- Ultrasound is used antenatally for screening.

Management

- Affected children will be getting treatment from a multidisciplinary team to address any associated physical, developmental, hearing, visual and learning difficulties that may occur in association with the neural tube defect.
- The newborn with an open neural tube defect should be kept warm and the defect covered with a sterile saline dressing.
- The baby should be positioned in the prone position to prevent pressure on the defect.
- Open neural tube defects should be closed promptly.
- *Hydrocephalus:* Ventriculoperitoneal shunt placed at the time of myelomeningocele closure.
- *Symptomatic Chiari malformations:* Suboccipital craniotomy and decompression of the posterior fossa and tonsils.
- Laminectomy and placement of a syringosubarachnoid stent to divert the CSF out of the central canal.

Complications

- Infections
- Associated motor and sensory problems, particularly lower limb
- Associated learning disability, developmental delay and hearing impairment
- Bladder and bowel dysfunction.

Prevention

- *Periconceptional folic acid supplementation* can prevent most neural tube defects if widely used. Supplementation must begin before conception, for it to be effective.
- To prevent first occurrence, women who are planning to become pregnant should take 400 mcg folic acid daily before conception and during first 12 weeks of pregnancy. However, women who have had a previous NTD pregnancy are recommended to take an even higher dosage of folic acid prior to planning a pregnancy. They should increase the daily dose of folic acid from 0.4 to 4.0 mg, one month prior to conception through the first three months of pregnancy. The 4.0 to 0.5 mg of folic acid should only be obtained through a prescription from the doctor.
- Food fortification with the addition of folate to grain products is considered the most effective method of ensuring adequate intake of folic acid in pregnant women.

Role of Nurses

- Provide proper position to child to prevent further neurological damage.
- Ensure infection control measures in every contact with child to prevent infection.
- Keep the defect covered with sterile wet gauze to prevent infection.
- Involve the parents in care of child, ask parents to hold the chills and look to enhance parent-child relationship.
- The parents of a child with congenital defects must be provided a high level of support and effective nurse parents relationship is essential for effective outcome of total health care.
- Encourage the patients to ask as many as questions and provide answers for every question in simple and positive language, by providing expected hope.
- Discussion with parents about causes of disorder and expected outcome and prognosis based on severity of neural tube defect.
- Discuss about possible treatment modalities.
- Take or assist physical to take required sample to detect associated chromosomal abnormalities.
- Plan about discharge, provide discharge teaching and discuss about follow-up care.

DOWN SYNDROME

It is a common genetic disorder characterized by mental retardation, dysmorphic facial features and a host of structural abnormalities. It is so called after John Langdon Haydon Down, an English physician, 1828–1896. It is also known as Mongolism or trisomy 21chromosome.

One of the commonest genetic disorders, affecting 1 in 800 live births. Down syndrome is a chromosomal condition related to chromosome 21. Most cases of Down syndrome result from trisomy 21, which means each cell in the body has three copies of chromosome 21 instead of the usual two copies (Table 3.12). The extra genetic material disrupts the normal course of development, causing the characteristic features of Down syndrome. A small percentage of cases occur when only some of the body's cells have an extra copy of the chromosome. These cases are called mosaic Down syndrome. Although uncommon, Down syndrome also can occur when part of chromosome 21 becomes attached (translocated) to another chromosome before or at conception. Affected people have two copies of chromosome 21, plus extra material from chromosome 21 attached to another chromosome. These cases are called translocation Down syndrome. Incidence of Down syndrome cases are observed as following (Fig. 3.13):

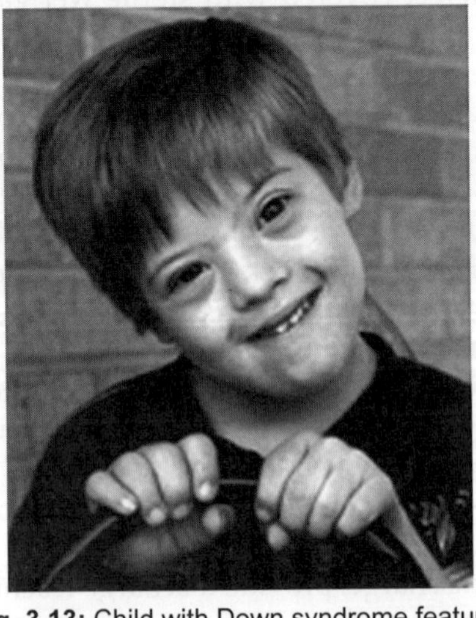

Fig. 3.13: Child with Down syndrome features

- The underlying genetic defect is trisomy 21 in 94% of cases.
- Mosaicism (2.4%) and translocations (3.3%) also occur.
- 75% of these translocations are *de novo* errors.

Risk Factors

- Family history
- Age of mother:
  - 1:385 risk at 35
  - 1:106 at 40
  - 1:30 at 45 years

Clinical Manifestation

At birth there are a wide range of associated physical features. Not all babies have typical facies. Frequently the first feature noticed is hypotonia.

Table 3.12: Neonatal features of Down syndrome

• Brachycephaly • Oblique palpebral fissures • Gap between hallux and second toes • Loose skin on nape of neck • Hyperflexibility • Ears set low, folded or stenotic meatus	• Epicanthic folds • Ring of iris speckles-Brushfield spots • Short little finger • In-curved little finger • Short broad hands
• Protruding tongue (small narrow palate) • Flat nasal bridge • Muscular hypotonia	• High arched palate • Single palmar crease • Congenital heart defects (CHD) • Transient myelodysplasia of the newborn* • Duodenal atresia*

*Highly specific for Down syndrome

Soon after birth all babies with Down syndrome should be assessed for congenital heart disease by echocardiogram. They should also have auditory evoked potential testing (before age 6 months) to check for hearing loss, and also be checked for congenital cataracts and glaucoma (Table 3.13).

Table 3.13: Associated conditions in a child with Down syndrome

Cardiological disorders	***Hematological disorders***
• Atrioventricular canal defects	• Impaired cellular immunity (greater risk of infections, e.g. pneumonia)
• Ventricular septal defect • Isolated secundum atrial septal defects • Isolated persistent patent ductus arteriosus • Tetralogy of Fallot	• Increased risk of acute leukemia • Polycythemia and transient myeloproliferative disorder
Orthopedic disorders	***Ophthalmological disorders***
• Atlantoaxial instability • Hyperflexibility • Scoliosis • Hip dislocation after 2 years • Patellar subluxation or dislocation • Foot deformities	• Cataracts • Refractive errors • Strabismus • Nystagmus • Congenital glaucoma • Keratoconus
Gastrointestinal disorders	***Neurological disorders***
• Esophageal atresia or tracheo-esophageal fistula • Duodenal atresia • Pyloric stenosis • Meckel's diverticulum • Hirschsprung's disease • Imperforate anus • Gastroesophageal reflux • Dental problems • Celiac disease	• Mental retardation (Severe retardation to 'low normal') • Behavioral problems • Seizures occur in 5–10% • In older patients an Alzheimer's type picture develops in > 60% of those over 60 years of age.
ENT disorders	***Endocrine disorders***
• Conductive, sensorineural, or mixed hearing loss • More susceptible to otitis media, sinusitis and pharyngitis Obstructive sleep apnea	• Hypothyroidism

Prenatal Screening and Diagnosis

- There is a large amount of published research on Downs syndrome screening. It looks at combinations of markers ± ultrasound (Nuchal translucency scans measure the thickness of skin at the nuchal fold at around 10 to 12 weeks gestation), used in the first or second trimesters. Screening aims to identify women at higher risk, than that predicted on the basis of age alone. If the woman chooses to, after counseling on associated risks, she may proceed to invasive testing, e.g. chorionic villus sampling or amniocentesis, to establish fetal karyotype.

- The Integrated test offers the most effective and safe method of screening for women who attend in the first trimester. This test comprises Nuchal translucency scanning and pregnancy associated plasma protein-A [PAPP-A] at 11 completed weeks of pregnancy, and alpha-fetoprotein, unconjugated oestriol [uE3], free beta or total human chorionic gonadotrophin (hCG) and inhibin-A in the early second trimester. With this method at an 85% detection rate, it has been estimated that there would be six amniocentesis-caused miscarriages of unaffected fetuses per 100,000 women screened, compared with 35 using the Combined test or 45 with the Quadruple test.
- If PAPP-A, hCG and nuchal translucency scanning (NT) are used as a first-trimester screening test, it is commonly referred to as the combined test.
- When hCG and AFP are used between 14 and 20 weeks as a screening test, this is often called the double test.
- If uE3 is added to the double test combination, it becomes known as the triple test.
- The addition of inhibin A to the triple test comprises the quadruple test.

- First trimester prenatal screening using a combination of maternal serum biochemistry and fetal nuchal translucency thickness, has been shown to achieve detection rates over 90%.
- A Disintegrin And Metalloprotease 12 (ADAM 12) is a glycoprotein synthesised by placenta. It has been shown to be a potential first-trimester maternal serum marker for Down syndrome (DS). ADAM 12 and PAPP-A measured at 8 to 9 weeks and combined with NT and free beta-hCG measured at 12 weeks has been predicted to give a detection rate of 97% at a 5% false-positive rate.
- First trimester screening for trisomy 21 in twin pregnancies is possible and practical using a combination of nuchal translucency thickness and maternal serum biochemistry.

- Amniocentesis (at 14–16 weeks) is 99.5% accurate. Chorionic villus sampling (CVS) can be performed earlier (10–13 weeks) but accuracy is less (96–98%). Both procedures have an operator specific miscarriage risk.

Role of Nurses

- The parents of a child with Down syndrome must be provided a high level of support and nursing interventions which are essentials for effective outcome of total health care.
- Conduct a counseling sessions with parents in presence of expert counselor.
- Encourage the patients to ask as many as questions and provide answers for every question in simple and positive language, by providing expected hope.
- Ensure that parents hold and be with child, to enhance early parent-child bond.
- Help the parents to learn about available community resources and association, which can help them to care for child.
- Teach the parents about care of child at home.
- Discuss about further diagnosis of associated health problems.
- Plan about discharge, provide discharge teaching and discuss about follow-up care.
- Offer counseling about future pregnancy and needed prenatal testing.

REVIEW QUESTIONS

Short-note Questions

1. Neural tube defects.
2. Effects of Radiation on Fetal development.
3. Down syndrome.
4. Prenatal testing and diagnosis of genetic diseases.
5. Effect of maternal drug therapy in the development of genetic diseases.
6. Role of folic acid in lowering the risk of neural tube defects.
7. Radiation induced genetic damage.
8. Effects of maternal infection on fetal outcome of pregnancy.

9. Advanced maternal age and effect on pregnancy.
10. Genetic causes of spontaneous abortion.
11. Genetic basis of infertility.
12. Prenatal diagnosis.
13. Relationship between maternal nutrition and fetal health. Mention the birth defects due to maternal folic acid deficiency.
14. External agents affecting embryogenesis.
15. Spontaneous abortion.

Short-answer Questions

1. Define prenatal diagnosis.
2. Prenatal genetic analysis.
3. Mention two features of Down syndrome.
4. Mention two merits of chorionic villus biopsy.
5. Mention two uses of Ultrasound in prenatal diagnosis.

Multiple Choice Questions (MCQs)

1. **For prenatal screening Alpha fetoprotein in maternal serum is best detected in:**
   a. 12–14 weeks b. 16–18 weeks
   c. 16–20 weeks d. 8–12 weeks
2. **Which of the following stage of human development may have highest risk of chromosomal/Genetic damage due to toxic environment?**
   a. Embryonic b. Fetal
   c. Infancy d. Childhood
3. **Down syndrome is characteristics by:**
   a. 19 trisomy
   b. 21 trisomy
   c. 13 trisomy
   d. Only one X chromosome
4. **Down's syndrome is due to:**
   a. Crossing over
   b. Linkage
   c. Sex-linked inheritance
   d. Nondisjunction of chromosomes

5. The following infection comes under the 'TORCH' except:
   a. Ruballa
   b. Varicella
   c. Toxoplasmosis
   d. Hepatitis-B virus

6. How much is possibility of sharing the proportion of genes among the second degree close blood relatives?
   a. 50%
   b. 75%
   c. 25%
   d. 10%

7. Consanguious marriages are common in which of the following community in India?
   a. Sikhs
   b. North Indian Hindus
   c. Muslims
   d. Christians

8. Which of the following foods is believed to be avoided during pregnancy to avoid the allergies among children?
   a. Peanuts
   b. Eggs
   c. Banana
   d. Apple

9. Which of the supplementation in pregnant mothers may reduce the risk of mitral valve prolapsed among their children:
   a. Sodium   b. Magnesium
   c. Potassium   d. Zink

10. Neural Tube Defect is associated with deficiency of which of the following:
   a. Magnesium   b. Folic acid
   c. Potassium   d. Zink

11. Chorionic Villus Sampling (CVS) prenatal genetic test is ideally performed during time of pregnancy:
   a. 6–8 weeks   b. 10–13 weeks
   c. 15–20 weeks   d. 25–30 weeks

12. **The low level of Alpha-fetoprotein in maternal serum indicates which of the following condition?**
    a. Trisomy 13, 18 or 21
    b. Neural tube defect
    c. Multiple gestation
    d. Rh-isoimmunization

13. **Which of the following is the most appropriate time to perform the fetal tissue sample prenatal genetic test?**
    a. 10–12 weeks
    b. 16–22 weeks
    c. 25–29 weeks
    d. 30–32 weeks

14. **Which of the following may be considered latest true objective criteria of spontaneous abortion that the expulsion of intrauterine product:**
    a. Before 20 weeks
    b. After 22 weeks
    c. Before 28 weeks
    d. After 24 weeks

15. **Which of the following genetic condition could be main cause of male genetic infertility?**
    a. Hemochromatosis
    b. Klinefelter's syndrome
    c. Tay-sachs disease
    d. Huntington disease

ANSWER KEY

1. b	2. a	3. b	4. d	5. d	6. c	7. c
8. a	9. b	10. b	11. b	12. a	13. b	14. a
15. b						

FURTHER READING

1. ACOG Technical Bulletin: HIV Infection. No. 165, March; 1992.
2. Alfirevic Z, Gosden CM, Neilson JP. Chorion villus sampling versus amniocentesis for prenatal diagnosis. Cochrane Database Syst Rev. 2000;(2):CD000055.

3. Alfirevic Z, Sundberg K, Brigham S. Amniocentesis and chorionic villus sampling for prenatal diagnosis. Cochrane Database Syst Rev. 2003;(3):CD003252.
4. Alfirevic Z, von Dadelszen P. Instruments for chorionic villus sampling for prenatal diagnosis. Cochrane Database Syst Rev. 2003;(1):CD000114.
5. Alteneder RR, Kenner C, Greene D, et al. The lived experience of women who undergo prenatal diagnostic testing due to elevated maternal serum alpha-fetoprotein screening. MCN Am J Matern Child Nurs 1998;23:180-6.
6. American Academy of Pediatrics Committee in Infectious Diseases (1990): Parvovirus, erythema infectiosum, and pregnancy. Pediatrics 85:131.
7. Amniocentesis Guideline, Royal College of Obtetricians and Gynecologists (2005)
8. Antenatal care - Routine care for the healthy pregnant woman, NICE Clinical guidance (2003)
9. Baird PA, Sadovnick AD; Life tables for Down syndrome. Hum Genet. 1989;82(3):291-2.
10. Bender PL: Genetic family history assessment. AACN Clinical Issues 1998;9:467-83.
11. Birnbacher R, Messerschmidt AM, Pollak AP. Diagnosis and prevention of neural tube defects. Curr Opin Urol. 2002;12(6):461-4.
12. Blackburn ST. Assessment and management of neurologic dysfunction. In Comprehensive Neonatal Nursing Care: A Physiologic Perspective, ed 2. Philadelphia, WB Saunders, 1998: 564-607.
13. Brambati B, Tului L. Chorionic villus sampling and amniocentesis. Curr Opin Obstet Gynecol. 2005;17(2):197-201.
14. Breeze AC, Lees CC, Kumar A, et al. Palliative care for prenatally diagnosed lethal fetal abnormality. Arch Dis Child Fetal Neonatal Ed. 2007 Jan;92(1):F56-8. Epub 2006 May 16.
15. Burke SS, Matsumoto AR. Pastoral care for perinatal and neonatal health care providers. Journal of Obstetric, Gynecologic, and Neonatal Nursing 1999;28:137-41.
16. Busby A, Abramsky L, Dolk H, et al. Preventing neural tube defects in Europe: population based study. BMJ. 2005;330(7491):574-5.
17. Caughey AB, Hopkins LM, Norton ME. Chorionic villus sampling compared with amniocentesis and the difference in the rate of pregnancy loss. Obstet Gynecol. 2006;108(3 Pt 1):612-6.
18. Centers for Disease Control. Risks Associated with Human Parvovirus B19 Infection. Morbidity and Mortality Weekly Report. 1989;38:81-7.

19. Centini G, Rosignoli L, Kenanidis A, et al. A report of early (13 + 0 to 14 + 6 weeks) and mid-trimester amniocenteses: 10 years' experience. J Matern Fetal Neonatal Med. 2003;14(2):113-7.
20. Chen H. Down's Syndrome. e-Medicine; *January,* 2006
21. Chi C, Hyett JA, Finning KM, et al. Non-invasive first trimester determination of fetal gender: a new approach for prenatal diagnosis of haemophilia. BJOG. 2006;113(2):239-42.
22. Chitty LS, Kagan KO, Molina FS, et al. Fetal nuchal translucency scan and early prenatal diagnosis of chromosomal abnormalities by rapid aneuploidy screening: observational study. BMJ. 2006 Feb 25;332(7539):452-5. Epub 2006 Feb 13.
23. Cochrane DD, Wilson RD, Steinbok P, et al. Prenatal spinal evaluation and functional outcome of patients born with myelomeningocele: information for improved prenatal counselling and outcome prediction. Fetal Diagn Ther. 1996 May-Jun;11(3):159 68.
24. Conover E. Hazardous exposures during pregnancy. Journal of Obstetric, Gynecologic, and Neonatal Nursing 1994;23:524-32.
25. Coulson CC, Katz VL, Kuller JA. Triple-marker screening for aneuploidy. In Kuller JA, Chescheir NC, Cefalo RC (eds): Prenatal Diagnosis and Reproductive Genetics. St. Louis, Mosby, 1996: 8495.
26. Delisle MF, Wilson RD; First trimester prenatal diagnosis: amniocentesis. Semin Perinatol. 1999;23(5):414-23.
27. Dhallan R, Guo X, Emche S, et al. A non-invasive test for prenatal diagnosis based on fetal DNA present in maternal blood: a preliminary study. Lancet. 2007;369(9560):474-81.
28. Driscoll KM. The application of genetic knowledge: Ethical and policy implications. AACN Clinical Issues 1998;9:588-99.
29. Dwyer ML. Genetic research and ethical challenges: Implications for nursing practice. AACN Clinical Issues 1998;9:600-5.
30. Felblinger DM, Akers MC: Marfan's syndrome in pregnancy: Implications for advanced practice nurses. AACN Clinical Issues 2000;9:563-8.
31. Fischbach F. A Manual of Laboratory and Diagnostic Tests, ed 5. Philadelphia, lB Lippincott, 1996.
32. Foley SM, Sommers MS. Molecular genetics: From bench to bedside. AACN Clinical Issues 1998;9:491-8.
33. Fowler K, Stango S, Pass R, et al (1992). The Outcome of Congenital Cytomegalovirus Infection in Relation to Maternal Antibody Status. N Engl J Med 326:663-7.
34. Haddow JE. Antenatal screening for Down's syndrome: Where are we and where next? Lancet 1998;352:336-7.

35. Hanshaw J, Dudgeon J, Marshall W (1985). 'Viral Diseases of the Fetus and Newborn.' 2nd edition, W.B. Saunders.
36. Hiatt PW, Grace SC, Kozinetz CA, et al. Effects of viral lower respiratory tract infection on lung function in infants with cystic fibrosis. Pediatrics 1999;103:619-26.
37. Hoffman DE, Wulfsberg EA. Testing children for genetic predispositions: Is it in their best interest? Journal of Law and Medical Ethics 1995;23:331-44.
38. Indian Journal of Human Genetics May-Aug. 2005;11(2): 108-10.
39. Jones KL, Johnson K, Chambers C (1994). Offspring of Women Infected With Varicella During Pregnancy: A Prospective Study. Teratology 49:29-32.
40. Kennedy SJ, Blough RA, Kenner CA, et al. An assessment of two training interventions designed to increase the knowledge of obstetrical nurses and nurse-midwives about the maternal serum triple screen. Prenat Diagn 1998;18:713-20.
41. Kenner C, Dreyer L, Amlung Newborn genetic screening: Blessing or curse? Neonatal Network 1999;18:11-20.
42. Kenner C. National Coalition for Health Professional Education in Genetics. AACN Clinical Issues 1998;9:582-7.
43. Koren G (ed). Maternal-fetal toxicology, a clinician's guide. Marcel Dekker:New York (2nd ed), 1994.
44. Koren G, Pastuszak A, Ito S. Drugs in pregnancy. N Engl J Med 1998; 338: 1128-37.
45. Kramer MS. The epidemiology of adverse pregnancy outcomes: an overview. J Nutr. 2003;133(5 Suppl 2):1592S-6S.
46. Kuller JA, Chescheir NC, Cefalo RC. Prenatal Diagnosis and Reproductive Genetics. St. Louis, Mosby, 1996.
47. Kunk RM. Expanding the newborn screen: Terrific or troubling? MCN Am J Matern Child Nurs 1998;23:266-71.
48. Laigaard J, Spencer K, Christiansen M, et al. ADAM 12 as a first-trimester maternal serum marker in screening for Down syndrome. Prenat Diagn. 2006;26(10):973-9.
49. Lashley FRC. Clinical Genetics in Nursing Practice, ed 2. New York, Springer, 1998.
50. Laurent C. Antenatal screening and counseling: The midwife's role. Nursing Times 1998;94:52-5.
51. Lea DH, Jenkjp JF, Francomano CA. Genetics in Clinical Practice: New Directions for Nursing and Health Care. Sudbury, MA, Jones and Bartlett, 1998.

52. Mangels KJ, Tulipan N, Tsao LY, et al. Fetal MRI in the evaluation of intrauterine myelomeningocele. Pediatr Neurosurg. 2000;32(3):124-31.
53. Mann K, Fox SP, Abbs SJ, et al. Development and implementation of a new rapid aneuploidy diagnostic service within the UK National Health Service and implications for the future of prenatal diagnosis. Lancet. 2001;358(9287):1057-61.
54. March of Dimes Birth Defects Foundation: Statbook: Statistics for Monitoring Maternal and Infant Health. White Plains, NY, March of Dimes Foundation, 1997.
55. McCombs J, Cramer MK. Pregnancy and lactation: therapeutic considerations. In: DiPiro JT, Talbert RL, Yee GC, et al. (eds). Pharmacotherapy. A pathophysiologic approach p1298-312. Appleton & Lange:Stamford (4th ed), 1999.
56. NBDPN. Advances and Opportunities for Birth Defects Surveillance, Research, & Prevention 1999: 123-30.
57. Pastuszak A, Levy M, Schick B, et al. (1994). Outcome After Maternal Varicella Infection in the First 20 Weeks of Pregnancy. N Engl J Med 330:901-5.
58. Penticuff J. Ethical issues in genetic therapy. Journal of Obstetric, Gynecologic, and Neonatal Nursing 1994;23:498-501.
59. Philip J, Silver RK, Wilson RD, et al. Late first-trimester invasive prenatal diagnosis: results of an international randomized trial. Obstet Gynecol. 2004;103(6):1164-73.
60. Pickier RH, Munro CL. Blastomere analysis: Issues for discussion. Journal of Obstetric, Gynecologic, and Neonatal Nursing 1994;23:379-82.
61. Raff BA. Nursing and genetics for the 21st century. Journal of Obstetric, Gynecologic, and Neonatal Nursing 1994;23:477-86.
62. Raines DA: Ethical implications of genetic testing. Nurs Clin North Am 1998;33:275-86.
63. Remington J, Klein J (1990): 'Infectious Diseases of the Fetus and Newborn Infant.' W.B. Saunders, Co.
64. Rice E. The human genome project and gene therapy: A genetic counselor's perspective. J Prenat Neonatal Nurs 1998;12:16-25.
65. Richmond S, Atkins J. A population-based study of the prenatal diagnosis of congenital malformation over 16 years. BJOG. 2005;112(10):1349-57.
66. Roche ML, Kuller JA. Autosomal disorders: Cyctic fibrosis, Tay-Sachs disease, and Huntington disease. In Kuller JA, Chescheir NC, Cefalo RC (eds): Prenatal Diagnosis and Reproductive Genetics. St. Louis, Mosby, 1996: 53-63.

67. Rosenberg KD, Gelow JM, Sandoval AP. Pregnancy intendedness and the use of periconceptional folic acid. Pediatrics. 2003;111(5 Part 2):1142-5.
68. Ross U. Developmental disabilities: Genetic implications. Journal of Obstetric, Gynecologic, and Neonatal Nursing 1994;23:502-5.
69. Rubin P (ed). Prescribing in pregnancy. BMJ Publishing Group:London (2nd ed), 1995.
70. Saito H, Sekizawa A, Morimoto T, et al. Prenatal DNA diagnosis of a single-gene disorder from maternal plasma. Lancet. 2000; 30;356(9236):1170.
71. Schaap AH, van der Pol HG, Boer K, et al. Long-term follow-up of infants after transcervical chorionic villus sampling and after amniocentesis to compare congenital abnormalities and health status. Prenat Diagn. 2002;22(7):598-604.
72. Schardein JL. Chemically induced birth defects. Marcel Dekker:New York (2nd ed), 1993.
73. Seaver L, Hoyme HE (1992). Teratology on Pediatric Practice. Pediatric Clinics of North America 39.
74. Shaw C, Lammer EJ. Maternal periconceptional alcohol consumption and risk for orofacial clefts. J Pediatr 1999;134:298-303.
75. Sommers MS, Beery T. Foundations of genetics: Genetic structure, function, and therapeutics. AACN Clinical Issues 1998; 9:467-8.
76. Spencer K, Nicolaides KH. Screening for trisomy 21 in twins using first trimester ultrasound and maternal serum biochemistry in a one-stop clinic: a review of three years experience. BJOG. 2003;110(3):276-80.
77. Spencer K, Spencer CE, Power M, et al. One stop clinic for assessment of risk for fetal anomalies: a report of the first year of prospective screening for chromosomal anomalies in the first trimester. BJOG. 2000;107(10):1271-5.
78. Spencer K, Spencer CE, Power M, et al. Screening for chromosomal abnormalities in the first trimester using ultrasound and maternal serum biochemistry in a one-stop clinic: a review of three years prospective experience. BJOG. 2003;110(3):281-6.
79. Stranc LC, Evans JA, Hamerton JL. Chorionic villus sampling and amniocentesis for prenatal diagnosis. Lancet. 1997; 8;349(9053):711-4.
80. Theis JWG, Koren G. Maternal and fetal clinical pharmacology. In: Speight TM, Holford NHG (eds). Avery's Drug Treatment, Adis International Limited:Auckland (4th ed), 1997.
81. Theorell CJ, Dengenhardt M. Assessment and management of metabolic dysfunction. In Comprehensive Neonatal Nursing Care: A Physiologic Perspective. Philadelphia, WB Saunders, 1998: 409-75

82. Troy ES. The genetic privacy act: An analysis of privacy and research concerns. Journal of Law and Medical Ethics 1997;25:256-72.

83. von Dadelszen P, Sermer M, Hillier J, et al. A randomised controlled trial of biopsy forceps and cannula aspiration for transcervical chorionic villus sampling. BJOG. 2005 May;112(5):559-66.

84. Wald NJ, Rodeck C, Hackshaw AK, et al. SURUSS in perspective. Semin Perinatol. 2005 Aug;29(4):225-35.

85. Waliman CM. Newborn genetic screening. Neonatal Network 1998;17:55-60.

86. Wapner RJ, Evans MI, Davis G, et al. Procedural risks versus theology: chorionic villus sampling for Orthodox Jews at less than 8 weeks' gestation. Am J Obstet Gynecol. 2002;186(6):1133-6.

87. Whitley R, et al. Predictors of Morbidity and Mortality in Neonates With Herpes Simplex Virus Infections. N Engl J Med 1991;423:450-54.

88. Williams JK. Genetic testing. Implications for professional nursing. J Prof Nurs 1998;14:184-8.

89. Wright L. Prenatal diagnosis in the 1990s. Journal of Obstetric, Gynecologic, and Neonatal Nursing 1994;23:506-15.

Chapter

4

Neonatal and Children Testing or Screening

Learning Objectives

This chapter is designed to enable the reader to:

- Understand the meaning and purposes of neonatal and children genetic testing and screening
- Identify the important elements of newborn screening and common disorders screened in newborns
- Recognize the approaches of genetic testing in children
- Discuss the meaning, types, causes, genetic tests/ screening and management of congenital abnormalities
- Describe the meaning, risk factors, warning signs and screening tests for developmental delay
- Explain the concept, types, etiology, common syndromes, and genetics tests of dysmorphic syndromes
- Explore the role of nurses in genetic testing for neonates and children.

Key Terms

- Neonatal Testing/Screening
- Childern Testing/Screening
- Newborn Screening
- Congenital Abnormalities
- Dysmorphism
- Developmental Delay
- Battelle Developmental Inventory
- Bayley Infant Neurodevelop-mental Screener
- Child Development Inventory
- Denver Developmental Screening Test

INTRODUCTION

Neonatal testing can be performed to diagnose disorder or screen for a potential pathologic condition among newborns. In some states of USA, four conditions are tested for, whereas other states require more than 20 different tests. The most common tests are homocystinuria, phenylketonuria, hypothyroidism, and galactosemia. Hemoglobinopathies have been added in several states. The rationale behind the state mandate is that the risk to the infant is minimal, whereas the lifelong benefit is tremendous. Because many of these conditions involve errors of metabolism (formerly referred to as inborn errors of metabolism), they have a distant possibility of causing mental retardation, organic failure to thrive, and even death, if undetected and untreated. The quality of life for the infant and the family can be impacted positively with early detection, and the cost to society is decreased related to less extraordinary services that are required when treatment is expeditious and successful.

Other neonatal tests focus on chromosomal changes such as those seen with trisomy conditions. These are conditions in which the infant has three of any one chromosome instead of the normal two. The total number of chromosomes should be 46; however, in the infant with a trisomy, there is an extra chromosome when the karyotype is examined. This extragenetic material may have no clinical impact or may be severe enough, as in the case of trisomy 13 (three of chromosome 13), that death is inevitable. The diagnosis of this condition may facilitate informed family decisions about treatment. For instance, the infant diagnosed with trisomy 21 (Down's syndrome), the diagnosis may allow parents to gain access to services to foster early growth and development to help the child reach maximum potential. In addition, a diagnosis of trisomy 21 early in life clues the health care professional to look for related problems, such as congenital leukemia and cardiac anomalies.

Meaning and Purpose

Neonatal and children testing may be offered or conducted within the context of general or targeted neonate and children population screening programs or be offered to specific children at risk, but the *term 'genetic testing' is commonly referred to the use of specific tests for individuals who are believed to be at increased risk for a specific genetic conditions, because of their family history or symptom manifestations.*

The task force on genetic testing defines a genetic test as 'the analysis of human DNA, RNA, chromosomes, protein and certain metabolites in order to detect heritable disease-related genotypes, mutations, phenotypes or karyotypes for clinical purpose.'

Genetic testing or screening may be done for:

- Detecting or diagnosing a present disease state
- Determining carrier state
- Determining disease susceptibility
- Detecting abnormalities in the fetus, and
- The prediction of disease in usually asymptomatic person that may include late onset or adult disorders.

Although there can be difference in the use of the term 'screening', an accepted definition is 'the presumptive identification of an unrecognized disease or defect in an apparently healthy individual' Genetic screening was more specifically defined by the committee for the study of inborn errors of metabolism (1975) of the National Academy of Sciences and this is the accepted definition. Essentially it is a search for:

- Child who poses genotypes that is associated with the development of genetic disease. The usual purpose is such that the treatment can be instituted or the natural course of the disease can be altered. An example of this is screening newborn for PKU in order to restrict their diet to prevent mental retardation.
- Personss with certain genotypes that are known to predispose the individual to illness. An example, of this is the identification of individuals with G6PD deficiency, who after being identified can avoid the precipitation of hemolytic anemia by avoiding certain foods and drugs.
- Person who are heterozygous carriers of recessive inheritance genes that in autosomal recessive disorders (in double dose) can cause genetic disease in their descendants. An example of this would be screening program for the detection of Tay-Sachs carriers. This type of screening provides information to an individual so that he or she can makes reproductive plan for the future genetic counseling, including reproductive options and the availability of prenatal diagnosis, is an essential component of this type of screening.
- Person with polymorphism (variability) is not known to be associated with a disease state. This allows for gathering the

information related to the genetic makeup of the population. This may begin as research and later have therapeutic value. A common example is in the observed variation of human blood groups.

NEWBORN SCREENING

Genetic knowledge from the human genome project and the development of new technologies have led to a new era in newborn screening; which is one of the great genetic public health success stories. Once phenylketonuria (PKU) was found to be associated with a type of mental retardation which could be prevented if a low phenylalanine diet was instituted soon after birth, a search began for a method to reliability test to detect PKU in a newborn. Eventually, Robert Guthrie developed such a test using blood taken from drops placed on filter paper and dried. Testing was based on a bacterial growth inhibition essay using the dried blood spot. This test became the base for screening; virtually for the entire newborn population. If an abnormal screening test was identified, a low phenylalanine (phe) diet could be initiated and effective treatment put in place for those whose diagnosis was confirmed. Recently, newer technology such as tandem mass spectrometry (MS/MS) and the expansion of molecular and DNA-based techniques have identified additional mutations that have expanded the scope of genetic screening among neonates and children.

The major reason for newborn screening is to identify apparently healthy newborn at risk through newborn screening programs, provide early treatment for certain disorders as soon as possible and thereby prevent serious health consequences, especially severe mental retardation.

Important Elements in Newborn Screening

- Inclusion of new neonates before hospital discharge according to state law guidelines.
- Provision to include neonates not tested before discharge and those born outside the hospital as possible.
- Education of parents about screening at appropriate educational level, considering cultural beliefs, religions, that involves as to how the test results will be communicated.
- Informed parental consent within state laws.

- Collection of appropriate specimen at proper time.
- Reliable, accurate, standardized testing in centralized laboratory is ideal.
- Provision for re-screening, if tested early; re-screening should be done at about 3 weeks of age for PKU.
- Communication of positive screening results to local physician and parents quickly (by telephone with letter of confirmation). Ideally have counseling and psychosocial support available to help parents and family with stressful situation.
- Follow up all newborns with positive screening test results.
- Insure means of accurate diagnosis are available for all with confirmed positive screening tests.
- Provision genetic and other counseling that is culturally competent and educationally appropriate.
- Provision for treatment and ongoing management of infant and family.

Common Disorders can be Screened in Newborns

- *Phenylketonuria (Hyperphenylalaninemia)*: Phenylketonuria (PKU) was the first disorder to be included in mass newborn screening in the early 1960s. Worldwide, more than 10 million newborns are now screened for PKU each year. The amino acid phenylalanine (phe) is essential for protein synthesis in humans. A complex reaction is involved in the hepatic conversion of phenylalanine to tyrosine and blockage causes elevations, collectively referred to as hyperphenylalaninemia. Need for education of parents, informed consent for testing and provision of genetic counseling services as integral part of treatment programs.
- *Congenital hypothyroidism:* Screening for congenital hypothyroidism was carried out by measuring thyroid stimulating hormone (TSH) on dried blood spots by fluoroimmunoassay using DELFIA kits.
- *Galactosemia:* Lactose (milk sugar) is a diasaccharide composed of glucose and galactose. Defects in enzyme involved in the metabolism of galactose can result in galactosemia.
- *Homocystinuria:* It is a disorder of amino acid metabolism. It may result from impaired activity or deficiency of cystethionine-B-synthetase (CBS) or methionine synthetase.

- *Maple syrup urine disease:* Also known as branched chain ketoaciduria because the basic defect is in the second step (decarboxylation) of the metabolism of leucine, isoleucine and valine, which are the amino acids having branched chain and the corresponding ketoacids.
- *Hemoglobinopathies and sickle cell disease*
- *Tyosinemia*
- *Biotinidase deficiency*
- *Congenital adrenal hyperplasia*
- *Medium-chain Acyl-COA dehydrogenase deficiency*
- *Cystic fibrosis*
- *Congenital hearing loss*
- *Other fatty acid oxidation defects, organ acidemia, aminoacidemias and other metabolic defects*
- *Other disorders like* diabetes mellitus, hyperlipidemia, familial hypercholestrolemia, neurobalstoma, fragile X-syndrome and other chromosomal diseases, alfa-1-antitrypsin deficiency, Duchenne muscular dystrophy, hemochromatosis, BRCA and other gene mutations predisposing for cancer, Tay-Sachs disease, tuberous sclerosis and Huntington disease.

GENETIC TESTING AND SCREENING IN CHILDREN

Of the 100,000 genes contained in the human genome, 15% have been localized through the efforts of the Human Genome Project (HGP). Within a short time, 100% of the human DNA sequence will be determined. This effort is comparable to reading an expansive book series that consists of 3 billion letters. Rapidly advancing technology allows new genes to be identified at an exponential rate. Newly characterized genes can cause children and adolescents to have or be more susceptible to cancer, neurodegenerative, cardiac, psychiatric, and immune disorders and dyslipidemias, deafness, skeletal dysplasias, and multiple system syndromes. A complete list today would be out of date tomorrow. Although identifying a disease causing gene mutation may initiate our understanding of the disorder it confers, our understanding of the possible psychological and social ramifications for the individual or family is far less clear. The gap between discovering genetic cause and dealing with the effects of genetic testing is monumental.

It is conceivable that in the near future, armed with a web page that lists all the disease-causing genes, a family could present to their health care provider and request to be tested for diseases X, Y, and Z. On the surface, requesting genetic testing seems harmless. It is as easy as obtaining blood for any medical test. But the testing of children imposes some inherent conflicts, some of which are subtle and others more controversial. Decisions about whether to provide genetic testing become increasingly murky for a professional as the requests advance from testing a child for carrier status for an autosomal recessive disorder to testing a girl for a sex-linked mutation, to test an asymptomatic child for a disease not expected to manifest itself until adulthood, to test a child for a susceptibility to a particular disorder (Fig. 4.1). The rapidly advancing ability to provide testing in the current environment makes careful consideration on the part of the providers imperative.

More straightforward ↓ More complex

- **Affected child: Immediate treatment/Preventional surveillance**
  - Phenylketonuria (PKU)
  - Multiple endocrine neoplasia (MEN)
  - X-linked severe combined immune deficiency (XSCID)
  - Hyperlipidemias
  - Familial adenomatous polyposis (FAP)
- **Asymptomatic carrier: Testing to define reproductive risks**

  Sex-linked disorders
  - Hemophilia
  - Muscular dystrophy
  - XSCID

  Autosomal recessive disorders
  - Cystic fibrosis
  - Sickle cell disease
- **Healthy young person: Predisposition to develop disease**
  - Breast cancer (BRCA1, BRCA2)
  - Hereditary nonpolyposis colon cancer (HNPCC)
- **Healthy young person: Will develop disease**
  - Huntington's disease
  - Some forms of Parkinson's disease

Fig. 4.1: Categorization of genetic disorders in children

Approach to Genetic Testing in Children

In the past decade, the American Society of Human Genetics and the American College of Medical Genetics have developed guidelines for genetic testing in children. These guidelines have been endorsed by International Society of Nurses in Genetics. Currently, genetic testing of minors falls into several categories parallel to those shown in Figure 4.1.

Category I

- *Testing for a disorder for which there is immediate known benefit of treatment or preventive measures:* In this instance, greater harm occurs if testing is not done. Children at genetic risk of developing cancer may stand to gain tremendous benefits from testing that would allow preventive measures or detection early enough to achieve a cure. Those children who are known to have the gene for multiple endocrine neoplasia develop medullary thyroid cancer that can become clinically apparent between 2 to 30 months of age. In younger individuals, the tumor is more aggressive, with metastases to liver, lung, and bone. Affected children as young as 23 months have had life-preserving thyroidectomies. In this instance, genetic testing has replaced biochemical testing.

  Another identifiable gene with associated inheritable, childhood cancers is familial adenomatous polyposis. Familial adenomatous polyposis is manifested by multiple, premalignant adenomatous polyps in the colon and gastrointestinal tract. Untreated polyps develop into colorectal cancer. Individuals with familial adenomatous polyposis are also predisposed to adenomas that occur in the duodenum, brain, and thyroid, and these children are at increased risk of developing hepatoblastoma. Colonic visualization beginning at the age 2 years has been recommended to detect and remove polyps. Youngsters who are found not to have the gene can be spared from the invasive and costly endoscopic screening.

Category II

- *Testing for the benefit of future reproductive choice without immediate health benefit:* There are a number of questions coming to our mind, like what are the benefits or the harms of learning this information at this time? The burden to advocate about whether testing best serves the child is on the professional. What if parents request testing for a daughter of 12 or 15 years? There are obvious cognitive, developmental, and decision-making skills that differ between a 4-year-old child and an adolescent. A child who already has experienced the death of siblings, has heard the stories told by her mother and grandparents, or has participated as a marrow donor may weigh the confirmation of being a carrier much differently than a child without that experience. Potential consequences to individual and family dynamics as a result of DNA-based testing of children have been described. The alteration in parent-child bonding is possible if the parent misinterprets the meaning of the carrier status and withdraws from the child or the child is rejected because she shares carrier status with a rejected spouse. A minor may undergo changes in self-concept. Anxiety about dating or marriage may be increased. Will the parents be able to convey genetic results and implied risks accurately to the child? In contrast, testing may be justified if the family's anxiety is so high that the child is suffering. Perhaps bad news may be preferential to living in a dysfunctional environment caused by uncertainty. What about the child as a future adult who has the right to explore the potential risks and benefits of carrier testing for herself when she chooses? However, adolescents do not necessarily wait until the age of majority to become parents; knowing their carrier status as teenagers might influence their sexual behavior, but they might indulge in thinking 'It will never happen to me.

Category III and IV

- *Testing in the absence of medical benefits:* In this category, decision of whether to provide genetic testing becomes increasingly complex. Predisposition testing identifies a disease gene in an individual that increases the risk for that disorder in a person but does not confer 100% certainty that the disorder will occur. In fact, the individual who carries a predisposition gene may never become affected with that disorder. Examples of these disorders currently include familial breast cancer and hereditary nonpolyposis colon cancer. Identifying a predisposition gene in a family is not the same as knowing who will develop the disorder or how severe it will be. Other modifying genes or environmental influences determine the clinical manifestation of predisposition genes. Predisposition testing may have a role in identifying individuals who would benefit from increased surveillance and early detection. In children, however, little current evidence shows benefit for testing before the recommended age for initiating surveillance measures.

Presymptomatic testing identifies the gene alteration in an individual before the clinical manifestation of the disorder appears, with extremely high certainty that the disorder will manifest itself in adulthood. Huntington's disease, some forms of Parkinson's disease, and polycystic kidney disease are examples of disorders that can be identified by genetic testing before symptoms are clinically evident. Although treatments are under development, no current intervention arrests the progression or cures these disorders. If this testing is done on at risk family members who are minors, several harmful consequential events are conceivable. Insurability for the affected child in current environment in India could be compromised. Through stigmatization, the child may not be encouraged to meet his or her full potential or resources for educational pursuits could be diverted away from the child. Prospects for future employment might be threatened. Unrelated illnesses may be ignored, inadequately evaluated, or misdiagnosed because of the underlying assumption that symptoms are related to the genetic disorder for which the child is known to have the gene.

Many unanswered questions remain about the psychologic impact of genetic testing in children. Genetic testing may relieve uncertainty. Understanding how families manage uncertainty might help to identify which families would benefit from childhood testing. Improvement in the parents' ability to cope might benefit the child.

Should children be tested/screened?

Should children be tested for susceptibility to genetic diseases, presence of the genes for late-onset diseases and/or carrier state? The issue of genetic testing and screening of children has been an area of great controversy. Some centers and groups have condemned such testing and refused to provide such services to children even with parent's consent, while others are more liberal. Newborn screening already tests infants for some disorders that do have a direct therapeutic benefit. To be considered are personal issues such as medical, psychosocial, reproductive issue and issue with a broader impact such as those affecting insurance, career and future employment. A thought report by the ASHG/ACMG (1995) discusses many related issues. In a study in Great Britain, pediatricians were more likely than geneticists to allow such testing at the request of parents or adoption agencies. There was great variation according to condition. In a study by Tibben (1992), parents were more favorable towards genetic testing than were health professionals. Michie et al (1996) reported on a family in which testing for familial adenomatous polyposis was done for the 2 and 4 years old sisters. Their hypothesis was that 'complying with requests for predictive DNA testing…in parents wishing to reduce uncertainty about their children in future health is associated with good psychological outcome regardless of the test results'.

Reasons for considering testing in children commonly evolve from the diagnosis of a genetic disorder within a family, particularly one that has onset in late childhood, adolescence or adulthood rather than the necessity for diagnosis of a genetic disorder because of an immediate health implication. *Some reasons for such testing include:*

- The institution of preventive measures or therapy that can treat or ameliorate the severity or influence the natural history of the disease is a question (a direct timely medical benefit or evidence-based risk reduction program is the most compelling reason for testing).
- Sparing the child from the unpleasantness and trauma of continued testing for disorders such as familial cancer when a child may not possess the gene is question.
- Knowledge for the parents in terms of their own financial and reproductive planning gives the future outbreak for their present children.
- The elimination of the uncertainty of knowing whether or not they possess a gene of a serious disorder such as Huntington disease or disorder or adult polycystic kidney disease.

- The psychological benefit of a negative test for a positive result, the chance for parents to adjust to diagnose and plan ways to disease and cope with the news at the appropriate time for their child; and
- The opportunity for life planning based on this information, including choices related to education, career, lifestyle and reproductive decisions. For example, a child at risk for retinitis pigmentosa could choose a career that did not require visual activity or child with familial hypertrophic cardiomyopathy could receive early drug therapy for prevention of arrhythmia.

Some of the reasons given for not performing such testing include:

- The child may not be able to understand the ramifications of testing, such as future insurability risks and possible effects on education and employability.
- The child may not be able to give informed consent or even assent, thus taking away the child's right to decide.
- The potential psychological consequences of learning that one has genetic disorder or is a carrier, such as lowered self-esteem, changes in family dynamics and in parent-child bonding, loss of confidentiality of the child's condition since the parents will know the status.
- Stigmatization and labeling.
- The potential negative psychological consequences of learning that one does not have a disorder and developing 'survivor guilt' or feeling alienated from an affected sibling or family member.

Table 4.1: Qualities of an ideal screening test or procedure

• Rapid	• Accepted
• Inexpensive	• Valid
• Simple	• Uses easily available specimens and materials
• Sensitive	• Reproducible
• Specific	• Causes minimal discomfort
• Safe	

CONGENITAL ABNORMALITIES

A *congenital abnormality* (congenital anomaly, congenital malformation, birth defect) is a condition which is present at the time of birth which varies from the standard presentation. In other words, it is a type of congenital disorder which is primarily structural in nature.

About 3% of newborns have a 'major physical anomaly', meaning a physical anomaly that has cosmetic or functional significance. Congenital anomalies involving the brain are the largest group at 10 per 1000 live births, compared to heart at 8 per 1000, kidneys at 4 per 1000, and limbs at 1 per 1000. All other physical anomalies have a combined incidence of 6 per 1000 live births. Congenital anomalies of the heart have the highest risk of death in infancy, accounting for 28% of infant deaths due to congenital anomaly, while chromosomal anomalies and respiratory anomalies each account for 15%, and brain anomalies about 12%.

Types

- A limb anomaly is called a dysmelia. These include all forms of limb anomalies, such as amelia, ectrodactyly, phocomelia, polymelia, polydactyly, syndactyly, polysyndactyly, oligodactyly, brachydactyly, achondroplasia, congenital aplasia or hypoplasia, amniotic band syndrome, and cleidocranial dysostosis.
- Congenital anomalies of the heart include patent ductus arteriosus, atrial septal defect, ventricular septal defect, and tetralogy of Fallot. Helen Taussig has been a major force in research on congenital anomalies of the heart.
- Congenital anomalies of the nervous system include neural tube defects, such as spina bifida, meningocele, meningomyelocele, encephalocele and anencephaly. Other congenital anomalies of the nervous system include the Arnold-Chiari malformation, the Dandy-Walker malformation, hydrocephalus, microencephaly, megencephaly, lissencephaly, polymicrogyria, holoprosencephaly, and agenesis of the corpus callosum.
- Congenital anomalies of the gastrointestinal system include numerous forms of stenosis and atresia, and imperforate, etc.

Causes

- *Sporadic or unknown causes:* The cause of 40–60% of congenital anomalies in humans is unknown. These are referred to as sporadic, a term that implies an unknown cause, random occurrence regardless of maternal living conditions, and a low recurrence risk for future children. For 20–25% of anomalies, there seems to have a 'multifactorial' cause, meaning a complex interaction of multiple minor genetic anomalies with environmental risk factors.

- *Genetic causes* of congenital anomalies include inheritance of abnormal genes from the parents, as well as new mutations in one of the germ cells that gave rise to the fetus. Only 12–25% of anomalies have a purely genetic cause. Of these, the majority are chromosomal anomalies.
- *Environmental causes* of congenital anomalies are referred to as teratogenic. These are generally problems with the mother's environment. Teratogens can include dietary deficiencies, toxins, or infections. About 10–13% of anomalies have a purely environmental cause (e.g. infections, illness, or drug abuse in the mother). For example, dietary deficiency of maternal folic acid is associated with spina bifida. Ingestion of harmful substances by the mother (e.g. alcohol, mercury, or prescription drugs, such as phenytoin) can cause recognizable combinations of birth defects. Several infections (TORCH infection) which a mother can contract during pregnancy can also be teratogenic.

Genetic Testing/Screening

- Detailed physical examination
- Blood biochemistry of children
- Molecular genetic tests (Direct DNA testing)
- FISH (Fluorescence in situ hybridization)
- Ultrasonography
- Echocardiography
- ECG
- Radiological examination (X-rays, CT scan and MRI, etc.)

Management

Usually, surgery is required; howeve, it depends on the extent of congenital anomaly.

DEVELOPMENTAL DELAY

Child development refers to the process in which children go through changes in skill development during predictable time periods, called developmental milestones. Developmental delay occurs when children have not reached these milestones by the expected time period. For example, if the normal range for learning to walk is from 9 to 15 months, and a 20-month-old child has still not begun walking, this would be considered a developmental delay. Developmental delays can occur in all five areas of development or may just happen in one or more of those areas. Additionally, growth in each area of development is related to growth in the other areas. So, if there is a difficulty in one area (e.g. speech and language), it is likely to influence development in other areas (e.g. social and emotional).

'Developmental delay is a significant lag in a child's physical, cognitive, behavioral, emotional, or social development in compression to norms.' In other words, developmental delay refers to when a child's development lags behind established normal ranges for his or her age.

At least 8 percent of all children from birth to six years have developmental problems and delays in one or more areas of development. This includes delays in speech and language development, motor development, social-emotional development, and cognitive development. Some have global delays, which means they lag in all developmental areas.

Risk Factors for Developmental Delay

Risk factors for developmental problems fall into two categories:

- *Genetic factor:* Children are placed at genetic risk by being born with a genetic or chromosomal abnormality. A good example of a genetic risk is Down's syndrome, a disorder that causes developmental delay because of an abnormal chromosome.
- *Environmental factor:* Environmental risk results from exposure to harmful agents either before or after birth, and can include things like poor maternal nutrition or exposure to toxins (e.g. lead or drugs) or infections that are passed from mother to her baby during pregnancy (e.g. measles or HIV). Environmental risks also include a child's life experiences. For example, children who are born prematurely, face severe poverty, mother's depression, poor nutrition, or lack of care are at increased risk for developmental delays.

Risk factors have a cumulative impact upon development. As the number of risk factors increases, a child is put at greater risk for developmental delay.

Warning Signs of a Developmental Delay

There are several general 'warning signs' of possible delay. These include:

- *Behavioral Warning Signs*
  - Does not pay attention or stay focused on an activity for as long a time as other children of the same age
  - Focuses on unusual objects for long periods of time; enjoys this more than interacting with others
  - Avoids or rarely makes eye contact with others
  - Gets unusually frustrated when trying to do simple tasks that most children of the same age can do
  - Shows aggressive behaviors and acting out and appears to be very stubborn compared with other children
  - Displays violent behaviors on a daily basis
  - Stares into space, rocks body, or talks to self more often than other children of the same age
  - Does not seek love and approval from a caregiver or parent.
- *Gross Motor Warning Signs*
  - Has stiff arms and/or legs
  - Has a floppy or limp body posture compared to other children of the same age.
  - Uses one side of body more than the other
  - Has a very clumsy manner compared with other children of the same age.
- *Vision Warning Signs*
  - Seems to have difficulty following objects or people with her eyes
  - Rubs eyes frequently
  - Turns, tilts or holds head in a strained or unusual position when trying to look at an object
  - Seems to have difficulty finding or picking up small objects dropped on the floor (after the age of 12 months)
  - Has difficulty focusing or making eye contact
  - Closes one eye when trying to look at distant objects
  - Eyes appear to be crossed or turned
  - Brings objects too close to eyes to see
  - One or both eyes appear abnormal in size or coloring.

- *Hearing Warning Signs*
  - Talks in a very loud or very soft voice
  - Seems to have difficulty responding when called from across the room, even when it is for something interesting
  - Turns body so that the same ear is always turned toward sound
  - Has difficulty understanding what has been said or following directions after once she has turned 3 years of age
  - Does not startle to loud noises
  - Ears appear small or deformed
  - Fails to develop sounds or words that would be appropriate at her age.

Children usually acquire developmental milestones or skills during a specific time frame or 'window', we can predict when most children will learn different skills. If a child is not learning a skill that other children are learning at the same age, that may be a 'warning sign' that the child may be at risk for developmental delay.

Screening of Developmental Delay

A developmental screening test is a quick and general measurement of skills. Its purpose is to identify children who are in need of further evaluation. A screening test is only meant to identify children who might have a problem. The screening test may either over-identify or under-identify children with delay. As a result, simply using a screening test cannot make a diagnosis. If the results of a screening test suggest that the child may have a developmental delay, the child should be referred for a developmental evaluation to higher center.

The most popular developmental screening scale or procedures are based on pioneering work of Gessel and his colleagues. Some of the currently used popular developmental screening tools are:

- *Battelle Developmental Inventory Screening Test (BDIST):* The Battelle Developmental Inventory Screening Test (BDIST) can be used to screen children from age 12 to 96 months, using a combination of direct assessment, observation and parental interview.
- *Bayley Infant Neurodevelopmental Screener (BINS):* The Bayley Infant Neurodevelopmental Screener (BINS) is a recently developed test designed for screening high-risk infants aged

3 to 24 months. It uses 10 to 13 directly elicited items per 3 to 6 months range to assess neurodevelopmental skills and developmental accomplishments (measures motor and mental maturation).

- *Child Development Inventories (CDI):* The Child Development Inventory or CDI, formerly known as the Minnesota Child Development Inventory, was created to provide a systematic, standardized method for parents to report on their children's strengths, problems, and present development. The original 300-item instrument has been broken down into instruments that apply to 3 years of age intervals. The CDI measures a child's development in 8 areas: social, self-help, gross motor, fine motor, expressive language, language comprehension, letters, and numbers. It consists of a 300-item booklet and answer sheet for the parent to complete and a profile sheet for recording the results.
- *The Denver Developmental Screening Test (DDST):* The Denver Developmental Screening Test (DDST) was introduced in 1967. Research has consistently proved that it lacks sensitivity. In response to this criticism, a revised version, the Denver II, was released in 1992. The Denver II is the most commonly used developmental screening tool. It combines direct observation and parental report. The tool consists of 125 items, organized into 4 developmental domains: gross motor, fine motor/ adaptive, language, and personal/social.

The summary of the most important development milestone as *DDST* is shown in Table 4.2.

Table 4.2: Key developmental milestone

Gross motor		Fine motor	
Age	*Milestones*	*Age*	*Milestones*
3 months	Neck holding	4 months	Grasp a rattle or ring when placed in hand
5 months	Sitting with support	5 months	Reaches out to an object and holds it with both hands
8 months	Sitting without support		
9 months	Standing with support		
10 months	Walking with support		
11 months	Crawling (creeping)		

Contd...

Contd...

Gross motor		**Fine motor**	
Age	*Milestones*	*Age*	*Milestones*
12 months	Standing without support	7 months	Holding objects with crude grasp from palm *(palmer grasp)*
13 months	Walking without support		
18 months	Running		
24 months	Walking upstairs	9 months	Holding small objects, like a pellet between index finger and thumb *(pinchar grasp)*
36 months	Riding tricycle		
Language		***Personal/social***	
Age	*Milestones*	*Age*	*Milestones*
1 month	Turn head to sound	2 months	Social smile
3 months	Cooing	3 months	Recognizing mother
6 months	Monosyllables ('ma', 'ba')		
9 months	Bisyllables ('mama', 'baba')	6 months	Smile at mirror image
12 months	Two words with meaning	9 months	Wave 'bye-bye'
18 months	Ten words with meaning		
24 months	Simple sentences	12 months	Play a simple ball game
36 months	Telling a story	36 months	Knows gender

Early Intervention Services for Developmental Delay

Early intervention services include a variety of different resources and programs that provide support to families to enhance a child's development. These services are specifically tailored to meet a child's individual needs. Services include:

- Assistive technology (devices a child might need)
- Audiology or hearing services
- Counseling and training for a family
- Educational programs
- Medical services
- Nursing services
- Nutrition services
- Occupational therapy
- Physical therapy
- Psychological services
- Respite services
- Speech/Language.

DYSMORPHISM

'Any congenital structural or developmental defect is known as dysmorphism. This usually occurs due to abnormal embryogenesis or morphogenesis'.

Embryogenesis is the process by which the embryo is formed and develops. It starts with the fertilization of the ovum and egg, which, after fertilization, is then called a zygote. The zygote undergoes rapid mitotic division, the formation of two exact genetic replicates of the original cell, with no significant growth and cellular differentiation, leading to development of an embryo. Morphogenesis is one of the three fundamental aspects of developmental biology along with the control of cell growth and cellular differentiation. Morphogenesis is concerned with the shapes of tissue, organs and entire organism and the positions of the various specialized cell type. Therefore, abnormality in embryogenesis and morphogenesis may lead to dysmorphism.

Types of Dysmorphism

- *Major dysmorphism:* It is the several types of developmental defects, which produce functional disability and early life mortality. Incidence of these defects is about 2 to 3 percent in neonates.
- *Minor dysmorphism:* Nearly 10 to 12 percent newborns have such defects, which are basically cosmetic defects and did not produce any functional disability. For example, nevis, pigmentation, preauricular skin tags, etc.

Etiology

- *Chromosomal or genetic causes* of these anomalies include inheritance of abnormal genes from the parents, as well as new mutations in one of the germ cells that gave rise to the fetus.
- *Environmental causes* of dysmorphic anomalies are referred to as teratogenic. Teratogens can include dietary deficiencies, toxins, or infections. For example, dietary deficiency of maternal folic acid is associated with spina bifida. Ingestion of harmful substances by the mother (e.g. alcohol, mercury, or prescription drugs, such as phenytoin) can cause recognizable combinations of birth defects. Several infections (TORCH infection) which a mother can contract during pregnancy can also be teratogenic.

- *Unknown causes, in some situations, even a, cause can be established for a defect.*

Common Dysmorphic Syndromes

- *Syndromes with craniofacial dysmorphism*:
  - Moebius sequence
  - Frontonasal dysplasia sequence
  - Goldenhar syndrome
  - Craniosynostoses syndrome
  - Carpenter syndrome
- *Syndromes with physical overgrowth:*
  - *Fragile X syndrome*
  - *Marshall-Smith syndrome*
  - *Weaver-Smith syndrome*
- *Syndromes with CNS and neuromuscular defects:*
  - *Prader-Willi syndrome*
  - *Myotonic dystrophy syndrome*
- *Syndromes with chromosomal abnormalities:*
  - *Down's syndrome (trisomy 21)*
  - *Edward syndrome (trisomy 18)*
  - *Patau syndrome (trisomy 13)*
  - *Turner syndrome (Monosomy of X)*

Genetic Testing/Screening

- Detailed physical examination
- Blood biochemistry of children
- Molecular genetic tests (Direct DNA testing)
- FISH (Fluorescence in situ hybridization)
- Ultrasonography
- Echocardiography
- ECG
- Radiological examination (X-rays, CT scan and MRI, etc.)

Management

Depending on the extent of defect, it may not require any management or may require several surgeries.

Role of nurses in genetic testing for neonates and children:

- Nurses must take a thorough family history. This includes information about family history, exposures, and lifestyles, if clues are to be uncovered as to the relative risk a family may have for a specific condition. Asking about unaffected as well as affected family members can suggest an inheritance pattern for a specific problem.
- Nurses who work in neonatal and children areas have the responsibility to assist with testing procedures, support the client and family, and provide appropriate education and clarification of information.
- Nurses' awareness of how personal values may color personal perceptions of the family's situation is imperative to avoid imposing personal values on the family.
- As advocates, nurses translate complex genetic information to allow the family to be competent in the use and application of that information. Many health care professionals feel uncomfortable with genetic interpretations; yet the family feels so even more.
- If the neonate requires intensive care or if the condition is detected early in neonatal period, the family and the nurse may benefit from pastoral care. From the family's perspective, this element of spirituality, if important to them, may help them cope. For the health care professional, it may facilitate working with families whose beliefs and values may differ from their own.
- Offer detailed information and support both parents and child during testing.
- Provide referral and follow-up services, if required.

REVIEW QUESTIONS

Short-note Questions

1. Genetic Testing—Screening for congenital abnormalities.
2. Genetic testing and screening for dysmorphism.
3. Screening of developmental delays.
4. Newborn screening.

Short-answer Questions

1. Mention two causes of congenital abnormalities.
2. Mention two screening tests for detecting congenital abnormalities.
3. Name two causes of congenital anomaly.

Multiple Choice Questions (MCQs)

1. **Which of the following is the main purpose of performing the neonatal testing or screening?**
   a. Diagnosis of genetic disease in fetus.
   b. Screening potential genetic conditions in newborns.
   c. Screening of genetic conditions in children.
   d. All of the above.

2. **Which of the following is the most common condition which is screened among newborns in American states?**
   a. Aniridia and sickle cell disease.
   b. Klinfelter's syndrome and hemochromatosis
   c. Phenylketonuria and homocystinuria.
   d. All of the above

3. **Which of the following does most suitably define the genetic testing:**
   a. Genetic testing of DNA, RNA and chromosome for diagnosis of genetic diseases.
   b. Genetic screening of DNA, RNA and chromosome for prevention and diagnosis of genetic disorders.
   c. Analysis of human DNA, RNA, chromosomes, protein and certain metabolites in order to detect inheritable disease-related genotypes, mutations, phenotypes or karyotypes for clinical purposes.
   d. All of the above.

4. **Which of the following is NOT an important element of newborn screening?**
   a. Inclusion of new neonates before hospital discharge according to state law guidelines.
   b. Provision to include neonates not tested before discharge and those born outside the hospital as possible.

c. Education of parents about screening at appropriate educational level, considering cultural beliefs, religions, that involves how the test results will be communicated.
d. Conducting chorionic villous sampling for screening of genetics for identifying any genetic abnormality.

5. Which of the following may be considered as qualities of an ideal screening test?
a. Rapid
b. Acceptable
c. Valid
d. All of the above

6. Which of the following screening tools is used to assess the motor and mental maturation among high-risk infants?
a. Battelle development inventory screening test.
b. Bayley infant neurodevelopment screener.
c. Child development inventories.
d. Denver development screening test.

7. Which of the following genetic tests may be used for screening of congenital abnormalities among newborns?
a. Molecular genetic tests.
b. Fluorescence in situ hybridization (FISH).
c. Ultrasonography.
d. All of the above.

8. Which of the following conditions can be considered as craniofacial dysmorphism?
a. Fragile x-syndrome
b. Prader-Willi syndrome
c. Goldenhar syndrome
d. Marshall-Smith syndrome

9. Which of thc following conditions may be considered as CNS and neuromuscular dysmorphism?
a. Carpenter syndrome
b. Prader-Willi syndrome
c. Goldenhar syndrome
d. Marshall-Smith syndrome

10. Which of the following is the most priority nurse's intervention in genetic testing and screening of newborns and children?

a. Assist in genetic testing/screening procedure and support the patient and family
b. Assess the thorough personal and family history of the neonate and children.
c. Providing the appropriate education and clarification of information related to genetic testing/screening.
d. Providing referral and follow-up services, if required.

ANSWER KEY

1. b	2. c	3. c	4. d	5. d	6. b	7. d
8. c	9. b	10. b				

FURTHER READING

1. ASHG/ACMG: ASHG/ACMG report points to consider: Ethical, legal and psychosocial implications of genetic testing in children and adolescents. Am J Hum Genet 1995;57:1233-41.
2. Buckley RH, Schiff S, Schiff RI, et al: Hematopoietic stem-cell transplantation for the treatment of severe combined immunodeficiency. N Engl J Med 340:508-9, 1999
3. Clayton E: Genetic testing in children. J Med Philos 1997;22:233-51.
4. Collins F: Shattuck lecture: Medical and societal consequences of the Human Genome Project. N Engl J Med 1999;34:28-37.
5. Fanos J: Developmental tasks of childhood and adolescence: Implications for genetic testing. Am J Hum Genet 1997;71:22-8.
6. Garber J, Diller L: Screening children at genetic risk of cancer. Curr Opin Pediatr 1993;5:712-5.
7. Geiger J, Thompson NW: Thyroid tumors in children. Otolaryngol Clin North Am 1996;29: 711-9.
8. Gross, RH, et al: Early Management and Decision Making for the Treatment of Myelomeningocele. Pediatrics 1983;72(4),450-8.
9. *http://www.ncbi.nlm.nih.gov/Omim/searchomim.html*
10. Kennedy, F. The problem of social control of the congenital defective: Education, sterilization, euthanasia. American Journal of Psychiatry 1942;99,13-16.
11. Lessick M, Faux 5: Implications of genetic testing of children and adolescents. Holistic Nursing Practice 1998;12:38-46.

12. Petersen C, Francomano C, Kinzler K, et al: Presymptomatic direct detection of adenomatous polyposis coli (APC) gene mutation in familial adenomatous polyposis. Huts' Genet 1993;91:307-11.
13. Puck J: Molecular and genetic basis of X-linked immunodeficiency. J Clin Immunol 1994;14:81-88.
14. Raines D: Ethical implications of genetic testing. Nurs Clin North Am 1998;33:275-286.
15. Singer, P. Sanctity of life or quality of life? Pediatrics 1983;72 (1):128-9.
16. Strong L, Marteau T: Evaluating children and adolescents for heritable cancer risk.. J Natl Cancer Inst Monogr 1995;17:111-3.
17. Wertz D, Fanos JH, Reilly PR: Genetic testing for children and adolescents: Who decides? JAMA 1994;272:875-81.
18. Williams J, Lessick M: Genome research: Implications for children. Pediatr Nurs 1996;22:40-6.

Chapter

5

Genetic Conditions of Adolescents and Adults

Learning Objectives

This chapter is designed to enable the reader to:

- Understand the meaning of common genetic conditions of adolescents and adults.
- Discuss the meaning, genetics test and management of familial cancer.
- Classify the inborn errors of metabolism and mention their common clinical manifestations, diagnostic tests and management.
- Explore the meaning, clinical manifestations, screening tests and treatment of phenylketonuria, maple syrup urine disease and Gaucher' disease.
- Recognize the common hematological disorders.
- Explain the concept, pathogenesis, clinical manifestations, diagnostic tests and management of common hematological disorders.
- Identify the genetic basis, genetic testing and management of common mental illnesses and other genetic conditions of adolescents and adults.
- Describe the therapeutic approaches and nursing management for genetic disorders.

Key Terms

- Genetic Statistics
- Genetic Conditions
- Cancer Genetics
- Familial Cancer
- Inborn Errors Of Metabolism
- Phenylketonuria
- Hemophilia
- von Willebrand's Disease
- Genetic Hemochromatosis
- Huntington's Disease
- Mental Illness
- Maple Syrup Urine Disease

Contd...

Contd...

Key Terms

- Gauchers-Disease
- Blood Group Alleles
- Hematological Disorders
- Hemolytic Disease of Newborn
- G-6-PD Deficiency
- Hereditary Spherocytosis
- Thalassemia
- Sickle-cell anemia
- Blackfan-Diamond Anemia
- Congenital Amegakryocytic Thrombocytopenia

GENETIC STATISTICS

Some statistical terms are commonly used when describing genetic conditions and other disorders. These terms include:

- *Incidence:* The incidence of a gene mutation or a genetic disorder is the number of people who are born with the mutation or disorder in a specified group per year. Incidence is often written in the form '1 in [a number]' or as a total number of live births. About 1 in 200,000 people in India are born with syndrome A each year. An estimated 15,000 infants with syndrome B were born last year worldwide.
- *Prevalence:* The prevalence of a gene mutation or a genetic disorder is the total number of people in a specified group at a given time who have the mutation or disorder. This term includes both newly diagnosed and pre-existing cases in people of any age. Prevalence is often written in the form '1 in [a number]' or as a total number of people who have a condition. Approximately 1 in 100,000 people in India have syndrome A at the present time. About 100,000 children worldwide currently have syndrome B.
- *Mortality:* Mortality is the number of deaths from a particular disorder occurring in a specified group per year. Mortality is usually expressed as a total number of deaths. An estimated 12,000 people worldwide died from syndrome C in 2002.
- *Lifetime risk:* Lifetime risk is the average risk of developing a particular disorder at some point during a lifetime. Lifetime risk is often written as a percentage or as '1 in [a number]'. It is important to remember that the risk per year or per decade is much lower than the lifetime risk. In addition, other

factors may increase or decrease a person's risk as compared with the average. Approximately 1 percent of people in India develop disorder D during their lifetimes. The lifetime risk of developing disorder D is 1 in 100.

NAMING GENETIC CONDITIONS

Genetic conditions are not named in one standard way (unlike genes, which are given an official name and symbol by a formal committee). Doctors who treat families with a particular disorder are often the first to propose a name for the condition. Expert working groups may later revise the name to improve its usefulness. Naming is important because it allows accurate and effective communication about particular conditions, which will ultimately help researchers to find new approaches for treatment.

Disorders' names are often derived from one or a combination of sources:

- The basic genetic or biochemical defect that causes the condition (for example, alpha-1 antitrypsin deficiency);
- One or more major signs or symptoms of the disorder (for example, sickle-cell anemia);
- The parts of the body affected by the condition (for example, retinoblastoma);
- The name of a physician or researcher, often the first person to describe the disorder (for example, Marfan's syndrome, which was named after Dr Antoine Bernard-Jean Marfan);
- A geographic area (for example, familial Mediterranean fever, which occurs mainly in populations bordering the Mediterranean Sea); or
- The name of a patient or family with the condition (for example, amyotrophic lateral sclerosis, which is also called Lou Gehrig disease after a famous baseball player who had the condition).

Disorders named after a specific person or place are called eponyms. There is debate as to whether the possessive form (e.g. Alzheimer's disease) or the nonpossessive form (Alzheimer disease) of eponyms is preferred. As a rule, medical geneticists use the nonpossessive form, and this form may become the standard for doctors in all fields of medicine. Genetics Home Reference uses the nonpossessive form of eponyms.

Genetics Home Reference consults with experts in the field of medical genetics to provide the current, most accurate name for each disorder. Alternate names are included as synonyms.

Common Genetic Conditions Discussed in the Chapter

- Cancer genetics: familial cancer
- Inborn errors of metabolism
- Blood group alleles and hematological disorders
- Genetic hemochromatosis
- Huntington's disease
- Mental illness.

CANCER GENETICS: FAMILIAL CANCER

Cancer is a class of diseases or disorders characterized by uncontrolled division of cells and the ability of these to spread, either by direct growth into adjacent tissue through *invasion*, or by implantation into distant sites by *metastasis* (where cancer cells are transported through the bloodstream or lymphatic system). Cancer may affect people at all ages, but risk tends to increase with age.

Based on causative foundation (carcinogenesis), cancer is broadly classified into two major categories:

1. *Sporadic cancer:* Most of the cancers are caused by series of mutations that develop during a person's lifetime called 'acquired mutations'. Acquired mutations are caused by tobacco, overexposure to UV radiation and other toxins and chemicals. These mutations are not in every cell of the body and are not passed from parents to child. Cancer caused by this type of mutation is called 'sporadic cancer'.
2. *Familial cancer:* For various reasons, genes often undergo mutations. Some mutations have no effect on a cell, while other mutations are harmful or helpful to the cell. These are two basic kinds of genetic mutations. If mutation passes from one of the parents to the child, it is called 'germline mutation'. When a germline mutation is passed on from a parent to the

child, it is present in every cell of the child's body, including the reproductive cells. It is passed from generation to generation. Germline mutations are responsible for 5 to 10 percent of cancer cases. This is also called 'familial cancer'.

Familial Cancer

Most forms of cancer are 'sporadic', and have no basis in heredity. There are, however, a number of recognized syndromes of cancer with a hereditary component, often a defective tumor suppressor allele. Examples are: In medicine, the term 'syndrome' is the association of several clinically recognizable features, signs, symptoms, phenomena or characteristics which often occur together, so that the presence of one feature alerts the physician about the presence of the others.

It is believed that about 5 percent of the colorectal and breast cancer arise as a result of an inherited cancer susceptibility gene. There are a number of other features, which suggest an inherited cancer susceptibility syndrome in a particular family. Features include:

- Several first-or second-degree relatives show a common cancer.
- Several close relatives have related cancer, e.g. breast and ovary or bowel and endometrial cancer.
- An early age of onset.
- Tumors in two different organ systems in one person.
- Bilateral tumors in paired organs.
- Two family members may have the same rare cancer.

Family Cancer-predisposing Syndrome

Most cancer occurs at a specific site. There are some families in which the cancer occurs at different sites in various members of the family or at more than one site in an individual. The incidence is more common than would be expected. Such families are referred to have familial cancer-predisposing syndrome. Most of them are with dominant inheritance. Some of them are as follows (also summarized in Table 5.1):

- *Breast and ovarian cancer syndrome:* Certain inherited mutations in the genes *BRCA1* and *BRCA2* are associated with an elevated

Table 5.1: Inheritance of familial cancer-predisposing syndromes

Syndrome	Mutation in Gene	Chromo-somal location	Cancer	Inheritance
Breast and ovarian cancer	*BRCA1* and *BRCA2*	BRCA1-17q21 BRCA2-13q12–13	Breast, ovary	AD
Multiple endocrine neoplasia (MEN types 1, 2a, 2b)	MEN2a and 2b	10q	Thyroid, phe-nochromocy-toma	AD
Li-Fraumeni syndrome	p53	17q	Sarcoma of breast, brain, leukemia, adrenal cortex	AD
Turcot syndrome	–	–	Brain tumors, colonic polyposis	AD
Familial adenomatous polyposis	*APC* gene	5q	Colorectal, duodenal, thyroid	AD
Familial retinoblastoma	Rb1	13q	Retinoblas-toma	AD

risk of breast cancer and ovarian cancer. BRCA1 (named for breast cancer 1) is a human gene located on the long arm of the 17th chromosome (17q21). BRCA2 refers to either a gene [Breast-Cancer susceptibility gene 2, located on human chromosome 13, (13q12–13) or the protein coded for by that gene]. Breast cancer is cancer of breast tissue. Ovarian cancer is a malignant ovarian neoplasm (an abnormal growth located on the ovaries).

- *Multiple endocrine neoplasia (MEN types 1, 2a, 2b):* It refers to tumors of various endocrine organs. Multiple endocrine neoplasia (MEN) (or multiple endocrine adenomas, or multiple endocrine adenomatosis—MEA) consists of three syndromes featuring tumors of endocrine glands, each with its own characteristic pattern.

- *Li-Fraumeni syndrome:* Li-Fraumeni syndrome is a rare autosomal dominant hereditary disorder, which occurs due to mutations of p53. Various tumors seen in this disorder are osteosarcoma, breast cancer, soft-tissue sarcoma, and brain tumors. Osteosarcoma is a common primary bone cancer.
- *Turcot syndrome* (brain tumors and colonic polyposis). Turcot syndrome is the association between familial adenomatous polyposis and brain tumors. A brain tumor is any intracranial tumor created by abnormal and uncontrolled cell division, normally either found in the brain itself (neurons, glial cells, astrocytes, oligodendrocytes, ependymal cells, lymphatic tissue, blood vessels), in the cranial nerves (myelin-producing Schwann cells), in the brain envelopes (meninges), skull, pituitary and pineal gland.
- *Familial adenomatous polyposis* is an inherited mutation of the *APC* gene that leads to early onset of colon carcinoma, in which numerous polyps form mainly in the epithelium of the large intestine. Colorectal cancer includes cancerous growths in the colon, rectum and appendix.
- *Familial retinoblastoma* in young children is an inherited cancer. Retinoblastoma is a cancer of the retina.

Genetic Testing

Genetic testing for high-risk individuals is already available for certain cancer-related genetic mutations. Carriers of genetic mutations that increase risk for cancer incidence can undergo enhanced surveillance, chemoprevention, or risk-reducing surgery. Genetic testing allows the genetic diagnosis of vulnerabilities to inherited diseases, and can also be used to determine a person's ancestry.

Cancer types	Gene
Breast, ovarian, pancreatic	BRCA1, BRCA2
Colon, uterine, small bowel, stomach, urinary tract	MLH1, MSH2, MSH6, PMS, PMS2

Management of Familial Cancer

Cancer Gene Therapy

- *Cancer gene therapy* is one of the experimental areas in the field of cancer treatment. Some of the current areas of

research in cancer gene therapy include RNAi approaches, drug resistance, hematopoietic gene transfer, homologous recombination, ribozyme technology, antisense technology, tumor immunotherapy and tumor suppressors, translational research, gene delivery systems (viral and non-viral), anti-gene therapy (antisense, siRNA and ribozymes), apoptosis, mechanisms and therapies, vaccine development, immunology and immunotherapy, DNA synthesis and repair. Some of the successful cancer therapies are as follows:
  - Nanoparticle delivery of anti-metastatic NM23-H1 gene improves chemotherapy in a mouse tumor model.
  - Expression of HBX, an oncoprotein of hepatitis B virus, blocks reoviraus oncolysis of hepatocellular carcinoma cells.
  - Adoptive immunotherapy using human peripheral blood lymphocytes transferred with RNA encoding Her-2/neu-specific chimeric immune receptor in ovarian cancer xenograft model.
- *Chemoprevention:* For example, drug Tomoxifan can be given to a lady who is vulnerable to develop familial breast cancer.
- *Risk-reducing surgery*: For example, if someone is susceptible to breast cancer and the person finds a small lump during a regular breast self-examination (BSE), early breast surgeries can be performed.

INBORN ERRORS OF METABOLISM (IEM)

The term *inborn error of metabolism* was coined by a British physician, Archibald Garrod (1857–1936) in the early 20th century (1908). He is known for the 'one gene, one enzyme' hypothesis, which arose from his studies on the nature and inheritance of alkaptonuria.

Inborn errors of metabolism comprise a large class of genetic diseases involving disorders of metabolism. The majority are due to defects of single gene that code for enzyme that facilitate conversion of various substances (substrates) into others (products). In most of the disorders, problems arise due to accumulation of substances which are toxic or interfere with normal function, or due to the effects of reduced ability to synthesize essential compounds.

Inborn errors of metabolism are now often referred to as *congenital metabolic diseases or inherited metabolic diseases,* and these terms are considered synonymous.

In other words, *Inborn errors of metabolism (IEM)* are conditions due to genetic defects related to synthesis, metabolism, trasportation or storage of biochemical compunds.

Worldwide incidence of IEM has been estimated to be about 3–4/1000 live births. More than 300 such defects are known. Most of the IEMs are inherited in an autosomal recessive manner, some are through X-linked, though they can also arise out of spontaneous mutations.

Classification of Inborn Errors of Metabolism

Traditionally, the inherited metabolic diseases were categorized as disorders of *carbohydrate* metabolism, *amino acid* metabolism, *organic acid* metabolism, or *lysosomal storage diseases*. In recent decades, hundreds of new inherited disorders of metabolism have been discovered and the categories have proliferated. Following are some of the major classes of congenital metabolic diseases, with prominent examples of each class. Many others do not fall into these categories.

- *Disorders of carbohydrate metabolism,* e.g. glycogen storage disease
- *Disorders of amino acid metabolism,* e.g. phenylketonuria, maple syrup urine disease, glutaric acidemia type 1
- *Disorders of organic acid metabolism (organic acidurias),* e.g. alkaptonuria
- *Disorders of fatty acid oxidation and mitochondrial metabolism,* e.g. medium chain acyl dehydrogenase deficiency (glutaric acidemia type 2)
- *Disorders of porphyrin metabolism,* e.g. acute intermittent porphyria
- *Disorders of purine or pyrimidine metabolism,* e.g. Lesch-Nyhan syndrome
- *Disorders of steroid metabolism,* e.g. congenital adrenal hyperplasia
- *Disorders of mitochondrial function,* e.g. Kearns-Sayre syndrome

- *Disorders of peroxisomal function,* e.g. Zellweger syndrome
- *Lysosomal storage disorders,* e.g. Gaucher's disease, Niemann Pick disease.

Clinical Manifestations

Because of the enormous number of these diseases and wide range of systems affected, nearly every 'presenting complaint' to a doctor may have a congenital metabolic disease as a possible cause, especially in childhood. The following are examples of potential manifestations affecting each of the major organ systems:

Table 5.2: Systemwise clinical manifestations in IEM

System involved	Clinical features
General	Growth failure, failure to thrive, weight loss, unusual facial features, congenital malformations
Genital	Ambiguous genitalia, delayed puberty, precocious puberty
Neurological	Developmental delay, seizures, dementia, encephalopathy, stroke
Sensory	Deafness, blindness, pain, agnosia
Dermatology	Skin rash, abnormal pigmentation, lack of pigmentation, excessive hair growth, lumps and bumps
Hematological	Immunodeficiency, thrombocytopenia, anemia, enlarged spleen, enlarged lymph nodes
Gastrointestinal	Recurrent vomiting, diarrhea, abdominal pain
Hepatic	Hepatomegaly, jaundice, liver failure
Renal	Excessive urination, renal failure, dehydration, edema
Cardiovascular	Hypotension, heart failure, enlarged heart, hypertension, myocardial infarction
Respiratory	Excessive breathing (hyperventilation), respiratory failure
Musculoskeletal	Joint pain, muscle weakness, cramps
Endocrinal	Hypothyroidism, adrenal insufficiency, hypogonadism, diabetes mellitus
Behavioral	Abnormal behavior, depression, psychosis
Dental	Dental abnormalities
Others	Many forms of cancer

Diagnosis

Because of the multiplicity of conditions, many different diagnostic tests are used for screening. An abnormal result is often followed by a subsequent 'definitive test' to confirm the suspected diagnosis.

Common screening tests used:

- Ferric chloride test (turns colors in reaction to various abnormal metabolites in urine)
- Ninhydrin paper chromatography (detects abnormal amino acid patterns)
- Guthrie bacterial inhibition assay (detect a few amino acids in excessive amounts in blood). The dried blood spot can be used for multianalyte testing using Tandem Mass Spectroscopy (MS/MS)
- Quantitative plasma amino acids, quantitative urine amino acids
- Urine organic acids by mass spectrometry

Specific diagnostic tests (or focused screening for a small set of disorders):

- Tissue biopsy or necropsy: liver, muscle, brain, bone marrow
- Skin biopsy and fibroblast cultivation for specific enzyme testing
- Specific DNA testing.

Management

In the middle of the 20th century, the principal treatment for some of the amino acid disorders was restriction of dietary protein and all other care was simply management of complications. In the last two decades, enzyme replacement, gene transfer, and organ transplantation have become available and beneficial for many previously untreatable disorders. Some of the more common or promising methods are listed as follows:

- Dietary restriction, e.g. reduction of dietary protein remains a mainstay of treatment for phenylketonuria and other amino acid disorders
- Dietary supplementation or replacement, e.g. cornstarch several times a day helps prevent people with glycogen storage disease from becoming hypoglycemic as quickly

- Vitamins, e.g. thiamine supplementation benefits several types of lactic acidosis
- Intermediary metabolites, compounds, or drugs that facilitate or retard specific metabolic pathways
- Dialysis
- Enzyme replacement
- Gene therapy
- Bone marrow or organ transplantation
- Treatment of symptoms and complications
- Prenatal diagnosis and avoidance of pregnancy or abortion of an affected fetus.

Only commonly occurring inborn errors of metabolism are discussed in this chapter.

PHENYLKETONURIA

Phenylketonuria (PKU) is an autosomal recessive genetic disorder characterized by a deficiency in the autozome phenylalanine hydroxylase (PAH). This enzyme is necessary to metabolize the amino acid phenylalanine to the amino acid tyrosine. When PAH is deficient, phenylalanine accumulates and is converted into phenylpyruvate (also known as 'phenylketone'), which is detected in the urine.

Left untreated, this condition can cause problems with brain development, leading to progressive mental retardation and seizures. However, PKU is one of the few genetic diseases that can be controlled by diet. A diet low in phenylalanine and high in tyrosine can be a very effective treatment. There is no cure. Damage done is irreversible, so early detection is crucial.

Clinical Manifestations

- Early symptoms include seizures, albinism (excessively fair hair and skin), and a 'musty odor' of the baby's sweat and urine (due to phenylacetate, one of the ketones produced).
- Untreated children are normal at birth, but fail to attain early developmental milestones, develop microcephaly, and demonstrate progressive impairment of cerebral function. Hyperactivity, EEG abnormalities and seizures, and severe

learning disabilities are major clinical problems later in life. A 'musty' odor of skin, hair, sweat and urine (due to phenylacetate accumulation), and a tendency to hypopigmentation and eczema are also observed.

Diagnosis (Screening)

Blood is taken from a two-week old infant to test for phenylketonuria. PKU is normally detected using the HPLC test, but some clinics still use the Guthrie test, part of national biochemical screening programs. Most babies in developed countries are screened for PKU soon after birth.

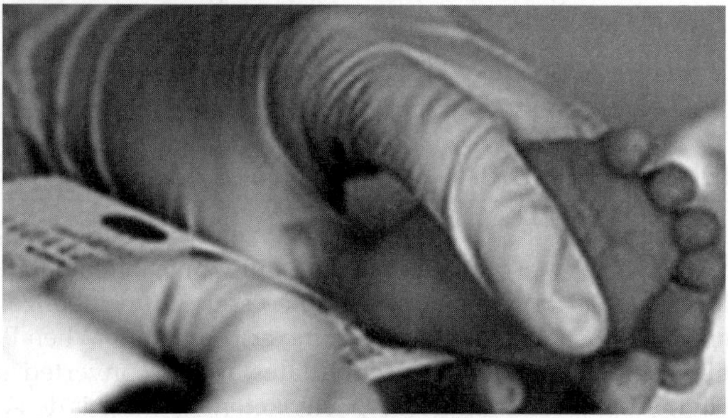

Fig. 5.1: HPLC test

Treatment

- Diet low in phenylalanine for the rest of his or her life.
- Avoiding foods high in phenylalanine, such as meat, chicken, fish, nuts, cheese, legumes and other dairy products.
- Starchy foods, such as potatoes, bread, pasta, and corn must be monitored.
- Infants may still be breastfed to provide all of the benefits of breastmilk, though the quantity must be monitored and supplementation will be required.
- Most of the foods and soft drinks that contain the sweetener aspartame must also be avoided, as aspartame consists of two amino acids: phenylalanine and aspartic acid.
- Supplementary infant formulas are used in these patients to provide the amino acids and other necessary nutrients that

would otherwise be lacking in a protein-free diet. These can continue in other forms as the child grows up, such as pills, formulas, and specially formulated foods. (Since phenylalanine is necessary for the synthesis of many proteins, it is required but levels must be strictly controlled, usually being limited to 10 grams of protein. More severe forms of PKU, such as CPKU, require patients to be restricted to less than 5. In addition, tyrosine, which is normally derived from phenylalanine, must be supplemented.)

- The oral administration of tetrahydrobiopterin (a cofactor in the oxidation of phenylalanine) can reduce blood levels of the amino acid in certain patients.
- There are a number of other therapies currently under investigation, including gene therapy, and an injectable form of PAH.
- Previously, PKU-affected people were allowed to go off diet after approximately 8, then 18 years of age. However, most physicians now agree that this special diet should be followed throughout life.

MAPLE SYRUP URINE DISEASE

Maple syrup urine disease (MSUD), also called *branched-chain ketoaciduria,* is an autosomal recessive metabolic disorder affecting branched-chain amino acids. It is a type of organic acidemia.

Clinical Manifestations

- From early infancy, symptoms of the condition include poor feeding, vomiting, dehydration, lethargy, hypotonia, seizures, ketoacidosis, and neurological decline.
- The disease is characterized in an infant by the presence of sweet-smelling urine, with an odor similar to that of maple syrup. Infants with this disease seem healthy at birth but, if left untreated, suffer severe neurological damage, and eventually die.

Diagnosis

Blood and urine biochemistry for presence of branched-chain amino acids (leucine, isoleucine, and valine) and their toxic by-products.

Management

- A diet with minimal levels of amino acids—leucine, isoleucine, and valine must be maintained in order to prevent neurological damage.
- As these three amino acids are required for proper metabolic function in all people, specialized protein preparations containing substitutes and adjusted levels of the amino acids have been synthesized and tested, allowing MSUD patients to meet normal nutritional requirements without causing harm.

GAUCHER'S SYNDROME

Gaucher disease is a lipid storage disease, characterized by the deposition of glucocerebroside in cells of the macrophage-monocyte system. Deficiency of a specific lysosomal hydrolase, acid beta-glucocerebrosidase, causes widespread accumulation of glucosylceramide-laden macrophages. Glucosylceramide accumulation is widespread and extends to the bone marrow, liver, spleen and lungs. Central nervous system involvement only occurs in patients with disease type 2 (acute neuronopathic) and type 3 (chronic neuronopathic) Gaucher's disease.

There are three clinical subtypes:

- *Type 1:* Non-neuronopathic form. Often presents in childhood with hepatosplenomegaly, pancytopenia, and skeletal disease. The severity of type 1 Gaucher disease is extremely variable, such that some patients present in childhood with virtually all the complications of Gaucher disease, while others are asymptomatic into the eighth decade. Patients diagnosed in the first 5 years of life are frequently non-Jewish and typically have a more malignant disease course.
- *Type 2 (rare):* Infantile form (acute neuronopathic). Causes rapidly progressive neurovisceral storage disease and death during infancy.
- *Type 3:* Juvenile or Norrbottnian form (chronic or subacute neuronopathic). Less rapidly progressive neurovisceral storage disease, causing death in childhood or early adulthood.

Clinical Manifestations

Type 1 Gaucher Disease

- May present with chronic fatigue, hepatomegaly, splenomegaly (may become massive), bone involvement (bone pain due to bone infarcts or pathological fractures due to osteopenia) and may bruise easily or present with nosebleeds, bruising and petechiae (because of thrombocytopenia).

- Short stature and wasting occasionally are found in patients with massive organomegaly.
- Occasionally present with pulmonary infiltration or portal hypertension.

Type 2 Gaucher Disease

- Presents in infancy, with increased tone, strabismus, and organomegaly. Failure to thrive and stridor (due to laryngospasm) are also common.
- Rapid neurodegenerative course with extensive visceral involvement and death (usually caused by respiratory problems) within the first 2 years of life.

Type 3 Gaucher Disease

- Presents in infancy or childhood. In addition to organomegaly and bony involvement, neurological involvement is present, including developmental delay and abnormal neurological findings, e.g. increased tendon reflexes.
- Has been further classified as type 3a (with progressive myotonia and dementia) and 3b (with isolated supranuclear gaze palsy) based on the extent of neurological involvement.

Diagnosis

- *Acid beta-glucosidase activity:* Diagnosis can be confirmed by measurement of acid beta-glucosidase activity in peripheral blood leucocytes. Heterozygotes have half-normal enzyme activity, but there is an overlap with nonaffected controls.
- *Acid beta-glucosidase genotyping:* Molecular diagnosis can be helpful, especially in Ashkenazi patients, in whom 4 mutations (N370S, 84GG, L444P, IVS 2 1) in the acid beta-glucosidase gene account for nearly 97% of disease alleles.
- *Bone marrow aspiration:* Diagnosis may be suggested by the presence of classic glycolipid-laden macrophages (Gaucher cells). Not now the initial diagnostic test as the blood enzyme test is sensitive, specific, and much less invasive.

General Assessment

- Full blood count and differential (assess the degree of pancytopenia), liver function tests (minor elevations of liver enzymes are common but jaundice is a poor prognostic indicator).
- Skeletal radiography can detect and evaluate skeletal manifestations of Gaucher disease. Chest X-ray to evaluate pulmonary manifestations.
- Ultrasonography of the abdomen: determine extent of organomegaly.
- MRI is more accurate in determining organ size and involvement.
- Patients with neuronopathic forms also need MRI scan of the brain, EEG and diagnostic brainstem-evoked responses.
- Dual-energy X-ray absorptiometry (DEXA) scanning: evaluation of osteopenia.

Complications

- Bone: Avascular necrosis of the hip, bone crises (secondary to infarcts).
- Splenic rupture (from trauma).
- Cirrhosis is rare.
- Rarely, pulmonary infiltration by Gaucher cells may lead to overt lung disease.
- Hematologic abnormalities (e.g. anemia, thrombocytopenia, and leucopenia) are common.
- Immunological abnormalities (e.g. hypergammaglobulinemia, T-lymphocyte deficiency in the spleen and impaired neutrophil chemotaxis) are also common.

Management

- *Enzyme replacement therapy (ERT)* with macrophage-targeted recombinant human glucocerebrosidase (imiglucerase) is administered as enzyme replacement therapy for non-neurological manifestations of type I or type III Gaucher disease. It is very effective in reversing the visceral and hematologic manifestations of Gaucher disease, but skeletal disease is slow to respond. In patients with established acute neuronopathic disease, enzyme replacement therapy has had little effect on the progressively downhill course.

- *Miglustat, an inhibitor of glucosylceramide synthase,* is licensed for the treatment of mild to moderate type I Gaucher disease in patients for whom imiglucerase is unsuitable. It has been shown to help with the symptoms of mild to moderate type 1 Gaucher disease. Responses to miglustat are slower and less robust than those observed with ERT, and miglustat may produce significant side effects. Miglustat is currently in trials in combination with ERT to assess whether it will help to reduce some of the neurological deterioration in type 3 Gaucher disease.
- *Bone marrow transplantation* may be an effective treatment for neurological involvement in this disorder. However, there is significant morbidity and mortality, and, therefore, not currently recommended in the current management of neuronopathic Gaucher disease.
- *Gene therapy* may offer the possibility of definitive therapy in the future.
- *Supportive treatment* for specific organ involvement.
- There is evidence that in neuronopathic Gaucher disease, complete or partial *splenectomy* is associated with increased severity and rate of progression of neurological and bone involvement and increased risk of infection.

BLOOD GROUP ALLELES AND HEMATOLOGICAL DISORDERS

Blood Group Alleles

This came in existence through the discovery by Landsteiner in Vienna. According to this, there are two antigens on the red blood cells. They are antigen A and antigen B. Their presence or absence give rise to four phenotypes. They are A, B, AB, and O. With the presence of an antigen, one can expect antibodies in the sera of these individuals. A person with blood group A has an antigen A on his red cells and antibody anti-B in his serum. An individual with 'O' blood group has neither A nor B antigen on his red cells. So, he possesses antibodies anti-A and anti-B in his serum.

The ABO system forms an example of multiple allelism. The alleles are A, B, and O genes located at ABO locus on long arm of chromosome 9. Please note that gene O is recessive to genes A and B, while A and B are dominant. If both A and B genes are present, then both antigens (A and B) will be formed. The O gene is an amorph, i.e. it has no effect, thus leaving H-substance unaltered. So far, numerous subtypes of A and B have been detected. Significant among them are A1 and A2. As a result of this, the AB group is also subdivided into A1B and A2B. Almost 85 percent of blood group A consists of A1. Other variations of A and B, although known, are rare.

Table 5.3: Alleles of the ABO blood group system

Alleles	Protein
A1	A1 transferase
A2	A2 transferase
B	B transferase
O	Nonfunctional

Landsteiner and Wiener discovered Rh blood group system in 1940. The Rh system claims its place because of its role in hemolytic diseases of the newborn. There are both Rh-positive and Rh-negative individuals. Rh-positive persons are homozygous or heterozygous for gene specifying an antigen D, while Rh-negative persons do not have antigen D. The Rh locus is on chromosome 1. Fisher and Race suggested that there are five Rh antigens designated as D, C, E, c, and e. There are eight alleles. Their antigenic determinants are shown in Table 5.4.

Table 5.4: Alleles of the Rh blood group system

Alleles	Antigen
R^o	D, c, e
R^1	D, c, e
R^2	D, c, E
R^z	D, C, E
r	c, e
r'	C, e
r"	c, E
r^y	C, E

HEMATOLOGICAL DISORDERS

The common hematological disorders, which have genetic or hereditary associations are as follows:

Hemolytic Anemia

- *Immune hemolytic anemia,* e.g. Hemolytic disease of newborn (Rh or ABO hemolytic disease).
- *Hereditary red cell enzyme deficiency,* e.g. Glucose 6-Phosphate dehydrogenase deficiency.
- *Hereditary defects of red cell membrane,* e.g. hereditary spherocytosis, hereditary elliptocytosis.
- *Ineffective erythropoiesis: e.g. Thalassemia (Beta or alfa).*
- *Hemoglobinopathies:* e.g. Sickle-cell anemia, hemoglobin C, D or E disease.
- *Paroxysmal nocturnal hemoglobinuria.*
- *Infantile pyknocytosis.*
- *Blackfan-Diamond anemia.*

Hereditary Coagulopathies

- *Hemophilia*
- *von Willebrand disease*
- *Congenital amegakaryocytic thrombocytopenia (CAMT).*

HEMOLYTIC DISEASE OF NEWBORN

In this disease, fetal red cells die earlier due to the action of antibodies formed by the mother against fetal Rh antigen. It begins in utero but continues after birth for about 3 months, the time taken by maternal antibodies to get cleared from newborn's circulation. Although it is based on genetically determined antigenic disparity between mother and fetus, it is an acquired hemolytic anemia, different from hereditary ones like hereditary spherocytosis.

Pathogenesis

In the natural course, there are no antibodies against Rh antigen in serum. During pregnancy, fetal and maternal blood pools are isolated by placental barrier. Towards the term, however, there are breaks occurring along this barrier. This permits transfer of fetal red cells to the mother's blood. When the mother is Rh-negative and fetus is Rh positive, this transfer of Rh-positive red cells of fetus shall evoke an antibody response in the mother. These antibodies may get transferred across placenta to fetus circulation. They get attached to fetal red cells. Such anti-Rh-coated cells are withdrawn from fetal circulation, rendering it anemic. To compensate this, a large number of immature red cells called 'erythroblasts' are poured into fetal circulation. This offers it the name erythroblastosis fetalis.

Clinical Manifestation

Hyperbilirubinemia may follow after birth because of the rapid destruction of red cells of the newborn. This leads to deposition of bilirubin in the brain and, if not prevented by replacement transfusion, may cause cerebral damage. This may lead to mental retardation.

Management

- Usually Rh sensitization occurs at the time of delivery within 72 hours of delivery with Rh-immune globulin.
- Replacement transfusion to newborn and phototherapy for management of increased bilirubin.
- Regular monitoring of serum bilirubin.
- Adequate hydration and infection prevention.

GLUCOSE-6-PHOSPHATE DEHYDROGENASE DEFICIENCY

G6PD deficiency is the most common human enzyme defect. *Glucose-6-phosphate dehydrogenase deficiency* is an X-linked recessive hereditary disease characterized by abnormally low levels of glucose-6-phosphate dehydrogenase *(G6PD)*, a metabolic enzyme involved in the pentose phosphate pathway, especially important in red blood cell metabolism. Individuals with the disease may exhibit nonimmune hemolytic anemia in response to a number of causes, most commonly infection or exposure to certain medications or chemicals.

G6PD is the most common human enzyme defect, being present in more than 400 million people worldwide. African, Middle Eastern and South Asian people are affected the most.

Signs and Symptoms

Symptomatic patients are almost exclusively male, due to the X-linked pattern of inheritance, but female carriers can be clinically affected due to lyonization, where random inactivation of an X-chromosome in certain cells creates a population of G6PD-deficient red blood cells coexisting with normal red cells. Abnormal red blood cell breakdown (hemolysis) in G6PD deficiency can manifest in a number of ways:

- Prolonged neonatal jaundice, possibly leading to kernicterus (arguably the most serious complication of G6PD deficiency)
- Hemolytic crises in response to:
  - Illness (especially severe infections)
  - Certain drugs (Antimalarial, sulfonamides, aspirin, non-sulfa antibiotics)
  - Certain foods, most notably broad beans
  - Certain chemicals
  - Diabetic ketoacidosis
- Very severe crises can cause acute renal failure.

Diagnosis

Generally, tests will include:

- Complete blood count and reticulocyte count; in active G6PD, Heinz bodies can be seen in red blood cells on a blood film;
- Liver enzymes (to exclude other causes of jaundice);
- Lactate dehydrogenase (elevated in hemolysis and a marker of hemolytic severity);
- Haptoglobin (decreased in hemolysis);
- A 'direct antiglobulin test' (Coombs' test) – this should be negative, as hemolysis in G6PD is not immune-mediated;
- Beutler fluorescent spot test (identify NADPH produced by G6PD under ultraviolet light)
- Direct DNA testing and/or sequencing of the G6PD gene.

Treatment

- Avoidance of the drugs and protein foods that cause hemolysis.
- Vaccination against some common pathogens (e.g. hepatitis A and hepatitis B) may prevent infection-induced attacks.

- In the acute phase of hemolysis, blood transfusions might be necessary.
- Dialysis in acute renal failure.
- Splenectomy, as this is an important site of red cell destruction.
- Folic acid should be used in any disorder featuring a high red cell turnover. Although vitamin E and selenium have antioxidant properties, their use does not decrease the severity of G6PD.

HEREDITARY SPHEROCYTOSIS

It is common cause of inherited disorder of red cell with varied clinical features that may present starting from the neonatal period to second decade of life. It is inherited as autosomal dominant with gene linked to short arm of chromosome 8 or 12.

Pathogenesis

Red cells' stromal protein spectrin and ankyrin are deficient because of reduced synthesis. Spectrin is also unstable and its binding to the red cell membrane is impaired. Due to this, red cells are sequestrated within the spleen. The stasis, hypoxia and metabolic acidosis decrease glycolysis of the red cells. As a result, less ATP is available. Phospholipids, cholesterol and protein are also lost. These metabolic changes cause loss of the red cell membrane, which reduces the surface area. As the cell volume does not concurrently decrease, the cells become more spheroidal or biconvex. Spheroidal cells are retained in the spleen and lyzed.

Clinical Manifestations

- Anemia
- Hyperbilirubinemia
- Pale and mild jaundice
- Spleen enlargement
- Hepatomegaly
- Mild growth and developmental retardation.

Diagnosis

- Peripheral blood smear shows microspherocytosis
- High reticulocyte count and indirect bilirubin level
- Excessive fragile red cells.

Management

- Phototherapy and exchange transfusion for newborns
- Blood transfusion to treat anemia in later childhood
- Folic acid to prevent megoloblastosis
- Splenectomy; preferable after 6 years of age to prevent risk of fulminating infection.

THALASSEMIA

Thalassemia is an inherited abnormality of hemoglobin production. It is also known as Mediterranean anemia and 'Cooley's anemia'. There are many forms and clinical severity varies enormously. The normal hemoglobin molecule has a hem base surrounded by 2 pairs of globin chains. The types of globin are called alpha, beta, gamma and delta. Most types of hemoglobin have 2 α chains and 2 other identical types.

- HbA, the commonest form of adult hemoglobin, has two α and two β chains.
- Fetal hemoglobin has 2 α and 2 γ components and is called HbF. This is the predominant type before birth.
- HbA2 is present in smaller amounts, with 2 α and 2 δ chains.

A decreased rate of production of any of these chains will lead to an imbalance between the amounts of the various forms of Hb in the erythrocytes leading to instability and hemolysis. The thalassemias are classified according to which chain of the globin molecule is affected. In α thalassemia, the production of α globin is deficient and in β thalassemia the production of β globin is defective. The classification of thalassemia major, thalassemia minor and sometimes thalassemia intermedia is based on clinical severity.

It is carried by 150 million or 3% of the world population. It is clinically apparent in 15 million people. The predominant type of thalassemia varies with geography. Beta thalassemia is the most common form around the Mediterranean, North Africa, the Middle East, India, and Eastern Europe. Alpha thalassemia is more common in Southeast Asia, India, the Middle East, and Africa.

Alpha Thalassemia

- Severe homozygous α thalassemia is usually lethal in utero. It should be considered when hydrops fetalis is diagnosed as rhesus incompatibility is a rare cause nowadays.
- Silent carrier α thalassemia is a fairly common type of subclinical thalassemia, usually found by chance among various ethnic African children being investigated for some other condition. There are two α genes on each chromosome 16, giving α thalassemia the unique feature of gene duplication. There is only one β-globin gene on chromosome 11. In the silent carrier state, one of the α genes is usually absent, leaving only 3 of 4 genes (aa/ao). Patients are hematologically normal, except for occasional low RBC indices. This diagnosis cannot be made on Hb electrophoresis, as results are usually normal in all α thalassemia traits. More sophisticated tests are necessary to confirm the diagnosis.
- α thalassemia trait is characterized by mild anemia and low RBC indices. This condition is typically caused by the deletion of 2 α (a) genes on one chromosome 16 (aa/oo) or one from each chromosome (ao/ao). It is found mainly in Southeast Asia, the Indian subcontinent, and some parts of the Middle East.
- Hb H disease results from the deletion or inactivation of three α globin genes (oo/ao). It represents a thalassemia intermedia, with mildly to moderately severe anemia, splenomegaly, jaundice, and abnormal RBC indices. When peripheral blood films stained with supravital stain or reticulocyte preparations are examined, unique inclusions in the RBCs are usually observed. These inclusions represent β chain tetramers (Hb H), which are unstable and precipitate in the erythrocyte, giving it the appearance of a golf ball. These inclusions are called 'Heinz bodies'.

Beta Thalassemia

- In β thalassemia, symptoms of anemia start when the γ chain production ceases and the β chains fail to form in adequate numbers. This is usually in the latter part of the first year of life but sometimes they are 3 to 5 years old because of delay in stopping HbF production.
- In most patients with either α or β thalassemia traits, there are no signs or symptoms.

Clinical Manifestations

- In more severe forms, such as β thalassemia major, the symptoms vary from extremely debilitating in nontransfused patients to mild or absent in those on regular transfusion regimes and closely monitored chelation therapy.
- Ineffective erythropoiesis creates a hypermetabolic state with fever and failure to thrive.
- Overall menifestations vary with severity. Thalassemia minor rarely has any physical abnormalities with Hb over 9g/dL. In patients with the severe forms, the findings on physical examination vary widely depending on how well the disease is controlled.
- Growth retardation is common even with well-controlled chelation therapy.
- Iron overload can cause endocrinopathy with diabetes, thyroid and adrenal disorders
- In severe, untreated cases there may be:
  - Hepatosplenomegaly
  - Bony deformities including frontal bossing, prominent facial bones, and dental malocclusion are striking.
  - Marked pallor and slight-to-moderate jaundice.
  - Severe anemia causes exercise intolerance, cardiac murmur, or even heart failure.

Diagnosis

Blood

- FBC shows a microcytic, hypochromic anemia.
- In the severe forms of thalassemia, the Hb level ranges from 2 to 8g/dL.
- WBC count is usually elevated from the hemolytic process.
- Platelet count may be depressed in splenomegaly.
- Hemoglobin electrophoresis usually gives the diagnosis.
- Serum iron level is elevated, with saturation as high as 80%.
- Ferritin is also raised.

Imaging

- Skeletal surveys show classical changes in the bones but only in patients who are not regularly transfused. They result from expansion of marrow spaces and usually disappear when marrow activity is reduced by regular transfusions.

- Plain skull X-ray shows the classical 'hair on end' appearance. The maxilla may overgrow, with overbite, prominence of the upper incisors, and separation of the orbit. These produce the characteristic facies of thalassemia major.
- Ribs, long bones, and flat bones may be deformed.
- Chest X-ray to see cardiac size and shape.
- CT or MRI scan can be used to evaluate the amount of iron in the liver in patients on chelation therapy.

Other Tests

- ECG and echocardiogram are used to monitor cardiac function.
- HLA typing is required where bone marrow transplantation is considered.
- Eye examinations, hearing tests, and renal function tests are needed to monitor deferoxamine therapy.
- Bone marrow aspiration is sometimes needed at the time of diagnosis to exclude other conditions that may present as thalassemia major.
- Liver biopsy is used to assess iron deposition and the degree of hemochromatosis.
- Measurement of excretion of iron in the urine after a challenge test of deferrioxamine evaluates the need for chelation therapy.

Staging

A staging system has been developed, based on history of blood transfusions and cardiac symptoms, to decide when to initiate chelation therapy.

- **Stage I** are patients who have received fewer than 100 units of packed RBCs. They are usually asymptomatic. The echocardiogram shows only slight left ventricular wall thickening, and both the radionuclide cineangiogram and the 24-hour ECG are normal.
- **Stage II** patients have received between 100 and 400 units of blood and may have some fatigue. Echocardiograms may show some left ventricular wall thickening and dilatation but the ejection fraction is normal. The radionuclide cineangiogram

findings are normal at rest but show no increase or fall in ejection fraction during exercise. Atrial and ventricular ectopic beats are usually found on the 24-hour ECG.

- **Stage III** patients have symptoms ranging from palpitations to congestive heart failure. The ejection fraction on echocardiography is decreased. There is normal or decreased ejection fraction on cineangiogram at rest, and it falls on exercise. The 24-hour ECG reveals atrial and ventricular premature beats, often in pairs or in runs.

Complications

- Iron overload is one of the major causes of morbidity in severe forms of thalassemia even if they are not transfused.
- Bleeding tendency, susceptibility to infection, and organ dysfunction are related to iron overload.
- Repeated transfusions increase the risk of bloodborne diseases. including hepatitis B and hepatitis C, although nowadays all blood is screened for these diseases.
- Infection with rare opportunistic organisms may cause pyrexia and enteritis in patients with iron overload. *Yersinia enterocolitica* thrives with the abundant iron. Unexplained fever, especially with diarrhea, should be treated with gentamicin and co-trimoxazole, even when cultures are negative.
- Osteoporosis is common and apparently multifactorial in etiology but pamidronate is an effective treatment.
- Hyperuricemia sometimes produces gout.
- With increasing length of survival, hepatocellular carcinoma is becoming an increasing problem.
- Deferrioxamine can cause toxicity.

Management

- *Blood transfusion:* Transfusion improves both quality and quantity of life in severe cases. The target is not to let Hb fall below 9 to 9.5g/dL. Transfused blood should be leucocyte poor. This is especially important if a bone marrow transplant is considered at some stage.
- *Neocyte transfusion:* Selecting and transfusion of younger red cells (neocytes), which will increase the interval between two transfusions and decrease the transfusion requirement.

- *Chelation therapy:* Desferrioxamine is given parenterally to aid iron excretion. The dose and means of delivery vary according to the needs of the patient. Oral chelating agents are being developed. Oral deferiprone used in combination with desferrioximine produces a greater effect than either alone. Together they increase iron excretion, decrease ferritin levels and improve glucose tolerance in borderline cases, suggesting some reversal of damage to the pancreas by iron. Folic acid and vitamin E deficiency may both need treating.
- *Splenectomy:* When hypersplenism occurs, splenectomy is often undertaken.
- Cure can be achieved with a bone marrow transplant from a compatible, usually related, donor.
- Recently, embryo selection has been used to produce an immunologically compatible sib. While this induces horror in the expected quarters, the child is not simply a tissue culture but will be a loved and wanted member of the family. The ethical and legal issues have been discussed.
- All families should be offered genetic counseling. In mild cases, no treatment is required but *anemia should not be treated with iron unless iron deficiency had been substantiated.*
- Avoid food rich in iron. Extra vitamin E, folic acid and some vitamin C may be beneficial. Tea and coffee can reduce the absorption of iron.
- *Gene manipulation and Gene therapy are under research.*

SICKLE-CELL ANEMIA

Sickle cell disease or *sickle-cell anemia* is a blood disorder characterized by red blood cells that assume an abnormal, rigid, sickle shape. Sickling decreases the red cells' flexibility and results in a risk of various other complications. Life expectancy is shortened, with studies reporting an average life expectancy of 42 and 48 years for males and females, respectively.

Sickle-cell anemia affects millions of people worldwide. Sickle cell disease occurs more commonly in people from parts of tropical and subtropical regions where malaria is or was common. It is particularly common among people whose ancestors come from

Africa, Mediterranean countries (such as Greece, Turkey, and Italy), the Arabian Peninsula, India, and Spanish-speaking regions (South America, Central America, and parts of the Caribbean).

Sickle-cell anemia is the most common inherited blood disorder in the United States, affecting 70,000 to 80,000 Americans. The disease occurs in approximately 1 in 500 African-American newborns and 1 in 1,000 to 1,400 Hispanic-American births.

Causes and Pathology of Sickle-cell anemia

- Sickle-cell anemia is caused by a point mutation in the β-globin chain of hemoglobin, causing the amino acid glutamic acid to be replaced with the hydrophobic amino acid valine at the sixth position. The β-globin gene is found on the short arm of chromosome 11. The association of two wild-type α-globin subunits with two mutant β-globin subunits forms hemoglobin S (HbS). Under low-oxygen conditions, the absence of a polar amino acid at position six of the β-globin chain promotes the non-covalent polymerization (aggregation) of hemoglobin, which distorts red blood cells into a sickle shape and decreases their elasticity.
- The loss of red blood cell elasticity is central to the pathophysiology of sickle cell disease. Normal red blood cells are quite elastic, which allows the cells to deform to pass through capillaries. In sickle cell disease, low-oxygen tension promotes red blood cell sickling and repeated episodes of sickling damage the cell membrane and decrease the cell's elasticity. These cells fail to return to normal shape when normal oxygen tension is restored. As a consequence, these rigid blood cells are unable to deform as they pass through narrow capillaries, leading to vessel occlusion and ischemia.
- Sickle-cell anemia is an inherited disease. People who have the disease inherit two copies of the sickle cell gene-one from each parent. The sickle cell gene causes the body to make abnormal hemoglobin. Two copies of the sickle cell gene are needed for the body to make the abnormal hemoglobin found in sickle-cell anemia.

Sickle cell Trait

If you inherit only one copy of the sickle cell gene (from one parent), you will not have sickle-cell anemia. Instead, you will have sickle-

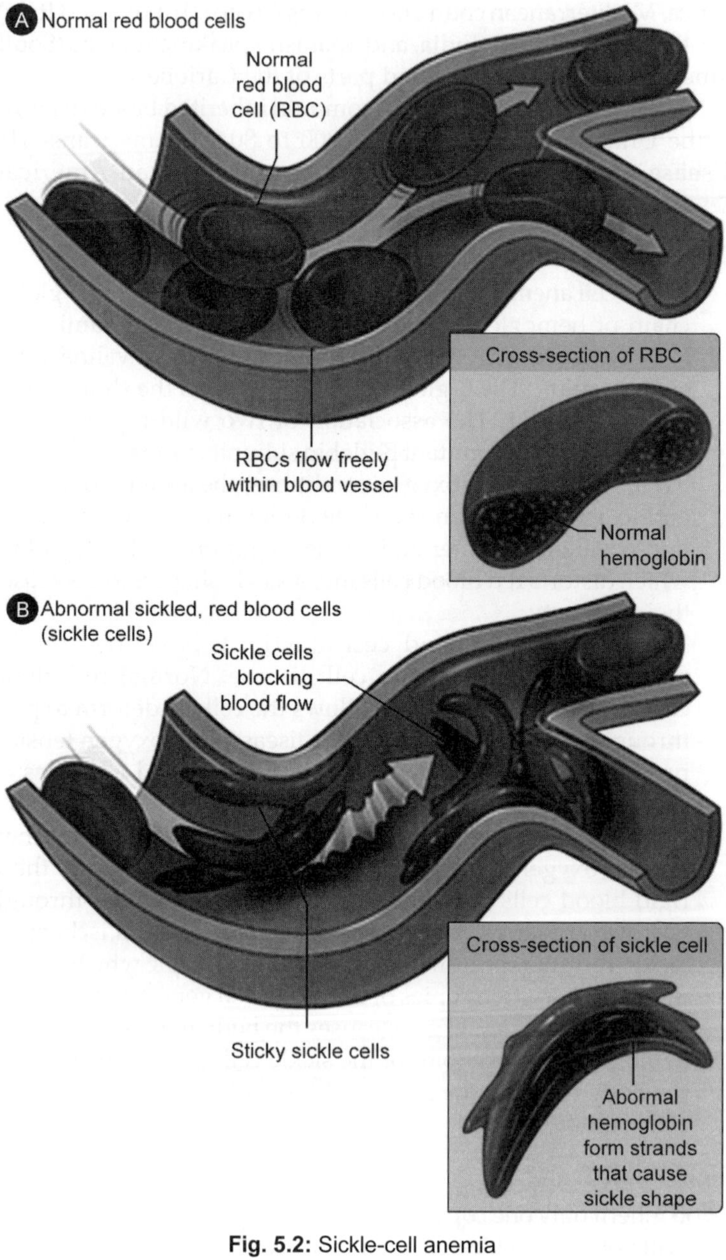

Fig. 5.2: Sickle-cell anemia

cell trait. People who have sickle cell trait usually have no symptoms and lead normal lives. However, they can pass the sickle cell gene to their children.

Inheritance Pattern

This condition is inherited in an autosomal recessive pattern, which means two copies of the gene in each cell are altered. Most often, the parents of an individual with an autosomal recessive disorder are carriers of one copy of the altered gene but do not show signs and symptoms of the disorder.

Clinical Manifestations

- The signs and symptoms of sickle-cell anemia vary.
- Some people have mild symptoms. Others have very severe symptoms and often are hospitalized for treatment. Sickle-cell anemia is present at birth, but many infants do not show any signs until after 4 months of age.
- The most common signs and symptoms are linked to anemia and pain. The most common symptom of anemia is fatigue (feeling tired or weak). Other signs and symptoms of anemia include:
  - Shortness of breath
  - Dizziness
  - Headache
  - Coldness in the hands and feet
  - Pale skin
  - Chest pain
- *Sickle cell crisis:* Sudden pain throughout the body is a common symptom of sickle-cell anemia. Sickle cell crises often affect the bones, lungs, abdomen, and joints. A sickle cell crisis occurs when sickled red blood cells form clumps in the bloodstream. These clumps of cells block blood flow through the small blood vessels in the limbs and organs. This can cause pain and organ damage.
- Other signs and symptoms are linked to the disease's complications.

Diagnosis

- Prenatal screening through amniocentesis.
- Newborn screening/testing for sickle-cell anemia as part of routine screening. If the test shows some sickle hemoglobin, then a second blood test is done to confirm the diagnosis. The second test should be done as soon as possible and within the first month of life.
- Later diagnosis is usually based on clinical history and sickling in peripheral blood sample. Hemoglobin S is identified by electrophoresis and solubility studies. HbS moves slower than HbA on electrophoresis.
- DNA sequences can be amplified using PCR technique.

Complications of Sickle-cell anemia

- Hand-Foot Syndrome
- Splenic Crisis
- Acute Chest Syndrome
- Infections
- Pulmonary Arterial Hypertension
- Stroke
- Delayed Growth and Puberty in Children
- Eye Problems
- Ulcers on the Legs
- Priapism
- Multiple Organ Failure
- Gallstones

Management

Sickle-cell anemia has no widely available cure. However, treatments can help relieve symptoms and treat complications. The goals of treating sickle-cell anemia are to relieve pain; prevent infections, eye damage, and strokes; and control complications (if they occur).

- *Bone marrow transplants* may offer a cure in a small number of sickle-cell anemia cases.
- Researchers continue to look for new treatments for the disease. These include *gene therapy* and *improved bone marrow transplants*.

- *Pain management* through analgesics (NSAIDs, and narcotics) and fluid administration to prevent sickling of red cells. Hydroxyurea is used to prevent painful crises, not to treat them when they occur.
- *Blood transfusions* are commonly used to treat worsening anemia and sickle cell complications. A sudden worsening of anemia due to an infection or enlargement of the spleen is a common reason for a blood transfusion.
- Routine vaccination and prophylactic antibiotic administration for prevention of infection.
- New drugs under research are; Butyric acid, Nitric oxide, and Decitadine. Butyric acid is a food additive that may increase normal hemoglobin in the blood. Nitric oxide may make sickle cells less sticky and keep blood vessels open. People who have sickle-cell anemia have low levels of nitric oxide in their blood. Decitadine increases hemoglobin F levels (this type of hemoglobin carries more oxygen). It may be a good choice instead of hydroxyurea.
- *Treating Other Complications*
  - Acute chest syndrome is a severe and life-threatening complication of sickle-cell anemia. Treatment usually requires hospitalization and may include oxygen, blood transfusions, antibiotics, pain medicine, and checking the body's fluids.
  - If you have leg ulcers due to sickle-cell anemia, you may be given strong pain medicines. Ulcers can be treated with cleansing solutions and medicated creams or ointments. Skin grafts may be needed if the condition continues. Bed rest and keeping the legs raised to reduce swelling are helpful, although not always possible.
  - Gallbladder surgery may be needed if the presence of gallstones leads to gallbladder disease.
  - Priapism (a painful erection of penis in males) can be treated with fluids or surgery.

BLACKFAN-DIAMOND ANEMIA

Blackfan-Diamond Anemia (BDA) is a rare blood disorder that is caused by a failure of the bone marrow to generate enough red blood cells. It is characterized by deficiency of red blood cells at birth (congenital hypoplastic anemia) as well as slow growth, abnormal weakness and fatigue, paleness of the skin, characteristic facial abnormalities, protruding shoulder blades (scapulae), webbing or abnormal shortening of the neck due to fusion of certain bones in the spine (cervical vertebrae), hand deformities, congenital heart defects, and/or other abnormalities. The symptoms and physical findings associated with Blackfan-Diamond Anemia vary greatly from case to case.

HEMOPHILIA

Hemophilia is a hereditary genetic disorder, where there is congenital deficiency of plasma coagulation factor that impairs the body's ability to control blood clotting or coagulation. It is inherited in X-linked recessive pattern. Hemophilia is quite rare, with only about 1 instance in every 10,000 births (or 1 in 5,001 male births) for hemophilia A and 1 in 50,000 births for hemophilia B.

Types and Causes

- *Hemophilia A (Classic hemophilia)* is an X-linked genetic disorder involving a lack of functional clotting Factor VIII and represents 90% of hemophilia cases.
- *Hemophilia B (Christmas disease)* is an X-linked genetic disorder involving a lack of functional clotting Factor IX. It is less severe but more uncommon than Hemophilia A.
- *Hemophilia C* is an autosomal recessive genetic disorder involving a lack of functional clotting Factor XI.

Inheritance Pattern and Genetic Pathology

Females possess two X-chromosomes, whereas males have one X and one Y chromosome. Since the mutations causing the disease are recessive, a woman carrying the defect on one of her X-chromosomes may not be affected by it, as the equivalent allele on her other chromosome should express itself to produce the necessary clotting factors. However, the Y-chromosome in men has no gene for factors VIII or IX. If the genes responsible for production of factor VIII or factor IX present on a male's X-chromosome are deficient, there is no equivalent on the Y-chromosome. So, the deficient gene is not masked by the dominant allele and he will develop the illness.

Since a male receives his single X-chromosome from his mother, the son of a healthy female silently carrying the deficient gene will have a 50% chance of inheriting that gene from her and with it the disease; and if his mother is affected with hemophilia, he will have a 100% chance of being a hemophiliac. In contrast, for a female to inherit the disease, she must receive two deficient X-chromosomes, one from her mother and the other from her father (who must, therefore, be a hemophiliac himself). Hence, hemophilia is far more common among males than females. However it is possible for female carriers to become mild hemophiliacs due to lyonization (inactivation) of the X chromosomes. Hemophiliac daughters are more common than they once were, as improved treatments for the disease have allowed more hemophiliac males to survive to adulthood and become parents. Adult females may experience menorrhagia (heavy periods) due to the bleeding tendency. The pattern of inheritance is criss-cross type.

A mother who is a carrier has a 50% chance of passing the faulty X chromosome to her daughter, while an affected father will always pass on the affected gene to his daughters. A son cannot inherit the defective gene from his father.

As with all genetic disorders, it is, of course, also possible for a human to acquire it spontaneously through mutation, rather than inheriting it, because of a new mutation in one of their parents' gametes. Spontaneous mutations account for about 33% of all cases of hemophilia A. About 30% of cases of Hemophilia B are the result of a spontaneous gene mutation.

Clinical Manifestations

The major signs and symptoms of hemophilia are excessive bleeding and easy bruising.

- The extent of bleeding depends on the type and severity of the hemophilia. Children with mild hemophilia may not have symptoms until they have excessive bleeding from a dental procedure, an accident, or surgery. Males with severe hemophilia may bleed heavily after circumcision. Bleeding can be obvious (external bleeding) or hidden within the body (internal bleeding). Signs of excessive external bleeding include:
  - Bleeding in the mouth from a cut or bite or from cutting or losing a tooth

- Nosebleeds for no obvious reason
- Heavy bleeding from a minor cut
- Bleeding from a cut that resumes after stopping for a short time

- Signs of internal bleeding include blood in the urine (from bleeding in the kidneys or bladder) and blood in the stool (from bleeding in the intestines or stomach).
- *Bleeding in the brain:* Internal bleeding in the brain is a very serious complication of hemophilia that can happen after a simple bump on the head or a more serious injury. The signs and symptoms of bleeding in the brain include:
  - Long-lasting painful headaches or neck pain or stiffness
  - Repeated vomiting
  - Changes in behavior or being very sleepy
  - Sudden weakness or clumsiness of the arms or legs or difficulty walking
  - Double vision
  - Convulsions or seizures.

Diagnosis

- Blood tests for bleeding time, clotting time and
- Blood level of clotting factors. Hemophilia A and B are classified as mild, moderate, or severe, depending on the amount of clotting factor VIII or IX in the blood.

Mild hemophilia	5–30% of normal factor
Moderate hemophilia	1–5% of normal factor
Severe hemophilia	< 1% of normal factor

Management

- *Replacement therapy:* Giving or replacing the clotting factor that's too low or missing. Concentrates of clotting factor VIII (for hemophilia A) or clotting factor IX (for hemophilia B) are given slowly by intravenous dripp or injection.
- *Desmopressin:* Desmopressin (DDAVP) is a synthetic hormone used to treat people with mild to moderate hemophilia A. DDAVP cannot be used to treat hemophilia B or severe hemophilia A. It is administered intravenous or nasal spray, which stimulates the release of stored factor VIII.

- *Antifibrinolytic medicines:* Tablet ranexamic acid and aminocaproic acid may be used with replacement therapy. Usually given before dental work, for treatment of nasal or oral bleeding or mild intestinal bleeding.
- *Gene therapy:* Researchers are trying to develop ways to correct the defective genes that cause hemophilia to cure the disorder. But it is still under trial.
- Specific exercises to strengthen the joints, particularly the elbows, knees, and ankles, after an internal bleed occurs and on a daily basis to strengthen the muscles and joints to prevent new bleeding problems. Many recommended exercises include standard sports warm-up and training exercises, such as stretching of the calves, ankle circles, elbow flexions, and Quadriceps sets.
- Selected alternative therapies-like self-hypnosis and certain herbs.

von WILLEBRAND DISEASE (vWD)

von Willebrand disease is an inherited bleeding disorder that occurs due to qualitative or quantitative deficiency of von Willebrand factor (vWF), a multimeric protein that is required for platelet adhesion. In humans, the incidence of vWD is roughly about 1 in 100 individuals. Because most forms are rather mild, they are detected more often in women, whose bleeding tendency shows during menstruation. The actual abnormality (which does not necessarily lead to disease) occurs in 0.9–3% of the population. It may be more severe or apparent in people with blood type O.

Types of von Willebrand Disease

- *Type 1 vWD:* In this, person has a low level of the von Willebrand factor, and may have lower levels of factor VIII than normal. This is the mildest and most common form of the disease. About 3 out of 4 people who have vWD have type 1.
- *Type 2 vWD:* In this the von Willebrand factor does not work the way it is supposed to work. Type 2 is divided into subtypes: 2A, 2B, 2M, and 2N. Different gene mutations cause each type, and each is treated differently. This makes knowing the exact type of vWD that one has very important.

- *Type 3 vWD:* In this, usually person has no von Willebrand factor and low levels of factor VIII. Type 3 is the most serious form of vWD, but it is very rare.

Inheritance Pattern and Genetic Pathology

von Willebrand disease types I and II are inherited in an autosomal dominant pattern. von Willebrand disease type III (and sometimes II) is inherited in an autosomal recessive pattern. The vWF gene is located on chromosome twelve (12p13.2). It has 52 exons spanning 178kbp. Types 1 and 2 are inherited as autosomal dominant traits and type 3 is inherited as autosomal recessive. Occasionally, type 2 also inherits recessively.

Clinical Manifestations

The signs and symptoms of von Willebrand disease (vWD) depend on the type and severity of the disease. Many people have following mild-to-moderate bleeding symptoms in type-1 or type-2 vWD:

- Frequent large bruises from minor bumps or injuries
- Frequent or hard to stop nosebleeds
- Extended bleeding from the gums after a dental procedure
- Menorrhagia (Heavy or extended menstrual bleeding in women)
- Blood in your stools from bleeding in your intestines or stomach
- Blood in your urine from bleeding in your kidneys or bladder
- Heavy bleeding after a cut or other accident
- Heavy bleeding after surgery.

People with type 3 vWD may have all of the symptoms listed above, as well as severe bleeding episodes for no reason. These bleeding episodes can be life-threatening if not treated right away. They also may have bleeding into soft tissues or joints, causing severe pain and swelling.

Diagnosis

- Complete blood count (especially platelet counts)
- APTT (activated partial thromboplastin time), prothrombin time, thrombin time and fibrinogen level. Testing for factor IX may also be performed if hemophilia B is suspected.
- A platelet function assay.

- Blood plasma for quantitative and qualitative deficiencies of vWF.
- Clotting Factor VIII levels estimation.
- Testing for factor IX may also be performed if hemophilia B is suspected.
- Other coagulation factor assays may be performed depending on the results of a coagulation screen.

Management

Treatment is based on the type and severity of von Willebrand disease (vWD). Most cases of vWD are mild, and may need treatment only if have surgery, tooth extraction, or an accident.

Specific Treatments

- Desmopressin (DDAVP) is a synthetic hormone that is usually given by injection or nasal spray. It makes the body to release more von Willebrand factor and factor VIII into your bloodstream. DDAVP works for most patients who have type 1 vWD and for some who have type 2 vWD.
- von Willebrand factor replacement therapy is an infusion of a concentrate of von Willebrand factor and factor VIII. This treatment can be used if:
  - DDAVP is contraindicated or needs extended treatment
  - Type 1 vWD that does not respond to DDAVP.
  - In type 2 or type 3 vWD.
- Antifibrinolytic drugs help prevent the breakdown of blood clots. They are mostly used to stop bleeding after minor surgery, tooth extraction, or an injury. They may be used alone or together with DDAVP and replacement therapy.
- Fibrin glue is medicine that is placed directly on a wound to stop the bleeding.

Treatments for women: Treatments for women who have vWD with heavy menstrual bleeding include:

- *Combined oral contraceptives:* The contraceptives can increase the amount of von Willebrand factor and factor VIII in bloodstream and reduce menstrual blood loss.
- *A levonorgestrel intrauterine device:* This is a contraceptive device that contains progestin. It is placed in the uterus.

- *Aminocaproic acid or tranexamic acid:* These antifibrinolytic drugs can reduce bleeding by slowing the breakdown of blood clots.
- DDAVP.
- Endometrial ablation, who has completed the family.

CONGENITAL AMEGAKARYOCYTIC THROMBOCYTOPENIA (CAMT)

Congenital amegakaryocytic thrombocytopenia (CAMT) is a rare inherited disorder. The primary manifestations are thrombocytopenia and megakaryocytopenia, or low numbers of platelets and megakaryocytes, which may make a person potential for bleeding. There is an absence of megakaryocytes in the bone marrow with no associated physical abnormalities. The cause for this disorder appears to be a mutation in the gene for the TPO receptor, *c-mpl,* despite high levels of serum TPO. In addition, there may be abnormalities with the central nervous system including the cerebrum and cerebellum which could cause symptoms. The primary treatment for CAMT is bone marrow transplantation. Bone Marrow/Stem Cell Transplant is the only thing that ultimately cures this genetic disease. Frequent platelet transfusions are required to protect the patient from bleeding to death until transplant is done, although this is not always the case.

GENETIC HEMOCHROMATOSIS

'Hemochromatosis is a disorder that causes the body to absorb too much iron from the diet. The excess iron is stored in the body's tissues and organs, particularly the heart, liver, pancreas, and joints. Because humans cannot increase excretion of iron, the extra iron accumulates over time and eventually can damage the tissue or organ.'

Normally, an individual gets 10 to 20 milligrams of iron a day in diet. However, of that amount, the body typically only absorbs 1 to 2 milligrams. The rest of the iron is not absorbed, and some is lost in any skin cells that are shed. Individuals with hereditary hemochromatosis absorb 3 to 4 milligrams of iron through the intestine, and the body does not have any way to get rid of it. Over the decades, this iron accumulates in organs including the heart, liver, and pancreas. Iron accumulation results in organ damage and other conditions like diabetes and abnormal heart rhythms that indicate that the organs are sick.

It takes a long time for organs to sustain enough damage due to excess iron before they begin to malfunction. Excess iron accumulation in the organs begins in childhood, but the symptoms of this disorder do not usually appear until adulthood. Symptoms of hemochromatosis begin to occur when the body has stored 20 grams or more of iron, which can take 4 to 6 decades.

Etiology and Genetic Basis

The most common cause of hemochromatosis is *genetics,* known as hereditary hemochromatosis, By definition, hereditary hemochromatosis is an iron overload disorder that runs in families: An individual develops the condition by inheriting altered, or mutated, copies of the HFE gene (which regulates iron absorption in our bodies) from his or her parents. However, even though the disorder is clearly inherited, it is not always easy to spot a pattern of disease within families who have the mutation. This is because people can be carriers of a hemochromatosis mutation without having any symptoms or complications. Thus, the fact that no one in one's immediate or extended family has symptoms of hereditary hemochromatos does not mean he/she cannot develop this disorder.

In fact, everyone who carries mutated copies of the HFE gene does not develop disorder, but a far smaller number of people develop fully symptomatic hemochromatosis. Others who carry a mutation, but do not have symptoms of hemochromatosis, may be at increased risk for other disorders, such as cardiovascular problems.

Inheritance Pattern

Although approximately 1 out of every 200 people is a carrier of one of the genetic mutations that cause hereditary hemochromatosis, not nearly that many people actually develop symptoms or complications from the disorder. This is because hereditary hemochromatosis is passed through families in what is known as autosomal recessive fashion, which means that an individual must inherit a mutated copy of the HFE gene from both parents to develop the disorder. A person who has inherited only one defective gene will most likely be a carrier of hemochromatosis and will not have the disease. A carrier can pass the defective gene on to his or her children.

- If only one parent is a carrier of a defective gene, the child will not have hemochromatosis; however, there is a 50% chance that the child will be a carrier.
- If both parents are carriers, there is only a 25% chance that the child will have hemochromatosis, but a 50% chance that the child will be a carrier.

Clinical Manifestations

Over 30 different symptoms are associated with hemochromatosis. Symptoms may begin anywhere from age 30 to age 60, although in some rare cases they occur as early as 20. Many of the early symptoms of hemochromatosis are nonspecific, including:

- Weakness
- Fatigue
- Abdominal pain
- General muscle aches
- Loss of sex drive
- Impotence
- Cessation of monthly menstrual cycles
- Joint pain in the fingers
- Shortness of breath on exertion
- Increased skin pigmentation (a bronze color)
- Loss of body hair
- Hepatomegaly.

If untreated, or not diagnosed early enough, hemochromatosis can lead to diabetes, joint pain, dysarrhythmias, heart failure, cirrhosis of the liver, liver failure, or (rarely) liver cancer, impotence or decreased sex drive in men and early menopause in women.

Factors Affecting Clinical Presentation

Many factors affect clinical presentation of hemochromatosis.

- *Alcohol:* Because alcohol is an independent toxin to the liver, liver disease may be present earlier due to the combined effects of alcohol and iron.
- *Diet:* People who take vitamin supplements that contain iron, or take vitamin C, which increases the body's effectiveness

at absorbing iron, may have symptoms at a younger-than-average age.

- *Gender:* Men are twice as likely to go to their doctor with symptoms of hereditary hemochromatosis than women. In untreated men, symptoms usually begin between age 40 and 60. For women, the symptoms usually start later, between age 50 and 65. One reason is that women have regular episodes of blood loss through menstruation or childbirth.
- *Blood loss:* Individuals who lose iron through blood donation may also delay the onset of symptoms.
- *Mutation type:* There are two common mutations in a gene called HFE, which is known to cause hereditary hemochromatosis. One of these two mutations, H63D, is associated with a less severe and later onset form of hemochromatosis. People who have one or two copies of this mutation have a milder form of the disease compared to people who have two copies of the other common mutation (called C282Y).

Diagnosis

- *Screening diagnosis of hemochromatosis is done through:*
  - *Transferrin Saturation Test*: The transferrin saturation test determines how much iron is held by the protein that carries iron in the blood. A fasting transferrin saturation of 60 percent or higher in men, or 50 percent or higher in women, on at least two occasions, is considered a sign of iron overload. However, factors in addition to hemochromatosis can cause iron overload. Values of greater than 45 percent are considered suggestive of hemochromatosis and deserve further evaluation.
  - *Serum Ferritin Level Test:* The serum ferritin test acts as an indirect measure of iron storage in the liver. Serum ferritin levels are considered in the normal range for males and postmenopausal females if they are between 20 and 300 μg/L, or between 20 and 200 μg/L for premenopausal females. People with advanced hemochromatosis may have serum ferritin levels as high as 15,000 μg/L. However, other factors besides hemochromatosis can cause high serum ferritin levels, including liver disease, infection, cancer,

heart disease, AIDS, metabolic disorders, and inflammatory conditions, such as arthritis.

- If individuals have elevated serum ferritin levels, or fasting transferrin saturation levels, genetic testing for hemochromatosis may help to identify the reason for the increase in iron storage.
- *Liver Biopsy:* Before the availability of genetic testing for hemochromatosis, a liver biopsy with measurements of hepatic iron was considered the 'gold standard' for diagnosing hemochromatosis. A liver biopsy is now rarely needed to make the diagnosis, and is usually only used in cases of apparent iron overload with a negative genetic test result and no other family history of hemochromatosis. However, a liver biopsy is the only test that can tell whether cirrhosis is present, which is the only complication that affects the lifespan of someone with hemochromatosis, since it increases the risk for liver cancer. A liver biopsy should be recommended for anyone with hemochromatosis who is also:
  - Over 40 years old
  - Has a ferritin level over 1000 μg/L, or
  - Has abnormal liver function test results
- *HLA Antigen Testing:* Testing of HLA antigens was also once used to help make the diagnosis. This was because the gene for hemochromatosis was very close to the highly polymorphic HLA genes on chromosome six, and certain HLA gene alleles were often found in patients with hemochromatosis. This test had many false positive and false negative results, and is now obsolete (although still offered by some laboratories).
- *Genetic Testing:* To identify affected gene.

Management

Management includes:

- Weekly phlebotomy until iron levels reach normal
- *Chelation therapy:* The chelating agents deferoxamine and deferasirox bind to iron in blood and help to remove excess iron present in the body.

- Preventing further accumulation of iron through blood removal three to four times a year, and avoiding supplemental iron and high doses of vitamin C.
- Regular monitoring of the serum ferritin levels. For effective treatment, serum ferritin iron levels are less than 50 nanograms (ng) per milliliter and transferrin saturation levels are less than 50% should be maintained.

HUNTINGTON'S DISEASE

Huntington's disease, also called *Huntington's chorea, chorea major,* or *HD, is a genetic neurological disorder characterized after onset by uncoordinated, jerky body movements and a decline in some mental abilities.* These characteristics vary per individual, physical ones less so, but the differing decline in mental abilities can lead to a number of potential behavioral problems.

The disorder itself is not fatal, but as symptoms progress, complications reducing life expectancy increase. Research of HD has increased greatly in the last few decades, but its exact mechanism is unknown, so symptoms are managed individually. Globally, up to 7 people in 100,000 have the disorder, although there are localized regions with a higher incidence. Onset of physical symptoms occurs gradually and can begin at any age, although it is statistically most common in a person's mid-forties (with a 30-year spread). If onset is before age twenty, the condition is classified as juvenile HD.

The disorder is named after George Huntington, an American physician who published a remarkably accurate description in 1872. In 1983, a marker for the altered DNA causing the disease was found, followed a decade later by discovery of a single, causal, gene. As it was caused by a single gene, an accurate genetic test for HD was developed. This was one of the first inherited genetic disorders for which such a test was possible. Due to the availability of this test, and similar characteristics with other neurological disorders, the amount of HD research has increased greatly in recent years.

Genetic Basis

Huntington's disease is one of the several trinucleotide repeat disorders caused by the length of a repeated section of a gene exceeding the normal range. The huntingtin gene (HTT) normally provides the information to produce Huntingtin protein, but when affected, produces mutant Huntingtin (mHTT) instead.

The Huntingtin gene (*HTT*) is located on the short arm of chromosome 4 (4p16.3). *HTT* contains a sequence of three DNA bases—cytosine-adenine-guanine (CAG)—repeated multiple times (i.e. ...CAGCAGCAG...) on its 5′ end, known as a trinucleotide repeat. CAG is the genetic code for the amino acid glutamine. So, a series of them results in the production of a chain of glutamine known as polyglutamine or polyQ tract, and the repeated part of the gene, the *PolyQ region*.

A polyQ region containing fewer than 36 glutamines results in production of the cytoplasmic protein called huntingtin (HTT). Generally, people have less than 27 repeated glutamines. However, a sequence of 36 or more glutamines results in the production of form of HTT which has different characteristics. This altered form called mutant HTT or more commonly *mHTT*, increases the rate of neuronal decay in certain types of neurons, affecting regions of the brain with a higher proportion or dependency on them. Generally, the number of CAG repeats is related to how much this process is affected, and correlates with age at onset and the rate of progression of symptoms. For example, 36–39 repeats result in much later onset and slower progression of symptoms than the mean, such that some individuals may die of other causes before they even manifest symptoms of Huntington's disease, this is termed 'reduced penetrance'. With very large repeat counts, HD can occur under the age of 20 years, when it is then referred to as juvenile HD, akinetic-rigid, or Westphal variant HD and accounts for about 7 percent of HD carriers.

Table 5.5: Huntingtin gene repeat count and severity of disease

Repeat count	Classification	Disease status
< 27	Normal	Unaffected
27–35	Intermediate	Unaffected
36–39	Reduced penetrance	+/– Affected
> 39	Full penetrance	Affected

Inheritance Pattern

Huntington's disease is inherited autosomal dominantly, meaning that an affected individual typically inherits a copy of the gene with an expanded trinucleotide repeat (the mutant allele) from an affected parent. In this type of inheritance pattern, each offspring of an affected individual has a 50% chance of inheriting the mutant allele and, therefore, being affected with the disorder.

Homozygous individuals, who have two affected genes, are very rare except in large consanguineous families. While HD seemed to be the first disease for which homozygotes did not differ in clinical expression or course from typical heterozygotes, more recent analysis suggests that homozygosity affects the phenotype and the rate of disease progression but does not alter the age of onset, suggesting that the mechanisms for these factors differ.

Clinical Manifestations

- The most characteristic physical symptoms are jerky, random, and uncontrollable movements called 'chorea'. In a few cases, very slow movement and stiffness (called 'bradykinesia' and 'dystonia') occur instead, and often become more prominent than the chorea as the disorder progresses. Abnormal movements are initially exhibited as general lack of coordination, an unsteady gait and slurring of speech, but, as the disease progresses, any function that requires muscle control is affected, causing physical instability, abnormal facial expression, and difficulties chewing and swallowing. Eating difficulties commonly cause weight loss and may lead to malnutrition. Associated symptoms involve sleep cycle disturbances, including insomnia and rapid eye movement sleep alterations. Juvenile HD generally progresses faster, is more likely to exhibit rigidity and bradykinesia, instead of chorea, and commonly includes seizures.
- Selected cognitive abilities are impaired progressively. Especially affected are executive functions, which include planning, cognitive flexibility, abstract thinking, rule acquisition, initiating appropriate actions and inhibiting inappropriate actions. Psychomotor function, controlling

muscles, perception and spatial skills are also affected. As the disease progresses, memory deficits tend to appear. Memory impairments reported range from short-term memory deficits to long-term memory difficulties, including deficits in episodic (memory of one's life), procedural (memory of the body of how to perform an activity) and working memory.

- Psychiatric symptoms vary far more than cognitive and physical ones, and may include anxiety, depression, a reduced display of emotions (blunted effect), egocentrism, aggression, and compulsive behavior, which can cause, or worsen addictions, including alcoholism and gambling, or hypersexuality. Difficulties in recognizing other people's negative expressions have also been observed.

Diagnosis

- *Prenatal screening through:*
  - Preimplantation genetic diagnosis in the setting of in vitro fertilization.
  - Prenatal diagnosis in case of family history to decide about continuation of pregnancy.
- *Postnatal disease diagnosis through:*
  - A physical and/or psychological examination.
  - Presymptomatic testing is possible using a blood test which counts the numbers of CAG repeats in each of the HTT alleles, although a positive result is not considered a diagnosis, since it may be obtained decades before onset of symptoms. A negative blood test means that the individual does not carry the expanded copy of the gene.
  - A full pathological diagnosis can only be established by a neurological examination's findings and/or demonstration of cell loss in the areas affected by HD, supported by a cranial CT or MRI scan findings.

Management

- Antidepressants, sedatives, and low doses of antipsychotics for cognitive and psychological symptoms.
- There is limited evidence for specific treatments aimed at controlling the chorea and other movement abnormalities,

although tetrabenazine has been shown to reduce the severity of the chorea.

- High-calorie diet to maintain body weight.
- Thickening agents can be added to drinks as swallowing becomes more difficult, as thicker fluids are easier and safer to swallow.
- Percutaneous endoscopic gastrostomy, when eating becomes too hazardous or uncomfortable. A 'stomach PEG' greatly reduces the chances of aspiration of food, which can lead to aspiration pneumonia, and also increases the amount of nutrients and calories that can be ingested, aiding the body's natural defenses.
- As for any patient with neurologic deficits, a multidisciplinary rehabilitation approach is the key to limiting and overcoming disability.

MENTAL ILLNESS

Mental illness is a psychological or behavioral pattern that occurs in an individual and is thought to cause distress or disability that is not expected as part of normal development or culture. Mental illnesses are broadly classified as neurotic illness and psychotic illness. As such, there is not a single accepted or consistent cause of mental illnesses.

Almost regardless of pathologic state, it is widely accepted that genetic information has started to provide or will soon provide a profound change in diagnosis and therapy in medicine. The potential for revolutionary changes in clinical management is based on the detail with which genetics is revealing the molecular steps of the pathophysiologic process. In psychiatric illness, this is also true, but there is a strong argument for predicting an effect that is even more fundamental than it is in other disease states. It is long being known that certain diseases tend to run in families. In fact, most of our understanding of mental illness comes from family, adoption, and twin studies. Now, researchers have discovered a gene that can double the risk of depression, another that can increase the risk of schizophrenia, and others that may play a role in the risk of bipolar disorder.

Causes of Mental Illness

There are several factors associated with causation of mental illness. However, there is no single accepted or consistent cause currently established. Some of the hypothesized theories are:

- *Genetic causes:* A most common opinion about the causes of mental illnesses is genetic vulnerabilities precipitated by environmental stressors. Genetic studies have indicated that genes often play an important role in the development of mental illness, via developmental pathways interacting with environmental factors. The reliable identification of connections between specific genes and specific categories of disorders has proven more difficult. However, researchers have uncovered more information about how genetics can determine the risk of schizophrenia and manic depression. Genes 'DISC1', and phosphodiesterase 4B (PDE4B) are found to be associated with increased risk of mental illness.
- *Environmental causes:* Prenatal environment as well as postnatal environment found to be associated with increased risk of mental illness.
- *Biopsychosocial causes:* A number of biological, psychological and social factors are found behind the development of several mental illnesses. As biological factors, malfunctioning of selected neurotransmitters, such as serotonin, norepinephrine, dopamine and glutamate may cause mental illness.

Genetics of Depression

Each year an estimated 9.5% of American adults suffer from mood disorders. People suffering from depression experience symptoms of sadness, emptiness, or hopelessness that interfere with their lives. One of the questions scientists have been trying to answer is why some people become depressed in reaction to life stresses while others do not.

One study sheds some light on this question. Researchers followed 847 New Zealanders over five years and charted their reaction to different life stressors. Stressors included things like loss of job, death of a loved one, broken relationships, or prolonged illness. It was found by them that the participants with a short version of a particular gene were more likely to become depressed than those who had the long version of the same gene. Specifically, 43% of people with the short form of the gene developed depression, in contrast to 17% of those with the long form. The findings suggest that some people because of their genes are more vulnerable to depression when certain stressors activate the gene. Other researchers have found similar findings.

Genetics of Schizophrenia

The family link to schizophrenia is well established, but paring down the risk to one specific gene has proven difficult. For example, we each inherit two copies of the COMT (catecho-O-methyltransferase) gene, one from each parent. There are two COMT types possible: the *val* type (short for the amino acid valine) and the *met* type (short for the amino acid methionine). Research suggests that the *val* type may increase the susceptibility to schizophrenia by reducing dopamine activity.

One study tested the working memory of 181 schizophrenic patients, 219 of their well siblings, and 75 controls. The researchers found that individuals who had two copies of the *val* type gene performed worse than those with only one copy, and those with the *met* type gene performed best of all. What this suggests is that the *val* type gene may increase an individual's susceptibility to schizophrenia.

Genetics of Bipolar Disorder

Bipolar disorder is a disease that causes extreme shifts of mood from depression to mania to a mixed state. While family and twin studies have shown that bipolar disease can be inherited, they have not yet pinpointed a particular gene. In fact, evidence suggests that bipolar disorder is affected by the presence and interaction of many genes.

In another study, researchers found that patients with bipolar disorder had a significantly higher frequency of the COMT and short 5-HTT genes. Again, these findings suggest that genes may affect people's susceptibility to this condition.

Genetic Testing in Mental Illnesses

Despite the growing number of genetic tests available, there are no genetic tests for depression, schizophrenia, or bipolar disorder. Genetic testing also causes concerns among many people, particularly in regards to privacy. Therefore, as new tests are developed, people who choose to be tested must weigh the benefits against the risks of finding out what their genes contain.

As exciting as these discoveries may be, researchers are quick to note that mental illness, like other diseases, is an equation of sorts, with genetics being only one of the variables. For example, while the genes may increase the risk for a disease, other factors also play a role. These factors can be exposures to toxins, bacteria, and viruses during fetal development, as well as nutritional status, stress, emotional trauma, childhood development, environment, and a history of other medical conditions.

Management

There is no gene therapy used to treat mental illness. Some of the traditional treatment modalities include:

- Cognitive behavioral therapy
- Psychoanalysis
- Systemic or family therapy
- Milieu therapy
- Psycho-education
- Creative therapies
- Music therapy
- Art or drama therapy
- Psychiatric medications (antidepressants, anxiolytics, mood stabilizers, antipsychotics)
- Electro-convulsive therapy (ECT)
- Lifestyle adjustment and supportive therapy
- Dietary supplementations.

THERAPEUTIC APPROACHES FOR GENETIC DISORDERS

Although prevention is the ideal goal for genetic disorders, genetic disorders can be detected early or prevented through preimplantation genetic testing, prenatal testing, newborn screening, effective required antenatal micronutrient supplementation, etc.

However, various types of therapeutic management approaches are available, such management approaches depend on the nature of defect, and how well it is understood or graded at the genetic and biochemical levels and the practical feasibility of correction. In some conditions, certain management approaches are now tailored to the specific genotype. The client being treated may be the fetus, the infant, the child, or the adult. Treatment methods used in genetic disorders may involve surgical, cognitive/behavioral, pharmacological, dietary, environmental, avoidance, transfusion, plasma exchange, enzyme, and cell or gene therapy. They are basically aimed at:

- Limiting the intake of a substrate or its precursor.
- Depleting the accumulation or promoting the excretion of a substrate, precursor or product.
- Directly or indirectly replacing or stimulating production of the enzyme, gene product.
- Replacing, repairing or reprogramming the gene itself.

For example, diet therapy may be based on the principle of limiting the amount of a specific substrate, which cannot be adequately metabolized by the appropriate enzyme, as in phenylketonuria, or it might be aimed at providing a product needed in order to circumvent a metabolic pathway, as in the provision of uridine in orotic aciduria. Gene product replacement might involve the administration of the product directly (e.g. insulin in type-I diabetes mellitus) or indirectly by means of bone marrow transplantation (e.g. in severe combined immunodeficiency caused by adenosine deaminase deficiency). Toxic substances can be removed by chelation with drugs, plasmapheresis, or surgical bypass procedures. The administration of pharmacological doses of vitamins, supplies the needed cofactor for holoenzyme function in certain vitamin-responsive disorders.

Pharmacological approaches have taken advantages of underlying genetic mechanism in certain disorders, most notably in treating certain cardiac conditions and cancer. For example, it is known that for some disorders, multiple combinations of therapies are necessary. In Refsum disease (an autosomal recessive disorder with retinitis, pigmentation, ataxia, peripheral neuropathy and accumulation of phytanic acid), for example, both dietary restrictions of phytanic acid and plasmapheresis at weekly intervals are usual. Correction of birth defects such as craniofacial anomalies or limb anomalies usually involve multiple phases of surgical treatment at various stages of the development of the individual, along with the use of prosthetic devices and long rehabilitation, such interventions require a skilled treatment group, that is prepared to deal not only with the physical correction by surgery but with the nursing, psychological, speech, hearing and rehabilitative measures needed to achieve optimum results. Therapeutic approaches may range from a one-time surgical correction of a birth defect to a long-term special diet, to an infant stimulation program to improve maximum potential, to experimental gene replacement. Some of the common therapeutic approaches for genetic disorders are as follows:

- *Promoting excretion of toxins:* The excretion of certain toxin metabolites can be promoted by chelating agents. For example, penicillamine promotes excretion of copper in patients with Wilson, disease, or desferrioxamine can be used to chelate iron in cases of thalassemia and hemochromatosis.
- *Reducing accumulation of toxins:* The intake of substance, which cannot be metabolized by the body, should be reduced, especially if their accumulation is potentially toxic. For example, in galactosemia, galactose cannot be metabolized adequately. As lactose in the milk is hydrolyzed in the body to glucose and galactose, milk in the diet of the affected infant is substituted by non-lactose containing dietary formula to obviate damage due to excess of galactose in tissue. The phenylketonuric infant is placed on the low protein diet to prevent irreversible neurological damage. Certain drugs, e.g. allopurinol inhibits Xanthine oxidase and thus reduces the synthesis of uric acid and hence is useful in cases of gout.
- *Induction or stabilization of enzymes:* Certain enzyme systems, which may be immature or reduced at certain phases of life, may be induced or stabilized by the use of chemical agents. For example, Phenobarbitone is used for inducing the hepatic microsomal enzyme glucuronyl transferase, in cases of neonatal hyperbilirubinemia or Crigler-Najjar syndrome.
- *Administration of enzymes:* In a number of metabolic disorders, enzymatic block can be bypassed by administration of large quantities of the coenzyme. For example, pyridoxine in homocystinuria.

- *Avoiding drugs:* Certain drugs, which precipitate adverse symptoms in metabolic disorders, such as barbiturates in porphyria hepatica and oxidative agents in glucose-6 phosphate dehydrogenase deficiency, should never be administered in these patients.
- *Environmental protection:* Patients with hemophilia and osteogenesis imperfecta should be protected from trauma and other environmental hazards to prevent excessive bleeding and fractures respectively.
- *Surgery:* Surgery helps to reduce the structural, functional and cosmetic deformity in many of the congenital defects. For example, surgery is required for cleft lip and cleft palate or congenital heart defects.
- *Replacement therapy:* The deficiency of the metabolic end-product may be made up by replacement or administration of the product. Thus, thyroxine restores the thyroid function in familial goiterogenous cretinism, cortisone suppresses the adrenogenital syndrome and administration of factor VIII/IX prevents bleeding in cases of hemophilia. Enzyme replacement has been used in Gaucher's disease.
- *Gene therapy:* Gene therapy is the ultimate goal for genetic disorders. Though significant research has been done in this field, gene therapy has been effectively tried only for adenosine deaminase deficiency, familial hyperchrolesterolemia and some cancers. The aim is to introduced the normal gene in the affected individual. This is done by using viral or no-viral vectors for introducing normal functioning genes. The therapy can be in vivo (i.e. directly introduction in the body/tissue) or ex vivo (when cells with the normal functioning gene are grown outside and then introduced), which is the preferred mode. As the exact regulation of gene function of single gene disorder is very complex, so implementation of gene therapy is complicated.

NURSING MANAGEMENT IN GENETIC DISORDERS

Assessment

- *Family history:* Blood relatives share the most similar genetic information and are thus at risk for acquiring characteristics or disease present in family members. Therefore, while dealing with a genetic case, the first step is recording the family history of the index case/proband. Proband is an affected person who has brought the family to the attention of a clinician. Proband is also called 'propositus', if male or proposita if female. The procedure starts with gathering information of the person's socio-bio-demographic profile, information about disorder, age of onset, duration of complaints and any other major illness. The next step is to collect information regarding the first-degree relatives, i.e. parents, siblings and offsprings of the proband. Following need to be collected in family history:

- Does any relative suffer from similar trait? This will help in deciding the pattern of inheritance and subsequently working out the recurrence risk of the disorder.
- Does any relative show any other disease which is not present in proband? For example, in case of dissecting aneurysm caused by Marfan's syndrome, ask about cardiac anomalies, ocular malformations or skeletal abnormalities in relatives.
- Ask for any condition with which any of the relatives suffered or is suffering. Or a condition that might have been unnoticed. For example, a propositus of pheochromocytoma can be suspected of having von Recklinghausen's disease if patient's brother has scoliosis and mental retardation since both are manifestations of this disease.
- Is the proband an outcome of consanguineous marriage? Special attention should be given to this because consanguinity may lead to an autosomal recessive trait.
- What is the ethnic group of the family? This is important because certain traits are common in some ethnic groups. African blacks show hematological disorders, such as sickle-cell anemia, beta Thalassemia and conditions like G6PD deficiency with much greater frequency.
- Some specific points need to be emphasized during family history, like infant deaths, stillbirths and abortions to be noted with time of abortion, any obvious deformity in fetus or stillborn baby or in deceased infant, etc. This may significantly alter the risk to subsequent pregnancy.

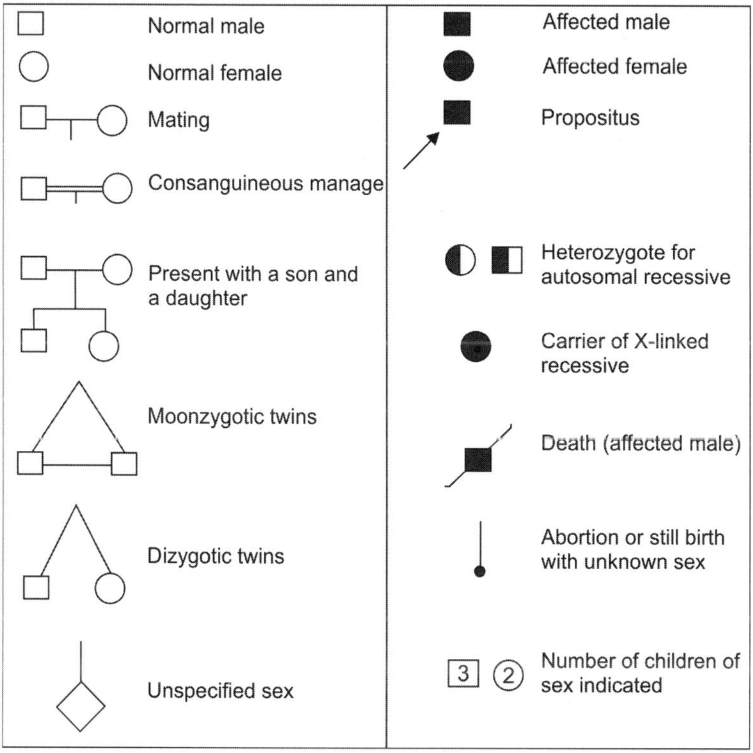

Fig. 5.3: Selected standardized symbols for use in drawing a pedigree

- *Preparing and analysis of family pedigree:* It depicts the family data. It is the shortest method of providing relevant information and also the mode of transmission of the disorders in the family. Furthermore, preparing a family pedigree is useful in identifying classic inheritance patterns and potential conditions for referral. A family pedigree using standardized documentation symbols indicating familial relationships, gender, and living or dead status should be part of the patient's medical record. Notes from the interview relevant to particular family members can be added to the pedigree. A three-generation display including the patient, parents, and grandparents is most useful in identifying patterns of inheritance. Pedigree symbols indicate whether the members are male or female, affected or unaffected by the disease of concern, and living or dead; lines denote relationship to the patient. A pedigree should also include marginal notes regarding current health status or diseases, age of onset for serious conditions, age of dead, cause of death, consanguinity, reproductive history, age of pregnant women, and ethnicity. There are standardized symbols used in drawing up a pedigree. Fig 5.3 shows symbols used in pedigree charting and Table 5.6 presents aspects of details about what should be included in pedigree.

Table 5.6: Specific facts and health information to be included in a pedigree

• Age/birth date or years of birth • Age of death (years, if known) • Cause of death • Age at diagnosis • Full sibling versus half or step-siblings • Pregnancy with gestational age (LMP) • Estimated date of delivery • Infertility versus no children by choice • Pregnancy complications with gestational age • Miscarriage	• Stillbirth • Pregnancy termination (TOP) • Relevant health information • Affected/unaffected status • Ethical background • Date pedigree taken or updated • Name of person who took pedigree • Key or legend

- Additional areas of assessment include:
  - Environmental factors (exposure to teratogens, triggers, radiation, and toxic substances)
  - Lifestyle factors (substance use and abuse, prescription drug use, and complementary therapies)
  - Nutrition
  - Psychosocial factors (emotional state, coping mechanisms, social support)
  - Family system (cohesion, communication styles, resources), and family support system.

Nursing Diagnosis, Outcomes, and Interventions

- Decisional conflict related to genetic testing or therapeutic interventions.
- Anticipatory grieving related to genetic disorder diagnosis.

- Anxiety related to genetic testing or therapeutic interventions.
- Disturbed body image related to genetic defects.
- Ineffective coping related to newly diagnosed genetic disorder.
- Interrupted family process related to genetic disorder to family member(s).
- Ineffective health maintenance related to poor social support and genetic disorder.
- Knowledge deficit related to genetic testing, interventions and inheritance pattern.
- Powerlessness related to structural, functional and behavioral genetic defects.
- Spiritual distress related to uncertainty of life secondary to genetic disorder.

Nursing diagnosis: *Decisional conflict related to genetic testing or therapeutic interventions.*

Expected outcomes: Patient will be able to make an effective decision about genetic testing or medical interventions.

Nursing Interventions:

- Provide relevant information about the genetic condition, associated genetic tests and interventions.
- Provide information about the alternatives of testing and not testing as a choice.
- Provide the information about consequences of having the genetic test and interventions or not having it.
- Provide specialized support.
- Recognize potential family resistance to pursuing genetic testing and interventions.
- Acknowledge the potential impact of information gathered from genetic tests on other family members.
- Acknowledge the risks of having genetic information after genetic tests as social, employment and insurance discrimination.
- Ensure active listening through paying a close attention to the verbal and nonverbal messages conveyed by the patient; clarify messages with follow-up questions.
- Provide for privacy and confidentiality during assessments and discussion.

- Provide information about alternatives and assist patient in identifying advantages and disadvantages of options.
- Facilitate discussions with other family members.
- Provide reassurance, acceptance, and encouragement during the decision-making process; be nonjudgmental and convey empathy.
- Arrange for services of a genetic counselor if desired; contact provider.

Nursing Diagnosis: *Anxiety related to genetic testing or therapeutic interventions.*

Expected outcomes: Patient will be able to have reduced anxiety state.

Nursing Interventions:

- Assess for the level of anxiety and factors responsible for precipitating and reducing the anxiety.
- Encourage the patient to verbalize the feelings.
- Clarify patients' doubts in simple language carefully.
- Provide diversional therapy through family discussion, music, reading tools, etc.

Nursing Diagnosis: *Anticipatory grieving related to genetic disorder diagnosis.*

Expected outcomes: Patient will be able to pass through normal grieving process.

Nursing Interventions:

- Assess the stage of grieving through which client is passing.
- Identify client's use of positive and negative defense mechanisms, boost positive defense mechanisms and discourage for negative mechanisms.
- Assess for support system available in family and community.
- Encourage the patient for ventilating the feeling loudly.
- Listen to the patient and family carefully and provide support as per need.
- Provide crisis interventions as therapeutic tolls to manage crisis situation.

Nursing Diagnosis: *Disturbed body image related to genetic defects.*

Expected outcomes: Patient will come to terms with altered body image as evidenced by ability to verbalize feelings, participating in self-care, and reintegrate into activities of daily living as capable.

Nursing Interventions:

- Note patient's ability to look at defect and reaction regarding the same.
- Note frequency and tone of critical remarks directed towards self, regarding appearance and/or functions.
- Assess perceived impact of actual change on activities of daily living (ADL), social behavior, personal relationship and/or occupational activities.
- Listen and share presence.
- Acknowledge normalcy of emotional response to actual or perceived change in body structure or function.
- Assist the patient in identifying frightening or worrisome potential situations; role-play responses.
- Encourage attendance at support group.

Nursing Diagnosis: *Ineffective coping related to personal vulnerability, secondary to genetic disorders.*

Expected outcomes: Patient will be able to identify own maladaptive coping behavior, available resources/support system and alternative coping strategies.

Nursing Interventions:

- Assess patient's ability to openly express feelings about disorder.
- Assess family and significant other's support system during disorder management.
- Set aside time to talk to patients when they are comfortable to do so.
- Assist the patient in understanding the chronicity of disorder(s) and the need to follow suggested testing and management instructions.
- Provide information on coping strategies.

- Establish a working relationship with patient through continuity of care.
- Involve social services, psychiatric liaison, and or pastoral care for additional and ongoing support resources.
- Inform patient and/or family about existing community resources.

Nursing Diagnosis: *Interrupted family process related to genetic disorder to family member.*

Expected outcomes: Family will identify resources available for problem-solving.

Nursing Interventions:

- Assess for precipitating events and family members' perception about a problem.
- Evaluate strengths, coping skills and current support system in their community.
- Provide opportunity to express concerns, fears, expectations and questions.
- Explore feelings, identify loneliness, anger, worry and fear.
- Encourage the family members to empathize with other family members.
- Assist family in setting realistic goals.
- Assist family in breaking down problems into manageable parts. Assist with problem-solving process, with delineated responsibilities and follow-through.
- Encourage family members to seek information and resources that increase coping skills.
- Refer family to social services or counseling.

Nursing Diagnosis: *Ineffective health maintenance related to presence of physical disabilities and mental retardation secondary to genetic disorder.*

Expected outcomes: Patient/family will describe positive health maintenance behavior, such as keeping scheduled appointments, making diet and exercise changes, improving home environment and using available resources effectively.

Nursing Interventions:

- Assess the patient's knowledge about health maintenance behavior.
- Determine patient's specific questions related to health maintenance.

- Assess for patient's economic, cultural and resources-related barriers for positive health maintenance.
- Compliment patient on positive accomplishments.
- Ensure regular follow-up programs.
- Involve family and friends in health planning discussion, so that later they can ensure adherence with advices.

Nursing Diagnosis: *Knowledge deficit related to genetic testing, interventions and inheritance pattern.*

Expected outcomes: Patient/family will verbalize understanding of condition, testing procedure, treatment and inheritance pattern.

Nursing Interventions:

- Assess understanding of genetic disorder(s) and usual expected genetic testing, management and their inheritance pattern.
- Teach about etiology, inheritance pattern, signs and symptoms and also discuss about medical and nursing management.
- Teach importance of genetic testing, continuous medical care and follow-ups.
- Instruct about dietary modifications and things to be avoided.

Nursing Diagnosis: *Powerlessness related to structural, functional and behavioral genetic defects.*

Expected outcomes: Patient will have improved power as evidenced by patient's accomplishment of self-care activities.

Nursing Interventions:

- Promote self-care and self-awareness.
- Advise the client to avoid coffee, tobacco and alcohol, and any of which increases fatigue further.
- Promote adequate sleep each day. Reduce amount of sleep cycle interruptions by preparing for sleep and keeping needed items at the bedside.
- Promote rest and activity by developing a written 24-hours schedule of daily activities that alternates short activities with rest periods.
- Identify activity priorities, such as eating breakfast and then resting before bathing in the morning, as opposed to the reverse.
- Evaluate the client's needs and point out ways to conserve energy, such as sitting down while dressing, shaving or preparing food, sitting on shower chair while bathing.

- Prepare an exercise schedule (immobilization may decrease endurance and increase fatigue) and plan exercise at peak of energy times (after a rest period). Follow exercise with rest.

Nursing Diagnosis: *Spiritual distress related to uncertainty of life secondary to genetic disorder.*

Expected outcomes: Patient/family will express hope in and value his/her own belief system and inner resources.

Nursing Interventions:

- Assess history of religious affiliation and desire for religious contact. Also assess cultural beliefs.
- Assess for hope and spiritual meaning of illness and treatment.
- Display an understanding and accepting attitude, encourage verbalization of feelings of anger or loneliness.
- Structure nursing interventions in terms of patient's belief system.
- Develop an ongoing relationship with patient and family.
- When requested by patient or family, arrange for clergy, religious ritual or display of religious objects, especially when the patient is hospitalized.
- Acknowledge and support patient's hope.
- Do not provide logical solutions for spiritual dilemmas.
- Facilitate communication between patient and family, clergy and other caregivers.

REVIEW QUESTIONS

Short-note Questions

1. Huntington's disease.
2. Sickle cell disease.
3. Role of heredity and genetics in cancer.
4. Hemophilia.
5. Thalassemia.
6. Genetics and mental diseases.
7. Inborn errors of metabolism.
8. Collagen vascular diseases.
9. Prenatal diagnosis of thalassemia.
10. Erythroblastosis fetalis (Hemolytic disease of the newborn).

Short-answer Questions

1. List any two inborn errors of metabolism.
2. Name any of the two family cancer-predisposing syndromes.

Multiple Choice Questions (MCQs)

1. **Hemophilia is more common in males because it is a:**
   a. Recessive character carried by Y-chromosome
   b. Dominant character carried by Y-chromosome
   c. Dominant trait carried by X-chromosome
   d. Recessive trait carried by X-chromosome.

2. **Branched chain ketoaciduria is characteristic of which metabolic disorder:**
   a. Alkaptonuria
   b. Phenylketonuria
   c. Maple syrup urine disease
   d. Gaucher's syndrome type 2.

3. **Which among the following disorders can be screened in neonates?**
   a. Nephrotic syndrome b. Asthma
   c. Phenylkeltonuria d. Huntington's disease

4. **Cancer is caused by:**
   a. Uncontrolled mitosis
   b. Uncontrolled meiosis
   c. Rupturing of cells
   d. Loss of immunity of cells

5. **A pedigree chart shows:**
   a. Genotype ratios of offspring
   b. The types of gametes produced by the parents
   c. The pattern of inheritance of a specific gene
   d. The genotypes of any parents.

6. **Huntington's disease is an:**
   a. X-linked recessive disorder
   b. X-linked dominant disorder
   c. Autosomal recessive disorder
   d. Autosomal dominant disorder.

7. **Cystic fibrosis is an example of an:**
   a. X-linked recessive disorder
   b. X-linked dominant disorder
   c. Autosomal recessive disorder
   d. Autosomal dominant disorder.

8. **Which of the following is known as Royal disease?**
   a. Sickle-cell anemia
   b. Hemophilia
   c. Alzheimer's disease
   d. Color blindness.

9. **Why is sickle cell disease so called?**
   a. Because it makes people sick
   b. It is named after a special type of white blood cell
   c. pH changes in the blood cells make them collapse into a sickle shape
   d. Because it is caused by an infectious microorganism that has sickle-shaped cells.

10. **BRCA1 gene mutation is associated with which of the following cancers?**
    a. Thyroid   b. Leukemia
    c. Lung   d. Breast

11. **Which of the following may contribute to causing cancer?**
    a. A mutation in a gene that slows the cell cycle
    b. Faulty DNA repair
    c. Loss of control over telomere length
    d. All of the above.

12. **Beta thalassemia disease is most commonly found among which of the following?**
    a. Indians   b. Nepalese
    c. Americans   d. Irish

13. **Genetic hemochromatosis is a disease caused by mutation in which of the following genes?**
    a. HFE gene   b. BRCA1 gene
    c. HTT gene   d. CFTR gene

14. **The symbol 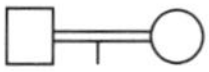 in pedigree is used for which of the following?**
    a. Monozygotic twin
    b. Dizygotic twin
    c. Consanguineous marriage
    d. Unspecified sex.

15. **After 9 years of marriage, a couple gave birth to the child, who is diagnosed with genetic hemochromatosis. The couple is crying and blaming the self and the God for this problem. Which of the following nursing diagnoses is most appropriate for the given scenario:**
    a. Decisional conflict Rt therapeutic interventions
    b. Anticipatory grief Rt genetic disorder diagnosis
    c. Ineffective coping Rt newly diagnosed genetic disorder
    d. Disturbed body image Rt genetic disorder.

ANSWER KEY

1. d	2. c	3. c	4. a	5. c	6. d	7. c
8. b	9. c	10. d	11. d	12. a	13. a	14. c
15. c						

FURTHER READING

1. American Society of Human Genetics/American College of Medical Genetics: Points to consider: Ethical, legal, and psychosocial implications of genetic testing in children and adolescents. Am J Hum Genet 1995;57:1233-41.
2. Beauchamp TL, Childress JF: Principles of Biomedical Ethics. New York, Oxford University Press, 1994.
3. Billings PR, Kohn MA, de Cuevas M, et al: Discrimination as a consequence of genetic testing. Am J Hum Genet 1992;50:476-82.
4. Borgna-Pignatti C, Vergine G, Lombardo T, et al: Hepatocellular carcinoma in the thalassemia syndromes. Br J Hematol. 2004 Jan;124(1):114-7.
5. Bove C, Fry ST, MacDonald DJ: Presymptomatic and predisposition genetic testing: Ethical and social considerations. Semin Oncol Nurs 1997;13:135-40.

6. Burke, W, et al: Hemochromatosis: genetics helps to define a multifactorial disease. Clin. Genet. 1998;54:1-9.
7. Cao A, Rosatelli C, Galanello R, et al: The prevention of thalassemia in Sardinia. Clin Genet. 1989 Nov;36(5):277-285.
8. Caspi A, Sugden K, Moffitt T, et al: Influence of life stress on depression: moderation by a polymorphism in the 5-HTT Gene. Science. 2003;301:386-9.
9. Clarke GM, Higgins TN (2000): 'Laboratory investigation of hemoglobinopathies and thalassemias: review and update'. Clin Chem. 46 (8 Pt 2):1284–90.
10. De Virgiliis S, Cossu P, Toccafondi C, et al: Effect of subcutaneous desferrioxamine on iron balance in young thalassemia major patients. Am J Pediatr Hematol Oncol. 1983 Spring;5(1):73-77.
11. Edwards, CQ, et al: Prevalence of hemochromatosis among 11,065 presumably healthy blood donors. New Engl J Med. 1988; 318: 1355-62.
12. Egan MF, Goldberg TE, Kolachana BS, et al: Effect of COMT Val108/158 Met genotype on frontal lobe function and risk for schizophrenia. Proceedings of the National Academy of Sciences of the United States of America. 2001;98:6917-22.
13. Egan MF, Kojima M, Callicott JH, et al: The BDNF val66met polymorphism affects activity-dependent secretion of BDNF and human memory and hippocampal function. Cell. 2003;112:257-69.
14. Farmaki K, Angelopoulos N, Anagnostopoulos G, et al: Effect of enhanced iron chelation therapy on glucose metabolism in patients with beta-thalassemia major. Br J Hematol. 2006 Aug;134(4):438-44.
15. Fucharoen S, Ketvichit P, Pootrakul P, et al: Clinical manifestation of beta-thalassemia/hemoglobin E disease. J Pediatr Hematol Oncol. 2000 Nov-Dec;22(6):552-7.
16. Gaba AM, Zhang K, Marder K, et al: (2005). 'Energy balance in early-stage Huntington disease'. Am. J. Clin. Nutr. 2005;81 (6): 1335–41.
17. Gill, JC; Endres-Brooks J, Bauer PJ, et al: (1987). 'The effect of ABO blood group on the diagnosis of von Willebrand disease'. Blood 1987;69 (6): 1691–5.
18. Gladwin MT, Sachdev V, Jison ML, et al (2004). 'Pulmonary hypertension as a risk factor for death in patients with sickle cell disease'. N Engl J Med 2004; 350(9):886–95.
19. Haldane JBS. The rate of mutation of human genes. In: Proceedings of the VIII International Congress on Genetics and Heredity. 1949; 267.

20. Hariri AR, Drabant EM, Munoz KE, et al: A susceptibility gene for affective disorders and the response of the human amygdala. Arch Gen Psychiatry . 2005;62:146-152.
21. Havens DMH, Kovner R: Genetic testing: How it is transforming the role of health professionals and the implications for pediatric nurse practitioners. Pediatr Health Care 1997;11:193-197.
22. Holtzman NA, Watson MS: Promoting Safe and Effective Genetic Testing in the United States: Final Report of the Task Force on Genetic Testing. Available http://www.nhgri.nih.gov/ELSI/TFGT_final. Accessed September, 1997
23. Imarisio S, Carmichael J, Korolchuk V, et al. 'Huntington's disease: from pathology and genetics to potential therapies'. Biochem J 2008; 412(2): 191–209.
24. James P, Notley C, Hegadorn C, et al. 'The mutational spectrum of type 1 von Willebrand disease: Results from a Canadian cohort study'. Blood 2007;109(1): 145–54.
25. Jenkins J: Educational issues related to cancer genetics. Semin Oncol Nurs 1997;13:141-44.
26. Johnson SA, Stout JC, Solomon AC, et al: 'Beyond disgust: Impaired recognition of negative emotions prior to diagnosis in Huntington's disease'. Brain 2007;130 (Pt 7): 1732–44.
27. Kieburtz K, MacDonald M, Shih C, et al: 'Trinucleotide repeat length and the progression of illness in Huntington's disease'. J Med Genet. 1994;31(11): 872–74.
28. Lippman-Hand A, Fraser FC: Genetic counseling: Provision and reception of information. Am J Hum Genet 1979;3:113-27.
29. Love RR: The accuracy of patient reports of a family history of cancer. Journal of Chronic Disease 1985;38:289-93.
30. Lucarelli G, Galimberti M, Polchi P, et al: Marrow transplantation in patients with thalassemia responsive to iron chelation therapy. N Engl J Med. 1993 Sep 16;329(12):840-44.
31. MacDonald DJ: The oncology nurse's role in cancer risk assessment and counselling. Semin Oncol Nurs 1997;13:123-28.
32. Matloff ET, Peshkin BN: Complexities in cancer genetic counseling: Breast and ovarian cancer. Principles and Practice of Oncology Updates 1998;12:1-11.
33. McDonnell, S, et al: A survey of 2,851 patients with hemochromatosis: symptoms and response to treatment. Am J Med 1999;106: 619-24.
34. Merikangans KR, Risch N. Will the genomics revolution revolutionize psychiatry?Am J Psychiatry. 2003;160:625-35.

35. Michie S, Bron F, Bobrow M, et al: Nondirectiveness in genetic counseling: An empirical study. Am J Hum Genet 1997;60:40-7.
36. National Society of Genetic Counselors: Code of Ethics 1992.
37. National Society of Genetic Counselors: Position Statements 1991
38. Offit K: Clinical Cancer Genetics: Risk Counseling and Management. New York, WileyLiss, 1998:249.
39. Olivieri NF, Brittenham GM, Matsui D, et al: Iron-chelation therapy with oral deferipronein patients with thalassemia major. N Engl J Med. 1995 Apr 6;332(14):918-22.
40. Pearson H. 'Sickle-cell anemia and severe infections due to encapsulated bacteria'. J Infect Dis 136 Suppl:S25–30.
41. Peters J, Stopfer J: Role of the genetic counselor in familial cancer. Oncology 1996;10:159-75.
42. Platt OS, Brambilla DJ, Rosse WF, et al (June 1994). 'Mortality in sickle cell disease. Life expectancy and risk factors for early death'. N Engl J Med. 330(23):1639–44.
43. Powars DR, Elliott-Mills DD, Chan L, et al (1991). 'Chronic renal failure in sickle cell disease: risk factors, clinical course, and mortality'. Ann Intern Med 115(8):614–620.
44. Powell, LW, et al: Diagnosis of hemochromatosis. Ann Int Med 1998;129:925-31.
45. Reilly PR, Boshar MF, Holzman SH. Ethical issues in genetic research: Disclosure and informed consent. Nat Genet 1997;15:16-20.
46. Rieger PT: Overview of cancer and genetics: Implications for nurse practitioners. Nurse Practitioner Forum 1998;9:122-33.
47. Rothenberg K, Fuller B, Rothstein M, et al: Genetic information and the workplace: Legislative approaches and policy changes. Science 1997;275:1755-7.
48. Rothenberg KH: Genetic discrimination and health insurance: A call for legislative action. J Am Med Womens Assoc 1997;52:43-4.
49. Rowland LP: Molecular basis of genetic heterogeneity: Role of the clinical neurologist. J Child Neurol 1998;13:122-32.
50. Sadler JE. 'A revised classification of von Willebrand disease. For the Subcommittee on von Willebrand Factor of the Scientific and Standardization Committee of The International Society on Thrombosis and Hemostasis'. Thromb Hemost. 1994;71 (4):520-5.
51. Salonen JT, Tuomainen, TP, and Kontula, K. Role of C282Y mutation in hemochromatosis gene in development of type 2 diabetes in healthy men: prospective cohort study. BMJ. 2000;320:1706-7.

52. Sandyk R. 'L-tryptophan in neuropsychiatric disorders: A review'. Int J Neurosci.1992;67(1-4):127–144.

53. Savage R, Armstrong D: Effect of a general practitioner's consulting style on patients' satisfaction: A controlled study. BMJ 1990;301:968-970.

54. Scanlon C, Fibison W: Managing genetic information: Implications for nursing practice. Washington, DC, American Nurses Association, 1995.

55. Schneider KA: Counseling About Cancer: Strategies for Genetic Counselors. Dennisport, MA, Graphic Illusions, 1994.

56. Shiloh S, Saxe L: Perception of risk in genetic counseling. Psychological Health 1989;3:45-61.

57. Thomas C; Preimplantation genetic diagnosis: Development and regulation. Med Law. 2006 Jun;25(2):365-78.

58. van Duijn E, Kingma EM, van der Mast RC. 'Psychopathology in verified Huntington's disease gene carriers'. J Neuropsychiatry Clin Neurosci 2007;19 (4):441–8.

59. Voskaridou E, Terpos E, Spina G, et al: Pamidronate is an effective treatment for osteoporosis in patients with beta-thalassemia. Br J Hematol. 2003 Nov;123(4):730-7.

60. Walker AP: Historical perspective and philosophical perspective of genetic counseling. In Emery AEH, Rimoin DL, Connor JM, et al (eds): Principles and Practice of Medical Genetics, ed 3. New York, Churchill-Livingstone, 1996.

61. Walker FO. 'Huntington's disease'. Lancet 2007;369 (9557): 218–28.

62. Wertz DC, Fanos JH, Reilly PR: Genetic testing for children and adolescents. Who decides? JAMA 1994;272:875 881.

63. Wong W, Powars D, Chan L, et. al. Smith WR, Penberthy LT, Bovbjerg VE, et al. 'Daily assessment of pain in adults with sickle cell disease'. Ann Intern Med 2008;148 (2): 94–101.

Chapter

6 Services Related to Genetics

Learning Objectives

This chapter is designed to enable the reader to:

- Understand the meaning and purposes of genetic testing
- Classify the types of genetic testing.
- Identify the benefits of genetic testing and interpretations of genetic test results.
- Recognize the ethical, legal and social issues in genetic testing.
- Appraise the role of nurses in genetic testing.
- Describe the meaning, importance, gaols, accomplishments, ethical, legal and social implications of human genome project and nurses role in it.
- Explore, significant advancements, negative and positive aspects of genomic era.
- Discuss the concept, types, approaches, facts, shortcoming, ethical issues of gene therapy and nurses' role in it.
- Mention concept, purposes and types of eugenic movement.
- Explain the meaning, purposes, beneficiaries, phases of genetic counseling and nurses' role in genetic counseling.
- Determine concept of pharmacogenomics.

Key Terms

- Genetic Testing
- Preimplantation Genetic Diagnosis
- Prenatal Testing
- Newborn Screening
- Predictive Genetic Testing
- Carrier Genetic Testing
- Diagnostic Genetic Testing
- Forensic Genetic Testing
- Genetic Research Testing

Contd...

Contd...

Key Terms

- Ethical, Legal and Social Issues
- Human Genome Project
- The Genomic Era
- Gene Therapy
- The Eugenic Movement
- Genetic Counseling
- Pharmacogenomics

INTRODUCTION

Genetic services provide genetic information, education and support to patient and families with genetic related health concerns. Genetics professionals, including medical geneticists, genetic counselors, and advanced practice nurses in genetics provide specific genetic services to patient and families who are referred by their primary health care providers. A team approach is often used by genetic specialists to obtain and interpret complex family history information, evaluate and diagnose genetic conditions, interpret and discuss complicated genetic tests results, support patients throughout the evaluation process and offer resources for additional professional and family support. Patient participates as team member and decision-maker throughout the process. Genetic services encompass an evaluation and communication process by which individuals and their families come to learn and understand relevant aspects of genetics, to make informed health decisions, and to receive support as they integrate personnel and family genetic information into daily living.

GENETIC TESTING

The task force on genetic testing defines a genetic test as 'The analysis of human DNA, RNA, chromosomes, protein and certain metabolites in order to detect heritable disease-related genotypes, mutations, phenotypes or karyotypes for clinical purpose'. Such purposes include predicting risk of disease, identifying carriers, establishing prenatal and clinical diagnosis or prognosis.

Genetic testing identifies changes in chromosomes, genes, or proteins. Most of the time, testing is used to find changes that are associated with inherited disorders. The results of a genetic test can confirm or rule out a suspected genetic condition or help determine a person's chance of developing or passing on a genetic disorder. Several hundred genetic tests are currently in use and more are being developed.

Genetic tests are performed on a sample of blood, hair, skin, amniotic fluid, or other tissue. The sample is sent to a laboratory where technicians look for specific changes in chromosomes, DNA, or proteins depending on the suspected disorder.

Some genetic tests are diagnostic while others are predictive or inform individual of an increased risk of acquiring a disease or condition. A 'positive' genetic test may indicate that the asymptomatic individual will develop a genetic condition, but a prediction of the onset or severity of the condition cannot be made. A negative test result cannot guarantee the disease or its development in the future, often because environmental influence cannot be measured or controlled. Also, the genetic test may have only been able to detect the most common gene mutations and not all of the disease-producing gene alterations are available for inclusion in clinical testing. Clients may learn they will develop a genetic condition, such as Huntington's disease, for which there is no treatment. Client may find out through testing that they are a carrier and they have unknowingly passed the altered disease-producing gene on to their children.

Purposes of Genetic Testing

Genetic tests can provide information about a person's genes and chromosomes from conception to throughout the life. Basically genetic testing may be used for clinical management, making personal decision or for assisting in reproductive choice. Some of the basic purposes of genetic testing is as following:

- Finding possible genetic diseases in unborn babies
- Finding out if person carry a gene for a disease and might pass it on to their children
- Screening embryos for disease
- Testing for genetic diseases in adults before they cause symptoms
- Confirming a diagnosis in a person who has disease symptoms.

Types of Genetic Testing

The nurses should understand that genetic testing can be classified into two categories: screening and diagnostic. A positive screening genetic test result notifies the client of an increased risk or probability but must always be confirmed by diagnostic testing. Screening genetic tests are most commonly completed in prenatal, newborn, and carrier circumstances. In contrast, a diagnostic test can definitively validate a genetic disorder in a symptomatic client and then direct clinical management.

Several categories of genetic tests included as subcategories of screening and diagnostic genetic tests follow:

Preimplantation genetic diagnosis (PGD)

- It involves the detection of disease-causing gene alteration in human embryo just after *in vitro* fertilization and before implantation in the uterus, thus providing an opportunity for preselection of unaffected embryo for implantation.
- This type of genetic testing is most often used by parents who are both carriers of a single gene recessive disorder and who wish to implant into the uterus only the embryo (s) without the disease causing alteration.
- PGD is usually very costly and is available at only a small number of centers and for only a small number of disorders.
- More recently it has also been used to determine tissue type for donation of tissue, such as bone marrow to a sibling or parent.

Prenatal testing

- Prenatal testing is used to detect changes in a fetus's genes or chromosomes before birth.
- This type of testing is offered to couples with an increased risk of having a baby with a genetic or chromosomal disorder.
- In some cases, prenatal testing can lessen a couple's uncertainty or help them decide whether to abort the pregnancy. It cannot identify all possible inherited disorders and birth defects.

Newborn screening

- It is carried out on large section of the newborn population and provides a means to identify infants who have an increased risk for developing a genetic disorder, such as phenylketonuria, congenital hypothyroidism and sickle cell disease or maple syrup urine disease.

- Newborn screening is used just after birth to identify genetic disorders that can be treated early in life to prevent disorders. For example, phenylketonuria with protein free diet.

Predictive genetic testing

- Predictive types of testing are used to detect gene mutations associated with disorders that appear after birth, often later in life.
- This is usually made available to the asymptomatic individual and includes both predispositional and presymptomatic testing.
- A positive predispositional testing results will indicate there is an increased risk that the individual might eventually develop the disease. For example, an individual with a mutation in *BRCA1* has a 65 percent cumulative risk of breast cancer, similarly hereditary nonpolyposis colorectal cancer.
- Presymptomatic testing can determine whether a person will develop a genetic disorder, such as hemochromatosis and hypercholesterolemia, before any signs or symptoms appear.
- The results of predispositional and presymptomatic testing can provide information about a person's risk of developing a specific disorder and help when making decisions about medical care. In addition, life planning and lifestyle choice can be influenced by predictive testing.

Carrier genetic testing

- This test is completed on asymptomatic individuals who may be carrier of one copy of a gene alteration that can be transmitted to future children in an autosomal recessive or X-linked pattern of inheritance.
- This may be part of couple's premarriage or preconception planning, if they belong to a particular ethnic group with known incidence to genetic disorders, such as sickle-cell anemia and Tay-Sachs disease.
- It may be necessary to determine the exact gene mutation from affected family member prior to carrier testing.
- This is often completed through lineage analysis.

Diagnostic genetic testing

- Diagnostic testing is used to diagnose or rule out a specific genetic or chromosomal condition.
- In many cases, genetic testing is used to confirm a diagnosis when a particular condition is suspected based on physical mutations and symptoms.
- Diagnostic testing can be performed at anytime during a person's life, but is not available for all genes or all genetic conditions.
- The results of a diagnostic test can influence a person's choices about health care and the management of the disease.

Forensic genetic testing

- Forensic testing uses DNA sequences to identify an individual for legal purposes.
- Unlike the tests described above, forensic testing is not used to detect gene mutations associated with disease. This type of testing can identify crime or catastrophe victims, rule out or implicate a crime suspect, or establish biological relationships between people (for example, paternity).

Genetic research testing

- Research testing includes finding unknown genes, learning how genes work and advancing our understanding of genetic conditions.
- The results of testing done as part of a research study are usually not available to patients or their health care providers.

Other genetic testing

- Other uses of genetic testing include organ transplantation tissue typing and pharmacogenetic testing, which involve predicting or studying the client's response to particular medication. For example, pharmacogenetic testing has shown that individuals who have Alzheimer's disease and carry two copies of a particular altered gene do not respond well to a drug frequently used in the treatment of Alzheimer's disease. However, if the individual only has one copy of the altered gene, the drug is effective in showing the progression of the disease.

Benefits of Genetic Testing

Provide for:

- Early screening and preventive measures
- Future planning and life preparation
- Lifestyle adaptations
- Decreased confusion, uncertainty and anxiety
- Psychological stress relief
- Reproductive choice
- Informed extended family members
- Cost medical follow-up reduced (if negative result).

Negative Outcomes of Genetic Testing

- Emotional, social, or financial consequences of the test results
- Angry, depressed, anxious, or guilty about their results.
- Tension within a family because the results can reveal information about other family members in addition to the person who is tested
- Genetic discrimination in employment or insurance
- Survivor guilt
- Loss of identity
- No treatment may exist
- Confusion about accessing health care and resources
- Risk for invasion of confidentiality and privacy
- Social stigmatization.

Table 6.1: Genetic test techniques

Type of genetic tests	Description	Examples of genetic conditions
Molecular genetic tests		
Direct deoxyribonucleic acid (DNA) testing	Tests for presences of genes known to cause disease	• Hemophilia • Huntington's disease • Polycystic kidney disease
Linkage testing	Tests genetic material from several family members for presence of genetic markers believed to be located near affected gene	• Familial adenomatous polyposis • Huntington's disease • Malignant hyperthermia susceptibility • Neurofibromatosis • Polycystic kidney disease

Contd...

Contd...

Type of genetic tests	Description	Examples of genetic conditions
Methylation studies	Examine attachment of methyl groups to DNA molecule	• Angelman's syndrome • Beckwith-wiedemann syndrome • Prader- willi syndrome • Rett syndrome
Protein truncation test (PTT)	Tests for proteins that have been shortened and whose function has been altered	• Breast cancer • Familial adenomatous polyposis
Uniparental disomy (UPD)	Tests for two chromosomes from same parent rather than one from each	• Angelman's syndrome • Prader-willi syndrome
X-inactivation studies	Tests for carrier status in women with some X-linked disorders	• Fragile X syndrome • Rett syndrome • X-linked severe combined immunodeficiency
Cytogenic test		
FISH (fluorescence in situ hybridization)	Identifies presence or absence of chromosome segments using fluorescein-tagged DNA probes	• Angelman's syndrome • Aniridia • Williams syndrome
Chemical genetic tests		
Analyte testing	Assesses presence of substance in body indicative of genetic disorder	Hemocystinuria
Enzyme assay	Measures rate of chemical reaction of an enyme in presence of a particular protein associated with genetic disorder; can identify affected individual or carrier	• Gaucher's disease • Lowe syndrome • Galactosemia
Protein analysis	Tests for structure of proteins known to be associated with genetic disorders	• Marfan syndrome • Spinocerebellar ataxia

Interpreting Genetic Test Results

- The results of genetic tests are not always straightforward, which often makes them challenging to interpret and explain. When interpreting test results, health care professionals consider a person's medical history, family history, and the type of genetic test that was done.
- *A positive test result* means that the laboratory found a change in a particular gene, chromosome, or protein of interest. Depending on the purpose of the test, this result may confirm a diagnosis, indicate that a person is a carrier of a particular genetic mutation, identify an increased risk of developing a disease (such as cancer) in the future, or suggest a need for further testing. Because family members have some genetic material in common, a positive test result may also have implications for certain blood relatives of the person undergoing testing. It is important to note that a positive result of a predictive or presymptomatic genetic test usually cannot establish the exact risk of developing a disorder. Also, health professionals typically cannot use a positive test result to predict the course or severity of a condition.
- *A negative test result* means that the laboratory did not find a dangerous copy of the gene, chromosome, or protein under consideration. This result can indicate that a person is not affected by a particular disorder, neither a carrier of a specific genetic mutation, or nor have an increased risk of developing a certain disease. It is possible, however, that the test missed a disease-causing genetic alteration because many tests cannot detect all genetic changes that can cause a particular disorder. Further testing may be required to confirm a negative result.
- In some cases, a negative result might not give any useful information. This type of result is called uninformative, indeterminate, inconclusive, or ambiguous. Uninformative test results sometimes occur because everyone has common, natural variations in their DNA, called polymorphisms, that do not affect health. If a genetic test finds a change in DNA that has not been associated with a disorder in other people, it can be difficult to tell whether it is a natural polymorphism or a disease-causing mutation. An uninformative result cannot confirm or rule out a specific diagnosis, and it cannot

indicate whether a person has an increased risk of developing a disorder. In some cases, testing other affected and unaffected family members can help clarify this type of result.

Ethical, Legal, and Social Issues in Genetic Testing

Advances in technology have presented numerous ethical challenges and concerns. Humans exist within the same society; however, subcultures with their own values, beliefs, and moral perspectives influence the individual's decision. Ethical questions raised by genetic testing, screening, and analysis vary considerably depending on the specific condition identified. Numerous issues exist in the obstetric and neonatal areas. Confidentiality in screening and counseling has become a major concern with regard to potential employer and insurance discrimination. Informed decision-making is another issue that arises frequently. At what point is an individual truly informed? When does the family understand the risk/benefit considerations? How is autonomy in decision-making most enabled? Some people ask why test if there is no intent to abort, whereas other people contend that genetic information facilitates adequate preparation or that knowing is better than not knowing. There is also concern about efficient resource allocation, potential for suffering, and the cost of maintaining life. Issues, such as pro-choice and pro-life are raised frequently along with issues of quality of life versus sanctity of life.

Currently genetic screening before implantation is possible with *in vitro* fertilization techniques using blastomere analysis. Such testing provides a couple with genetic information before transfer of the blastomere to the womb. The couple can make an informed decision whether to attempt pregnancy or stop at this point. Numerous legal and ethical issues have been raised regarding this practice. Who should pay for this service? Is this a form of legitimate diagnosis, prevention, and possible treatment of disease? Is this a vehicle for phenotype selection? If the pregnancy is continued are there grounds for a 'wrongful life' suit later if a genetic problem that should have been identified was not? Recently the concept of 'meaningful life,' meaning dependent on individual perception and cultural beliefs, also has been introduced. Also raised are issues concerning who has rights, the mother, father, fetus, extended family, or society?

Information from genetic testing can affect the lives of individuals and their families. In addition to personal and family issues, genetic disease or susceptibility may have implications for *employment* and insurance. Therefore, careful consideration in the *handling* of this information is very important. Critical issues include:

- *Privacy*: The rights of individuals to maintain privacy. Some genetic tests are required or strongly encouraged for developing fetuses and newborn babies. If an infant is found to be a carrier or likely to develop or be affected by an inherited disease, these findings may affect the future employability or insurability of the individual.
- *Informed consent:* Obtaining permission to do genetic testing. One must have knowledge of the risks, benefits, effectiveness, and alternatives to testing in order to understand the implications of genetic testing:
- *Confidentiality*: Acknowledgment that genetic information is sensitive and access should be limited to those authorized to receive it. Future access to a person's genetic information also should be limited.

Role of Nurses in Genetic Testing

- With knowledge available genetic tests and the many implications related to genetic testing, the nurses can assist client as they weigh choice regarding genetic testing.
- Nurses should inform about following aspects when considering a client for gentic testing;
  - The reason that testing is appropriate for this person.
  - What is being tested for?
  - How much can be predicted about disorder without genetic testing?
  - What the procedure being considered entails, including description, cost, length of time, where it is to be done?
  - What can and cannot be tested, if relevant, this should include the information that while some mutations will be looked for and detected, other rare ones might not be and that negative results refer only to whatever was being tested or screened for and to every genetic disorder for, e.g. if one is testing for Cystic Fibrosis (CF), the most common

mutations in that will be tested but not every rare mutation will be tested for.

- What would both positive and negative results means, including that negative results do not necessarily translate to a zero risk that a positive tested may result in fear and anxiety, were as negative results can also have emotional and relationship impact.
- The accuracy, validity and relationship of the test, including the likelihood of false negative or false positive results and the suitability of this test for the information the client is seeking.
- The possibility that testing will not yield additional risk information.
- The length of time between the procedure and when results will be obtained.
- How the result will be communicated to the client.
- What will be analyzed?
- What happens to the sample used for testing who own it, what uses are possible?
- A discussion of the possible risk of life and health insurance coverage and/ or employment discrimination after testing results are positive, although there may be benefit, such as if a person is free of a certain mutation, better insurance rates or coverage might result.
- The level of confidentiality of results and what this means (who can know or find out the results).
- Risk of psychological distress and negative impact not only on the individual but also on the family including stigmatization and altered self-image.
- Risk of passing on the mutation in the disorder being tested to children and the meaning of the risk.
- What discloser might the client consider for other family members.
- Provision for referral for periodic surveillance, further testing, lifestyle changes and or treatment after testing, if needed.
- What these mean in the context of both positive and negative test results?

- The nurses are responsible for alerting clients of their rights to make an informed decision prior to any genetic testing with considering of the special circumstances arising from the family, culture, and community life.
- All genetic testing should be voluntary and it is the nurse's responsibility to ensure that the consent process include discussion of the risk and benefit of the test, including any physical harm as well as potential psychological discrimination and emotional stress.
- Nurses need to ensure client's confidentiality and privacy of genetic testing.
- Nurses should address psychological, social and economic issues of person and family undergoing for genetic testing.

HUMAN GENOME PROJECT

The Human Genome Project was an international research effort to determine the sequence of the human genome and identify the genes that it contains. The Project was coordinated by the National Institutes of Health and the US Department of Energy. Additional contributors included universities across the United States and international partners in the United Kingdom, France, Germany, Japan, and China. The Human Genome Project formally began in 1990 and was completed in 2003, 2 years ahead of its original schedule.

The work of the Human Genome Project has allowed researchers to begin to understand the blueprint for building a person. As researchers learn more about the functions of genes and proteins, this knowledge will have a major impact in the fields of medicine, biotechnology, and the life sciences.

Meaning and Importance of Genome

- A genome is an organism's complete set of DNA, including all of its genes. Each genome contains all of the information needed to build and maintain that organism. In humans, a copy of the entire genome more than 3 billion DNA base pairs is contained in all cells that have a nucleus.
- Genes carry information for making all the proteins required by all organisms. These proteins determine, among other things,

how the organism looks, how well its body metabolizes food or fights infection, and sometimes even how it behaves.

- DNA is made-up of four similar chemicals (called bases and abbreviated A, T, C, and G) that are repeated millions or billions of times throughout a genome. The human genome, for example, has 3 billion pairs of bases.
- The particular order of As, Ts, Cs, and Gs is extremely important. The order underlies all of life's diversity, even dictating whether an organism is human or another species, such as yeast, rice, or fruit fly, all of which have their own genomes and are themselves the focus of genome projects. Because all organisms are related through similarities in DNA sequences, insights gained from nonhuman genomes often lead to new knowledge about human biology.

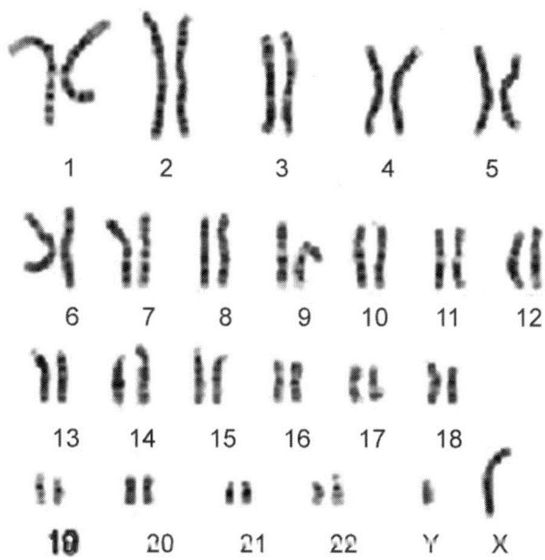

Fig. 6.1: Human genome karyotype

Goals of Human Genome Project

The main goals of the Human Genome Project were to:

- *Identify* all the approximately 20,000 to 25,000 genes in human DNA
- *Determine* the sequences of the 3 billion chemical base pairs that make-up human DNA.
- *Store* this information in databases.

- *Improve* tools for data analysis.
- *Transfer* related technologies to the private sector.
- *Address* the ethical, legal, and social issues (ELSI) that may arise from the project.

To help achieve these goals, researchers also studied the genetic make-up of several nonhuman organisms. These include the common human gut bacterium *Escherichia coli*, the fruit fly, and the laboratory mouse.

Accomplishments of Human Genome Project

In April 2003, researchers announced that the Human Genome Project had completed a high-quality sequence of essentially the entire human genome. This sequence closed the gaps from a working draft of the genome, which was published in 2001. It also identified the locations of many human genes and provided information about their structure and organization. The Project made the sequence of the human genome and tools to analyze the data freely available via the Internet.

In addition to the human genome, the Human Genome Project sequenced the genomes of several other organisms, including brewers' yeast, the roundworm, and the fruit fly. In 2002, researchers announced that they had also completed a working draft of the mouse genome. By studying the similarities and differences between human genes and those of other organisms, researchers can discover the functions of particular genes and identify which genes are critical for life.

The Project's Ethical, Legal, and Social Implications (ELSI) program became the world's largest bioethics program and a model for other ELSI programs worldwide. Some of the major tasks accomplished under Human Genome Project are:

Ethical, legal, and social implications of Human Genome Project: The Ethical, Legal, and Social Implications (ELSI) program was founded in 1990 as an integral part of the Human Genome Project. The mission of the ELSI program was to identify and address issues raised by genomic research that would affect individuals, families, and society. A percentage of the Human Genome Project budget at the National Institutes of Health and the US Department of Energy was devoted to ELSI research.

The ELSI program focused on the possible consequences of genomic research in four main areas:

1. Privacy and fairness in the use of genetic information, including the potential for genetic discrimination in employment and insurance.
2. The integration of new genetic technologies, such as genetic testing, into the practice of clinical medicine.
3. Ethical issues surrounding the design and conduct of genetic research with people, including the process of informed consent.
4. The education of health care professionals, policy makers, students, and the public about genetics and the complex issues that result from genomic research.

Table 6.2: Ethical, Legal and Social Issues (ELSI)

ELSI research areas identified as 'grand challenges' for the future of genomic research:
• Intellectual property issues surrounding access to and use of genetic information • Ethical, legal and social factors that influence the translation of genetic information to improved health • Issues surrounding the conduct of genetic research • Issues surrounding the use of genetic information and technologies in non-health care settings • The impact of genomics on concepts of race, ethnicity, kinship and individual and group identity • The implications for both individuals and society of uncovering genomic contributions to human traits and behaviors • How different individuals, cultures and religious traditions view the ethical boundaries for uses of genomics (adapted from National Human Genome Research Institute (2007a)

Future perspectives of genomic research: Discovering the sequence of the human genome was only the first step in understanding how the instructions coded in DNA lead to a functioning human being. The next stage of genomic research will begin to derive meaningful knowledge from the DNA sequence. Research studies that build on the work of the Human Genome Project are under way worldwide.

The objectives of continued genomic research include the following:

- Determine the function of genes and the elements that regulate genes throughout the genome.

- Find variations in the DNA sequence among people and determine their significance. These variations may one day provide information about a person's disease risk and response to certain medications.
- Discover the 3-dimensional structures of proteins and identify their functions.
- Explore how DNA and proteins interact with one another and with the environment to create complex living systems.
- Develop and apply genome-based strategies for the early detection, diagnosis, and treatment of disease.
- Sequence the genomes of other organisms, such as the rat, cow, and chimpanzee, in order to compare similar genes between species.
- Develop new technologies to study genes and DNA on a large scale and store genomic data efficiently.
- Continue to explore the ethical, legal, and social issues raised by genomic research.

Nursing and the Human Genome Project

Historically, the need for nurses to have genetic information has been well documented. Inadequate nursing knowledge of genetics was first documented in a nursing journal in 1979 (Cohen, 1979). Efforts to integrate genetics into nursing education began in the 1980s and accelerated in the mid-1990s, mirroring the progression of the HGP. Around the same time, the American Nursing Association (ANA) published a document summarizing a survey of nurses' knowledge and use of genetic information (Scanlon & Fibison, 1995).

In 1994 and 1995 two conferences were held to review the status of genetics in primary health care and to address ways to incorporate genetics into medical and nursing education (Touchette, Holtzman, Davis, & Feetham, 1997). During this time, Dr. Francis Collins, Director of the HGP, recognized that all health care providers, including nurses regardless of specialty, would need to integrate genetic knowledge into their routine practice (Collins, 1997).

In 2000, the Senior Clinical Advisor to the Director of the National Human Genome Research Institute, highlighted the relevance and importance of genetics to health care and described the implications of genetics for nursing education. The Clinical Advisor noted the need to add genetic content to the nursing curriculum and to make this information available to practicing nurses. Experts recognized early on the need for nurses to translate genetic information into understandable language for their patients. This would mean that all nurses would need to be familiar with genetic terminology and principles, along with genetic technology; even though the type of genetic knowledge might differ depending on the nurses' clinical focus and level of practice.

The complete sequencing of the human genome in 2003 has opened doors for new approaches to health promotion, maintenance, and treatment. Genetic research is now leading to a better understanding of the genetic components of common diseases, such as cancer, diabetes, and stroke, and creating new, gene-based technologies for screening, prevention, diagnosis, and treatment of both rare and common diseases. Nurses are on the forefront of care, and therefore will participate fully in genetic-based and genomic-based practice activities, such as collecting family history, obtaining informed consent for genetic testing, and administering gene-based therapies. This new direction in health care calls for all nurses to be able to effectively translate genetic and genomic information to patients with an understanding of associated ethical issues.

Table 6.3: Ethical challenges for nurses: seeds for thought

- Privacy and Confidentiality
  - Who should have access to genetic information? Who owns and controls it?
  - How can families resolve conflicts when some members want to be tested for a genetic disorder and others do not?
- Discrimination
  - Should employers be able to require job applicants to take genetic tests as a condition of employment?
- Equitable access to genomic technologies
  - Resource-poor nations, the uninsured, rural and inner city communities – How might genomic science and treatments be made available to those with fewer resources?
  - Rare genetic conditions – Who will fund the development of treatments for genetic disorders that affect a relatively small number of people?
- Impact of genetic information
  - How does a person's genetic information affect that individual and society's perception of that individual?

Contd...

Contd...

- How does genetic and genomic information affect members of minority communities?

(Adapted from human genome project information, 2007)

Table 6.4: Nursing competencies in professional responsibilities and practice domain for handling genetic- and genomic-related ethical issues

Professional responsibilities

- Recognize when one's own attitudes and values related to genetic and genomic science may affect care provided to clients.
- Advocate for the rights of all clients for autonomous, informed genetic-and genomic-related decision making and voluntary action.

Professional practice domain

- Identify ethical, ethnic/ancestral, cultural, religious, legal, fiscal, and societal issues related to genomic information and technologies.
- Define issues that undermine the rights of all clients for autonomous, informed genetic-and genomic-related decision making and voluntary action.
- Provide clients with accurate, appropriate, and current genetic and genomic information, resources, services, and/or technologies that will support and facilitate decision-making.

Adapted from: Essential nursing competencies and curricula guidelines for genetics and genomics (Consensus Panel, 2006)

THE GENOMIC ERA

The Genomic era can be said to have a precise birth date, it was in the midst of the appearance of the series, on April 14, 2003. That was when the international effort known as the Human Genome Project put a close to the pregenomic era with its announcement that it had achieved the last of the project's original goals, the complete sequencing of the human genome. The extent and pace of progress in genomics are suggested by the fact that this achievement occurred 11 days short of the 50th anniversary of the publication of Watson and Crick's seminal description of the DNA double helix. If science, technology, and medicine have consistently demonstrated anything, it is that they proceed at an ever-quickening pace. That we have gone in the past 50 years from the first description of the structure of our DNA to its complete sequencing gives some indication of how much the impact of genomic medicine on the health care of today's neonates will increase by the time they turn 50 years of age.

Significant Advancement in Genomic Era

However, it is not solely the next 50 years that will witness important advances in genomic medicine. Many such advances have already occurred, including the use of gene-expression profiling to assess prognosis and guide therapy, as in breast cancer; the use of genotyping to stratify patients according to the risk of a disease, such as the long-QT syndrome or myocardial infarction; the use of genotyping to shed light on the response to certain drugs, such as antiepileptic agents; and the use of genomic approaches in the design and implementation of new drug therapies, such as imatinib for the hypereosinophilic syndrome, and to improve our understanding of the role of specific genes in the causation of common conditions, such as obesity. During this same brief period, other notable genomics-based advances in our understanding of biology and of health have included the first comprehensive analysis of human chromosome 7, clarification of the male-specific region of the human Y chromosome, and the identification of the gene responsible for progeria.

Negative Aspects of Genomic Era

- In recent months, we have seen not only the promise of the genomic era with respect to medicine, but also its pitfalls. An example of the latter has been the revelation that confusion and misinformation have occasionally accompanied the counseling of persons who undergo screening for mutations in the cystic fibrosis transmembrane conductance regulator gene (*CFTR*) the gene responsible for cystic fibrosis. Different mutations in *CFTR* have different effects, leading to a range of phenotypes. Proper interpretation of screening results demands an understanding of the clinical implications of specific genotypes. For example, the relatively common 5T variant leads to the phenotype of classic cystic fibrosis only when it is accompanied by the R117H mutation on the same chromosome arm. However, there have been anecdotal reports of persons who were told that the presence of the 5T variant alone was indicative of a serious risk of cystic fibrosis. There is reason to believe that such problems are not intrinsic to genomic medicine and merely reflect the temporary difficulties of integrating virtually any new form of technology into health care. But this example, certainly points out the urgency with which genetic literacy must be achieved among all health care providers. In the genomic age, *primum non nocere* remains a useful aim.

- Genomics provide powerful means of discovering hereditary factors in disease. But even in the genomic era, it is not genes alone but the interplay of genetic and environmental factors that determines phenotype (i.e. health or disease). This point is not new, but it bears repeating. For example, a mutation in *CHE1* may be innocuous until a person carrying it is exposed to succinylcholine chloride anesthesia, when it leads to prolonged apnea. Conversely, substantial mutations in phenylalanine hydroxylase inevitably result in the sequelae of classic phenylketonuria, including profound mental retardation, unless the affected newborn is placed on a special diet, in which case essentially normal intellectual development can be expected. Recent reports further expand our knowledge of the complex interactions between genes and the environment. For instance, one such study suggests that common variations in the serotonin-transporter gene influence the likelihood of depression after exposure to stress.

Positive Aspects of Genomic Era

- Since it remains difficult to alter genes in humans (for both technical and ethical reasons), for the next couple of decades we will generally use personalized modifications of the environment, and not of genes, to translate genomics-based knowledge into improvements in health for most of our patients. Clinicians will much more frequently suggest to patients with hereditary hemochromatosis that they avoid iron supplementation than that they consider gene therapy. Women who carry mutations in *BRCA2* will profit more from taking tamoxifen than from manipulations of their genotype.
- With the end of the pregenomic era in sight, more than 600 experts recently collaborated to produce a vision for the future of genomic research and its applications to biology, health, and society. According to that vision, for instance, within a decade or two, it will be possible to sequence anyone's entire genome for a laboratory cost of less than $1,000. If this proves true, one can imagine how not only research, but also clinical

care, may change dramatically. However, as is true for so much of the application of genomics, ethical, legal, and social issues complicate this optimistic picture. Unless complex issues regarding the patenting and licensing of gene-based knowledge and techniques are dealt with more successfully than they are today, the '$1,000 genome' will remain a wish, not a reality. Even if the intellectual-property discussions are complex, the math is simple. Assuming that roughly half of the approximately 30,000 human genes are patented, if each patent holder were to charge only $1 per test to license his or her gene, the $1,000 genome would become the $16,000 genome, a very different economic, and thus clinical, reality.

While recognizing such challenges, we look forward with curiosity and real hope to the advances of the next 50 years; the first 50 years of the genomic era. As evidenced by the Genomic Medicine series, today's researchers and clinicians have already started to use the power of genomics to improve health, and we anticipate that this is but a hint of the progress to come.

GENE THERAPY

In gene therapy , a 'correct copy' or 'wild type' gene is provided or inserted into the genome. Generally, it is not an exact replacement of the 'abnormal,' disease-causing gene, but rather extra, correct copies of genes are provided to complement the loss of function. A carrier called a vector must be used to deliver the therapeutic gene to the patient's target cells. Currently, the most common type of vectors are viruses that have been genetically altered to carry normal human DNA. Viruses have evolved a way of encapsulating and delivering their genes to human cells in a pathogenic manner Scientists have tried to harness this ability by manipulating the viral genome to remove disease-causing genes and insert therapeutic ones. Target cells such as the patient's liver or lung cells are infected with the vector. The vector then unloads its genetic material containing the therapeutic human gene into the target cell. The generation of a functional protein product from the therapeutic gene restores the target cell, to a normal cell.

Gene therapy is the insertion of genes into an individual's cells and tissues to treat a disease, and hereditary diseases in which a defective mutant allele is replaced with a functional one. Although the technology is still in its infancy, it has been used with some success.

In other words gene therapy is the process of inserting genes into cells to treat disease. The newly introduced gene will encode proteins and corrrect the deficiency that occur in genetic diseases. Thus, gene therapy primarly involve genetic manipulation in animal or humans to correct a disease and keep the organism in good health.

Gene therapy is a technique for correcting defective genes responsible for disease development. Researchers may use one of several approaches for correcting faulty genes:

- A normal gene may be inserted into a nonspecific location within the genome to replace a nonfunctional gene. This approach is most common.
- An abnormal gene could be swapped for a normal gene through homologous recombination.
- The abnormal gene could be repaired through selective reverse mutation, which returns the gene to its normal function.
- The regulation (the degree to which a gene is turned on or off) of a particular gene could be altered.

Although gene therapy is a promising treatment option for a number of diseases (including inherited disorders, some types of cancer, and certain viral infections), the technique remains risky and is still under study to make sure that it will be safe and effective. Gene therapy is currently only being tested for the treatment of diseases that have no other cures.

Types of Gene Therapy

Basically gene therapy may be classified into the two types:

Somatic Gene Therapy

In the case of somatic gene therapy, theraputic genes are transferred into the somatic cells of a patient. Any modifications and effects will be restricted to the individual patient only, and will not be inherited by the patient's offspring.

Germ Line Gene Therapy

In the case of germ line gene therapy, germ cells, i.e. sperm or eggs, are modified by the introduction of functional genes, which are ordinarily integrated into their genomes. Therefore, the change due to therapy would be heritable and would be passed on to later generations. This new approach, theoretically, should be highly effective in counteracting genetic disorders. However, this option is prohibited for application in human beings, at least for the present, for a variety of technical and ethical reasons.

Approaches of Gene Therapy

- *Ex vivo gene therapy:* This is accomplished by transfer of genes in cultured cells (e.g. bone marrow cells) which then reintroduced into human body. In this approach following steps are followed:
  - Cells with genetic defect are isolated from patients
  - These cells are cultured to grow in laboratory
  - Introduction of therapeutic gene to correct gene defect
  - Select the genetically corrected cells and grow them fully
  - Ultimately transplant the modified cells into the patients.

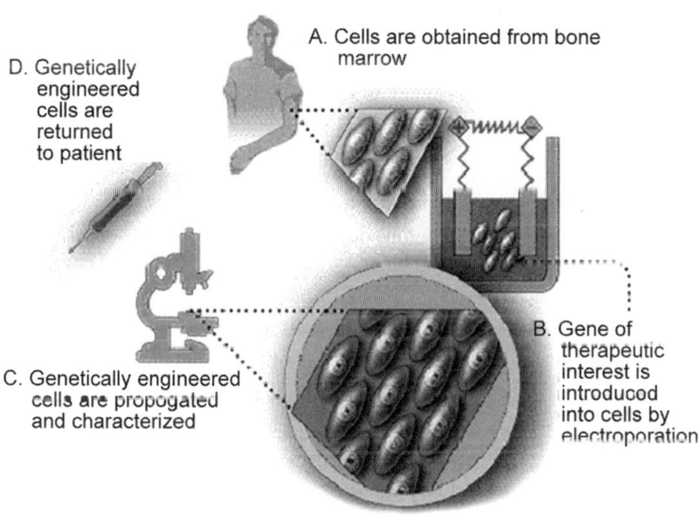

Fig. 6.2: *Ex vivo* gene therapy

- *In vivo gene therapy:* In this approach of gene therapy, therapeutic gene is directly delivered into target cell of particular tissue of a patient. Generally targeted tissues include liver, muscles, skin, spleen, lungs, brain, and blood cells. Gene delivery can be carried out by viruses or nonviral vector system. The success of *in vivo* therapy depends on:
  - The efficiency of the uptake of the therapeutic gene by the target cells
  - Intracellular degradation of the gene and its uptake by nucleus
  - The expression capability of the gene.

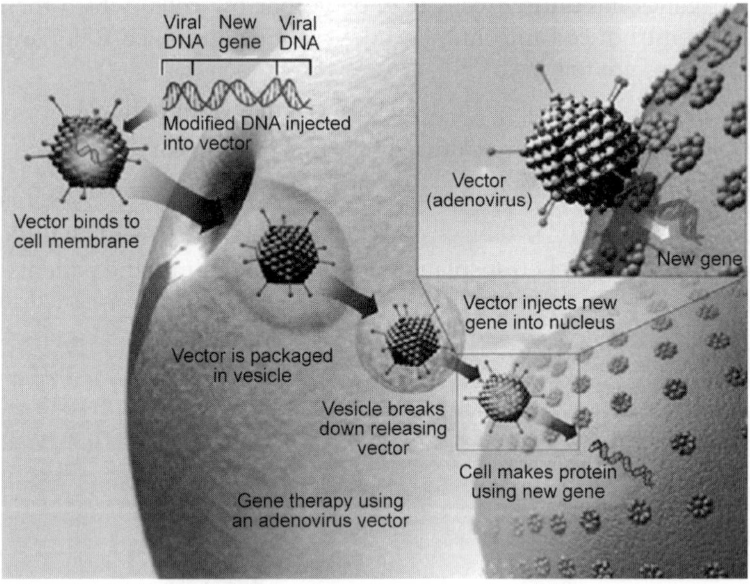

Fig 6.3: *In vivo* gene therapy approach
(A new gene is injected into an adenovirus vector, which is used to introduce the modified DNA into a human cell. If the treatment is successful, the new gene will make a functional protein)

Vectors Used in Gene Therapy

- *Viral vectors:* Some of the different types of viruses used as gene therapy vectors:

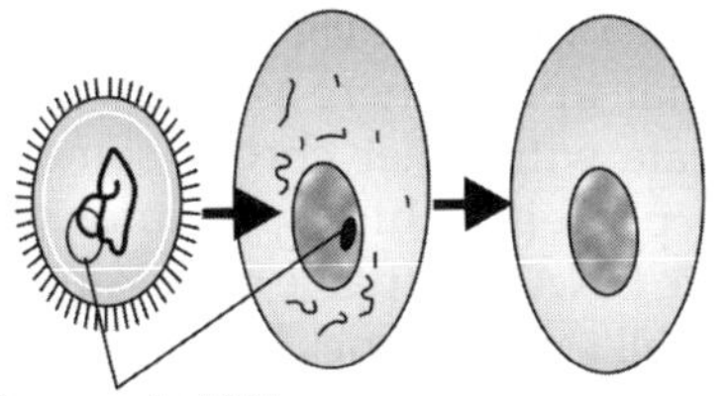

Fig 6.4: Process of replacing desired genetic material in a cell

- *Retroviruses:* A class of viruses that can create double-stranded DNA copies of their RNA genomes. These copies of its genome can be integrated into the chromosomes of host cells. Human immunodeficiency virus (HIV) is a retrovirus.
- *Adenoviruses*: A class of viruses with double-stranded DNA genomes that cause respiratory, intestinal, and eye infections in humans. The virus that causes the common cold is an adenovirus.
- *Adeno-associated viruses*: A class of small, single-stranded DNA viruses that can insert their genetic material at a specific site on chromosome 19.
- *Herpes simplex viruses*: A class of double-stranded DNA viruses that infect a particular cell type, neurons. Herpes simplex virus type 1 is a common human pathogen that causes cold sores.

• *Nonviral vectors:* Besides virus-mediated gene-delivery systems, there are several nonviral options for gene delivery.

Naked DNA. The simplest method is the direct introduction of therapeutic DNA into target cells. This approach is limited in its application because it can be used only with certain tissues and requires large amounts of DNA. This success, however, does not compare to that of the other methods, leading to research into more efficient methods for delivery of the naked DNA, such as electroporation, sonoporation, and the use of a 'gene gun', which shoots DNA coated gold particles into the cell using.

- *Human artificial chromosome:* It is synthetic chromosome (an artificial lipid sphere with an aqueous core), that can replicate with other chromosome besides encoding a human protein. This liposome, which carries the therapeutic DNA, is capable of passing the DNA through the target cell's membrane. As retrovirus as vector in gene therapy is associated with a heavy risks, these risks can be prevented with use of human artificial chromosome. However, this still under research.

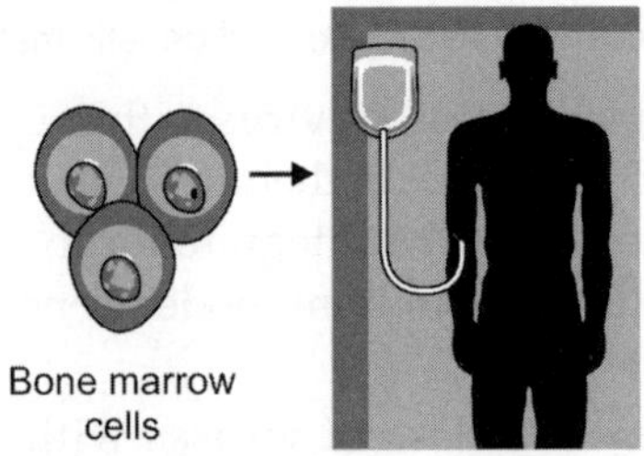

Fig 6.5: Genetically engineered bone marrow cell transfusion

- *Bone marrow cells:* Bone marrow contains totipotent embryonic stem cells. These cells are capable of dividing and differentiating into various cell type (e.g. red blood cells, platelets, macrophages, osteoclasts, B- and T-lymphocytes). For this reason, bone marrow stem cells are used a vector in ex-vivo gene therapy.
- *Oligonucleotides:* The use of synthetic oligonucleotides in gene therapy is to inactivate the genes involved in the disease process. There are several methods by which this is achieved. One strategy uses antisense specific to the target gene to disrupt the transcription of the faulty gene. Another uses small molecules of RNA called siRNA to signal the cell to cleave specific unique sequences in the mRNA transcript of the faulty gene, disrupting translation of the faulty mRNA, and therefore expression of the gene. A further strategy uses double stranded oligodeoxynucleotides as a decoy for the transcription factors that are required to activate the transcription of the target gene. The transcription factors bind to the decoys instead of the promoter of the faulty gene, which reduces the transcription of the target gene, lowering expression.

Additionally, single stranded DNA oligonucleotides have been used to direct a single base change within a mutant gene.

 - *Lipoplexes and polyplexes:* To improve the delivery of the new DNA into the cell, the DNA must be protected from damage and its entry into the cell must be facilitated. To this end new molecules, lipoplexes and polyplexes, have been created that have the ability to protect the DNA from undesirable degradation during the transfection process.

- *Hybrid methods:* Due to every method of gene transfer having shortcomings, there have been some hybrid methods developed that combine two or more techniques. Virosomes are one example; they combine liposomes with an inactivated HIV or influenza virus. This has been shown to have more efficient gene transfer in respiratory epithelial cells than either viral or liposomal methods alone. Other methods involve mixing other viral vectors with cationic lipids or hybridising viruses.

Shortcomings of Gene Therapy

- *Short-lived nature of gene therapy*: Before gene therapy can become a permanent cure for any condition, the therapeutic DNA introduced into target cells must remain functional and the cells containing the therapeutic DNA must be long-lived and stable. Problems with integrating therapeutic DNA into the genome and the rapidly dividing nature of many cells prevent gene therapy from achieving any long-term benefits. Patients will have to undergo multiple rounds of gene therapy.
- *Immune response*: Anytime a foreign object is introduced into human tissues, the immune system is designed to attack the invader. The risk of stimulating the immune system in a way that reduces gene therapy effectiveness is always a potential risk. Furthermore, the immune system's enhanced response to invaders it has seen before makes it difficult for gene therapy to be repeated in patients.
- *Problems with viral vectors*: Viruses, while the carrier of choice in most gene therapy studies, present a variety of potential problems to the patient like toxicity, immune and inflammatory responses, and gene control and targeting issues. In addition, there is always the fear that the viral vector, once inside the patient, may recover its ability to cause disease.

- *Multigene disorders*: Conditions or disorders that arise from mutations in a single gene are the best candidates for gene therapy. Unfortunately, some the most commonly occurring disorders, such as heart disease, high blood pressure, Alzheimer's disease, arthritis, and diabetes, are caused by the combined effects of variations in many genes. Multigene or multifactorial disorders, such as these would be especially difficult to treat effectively using gene therapy.

Facts of Gene Therapy

Gene therapy is under study to determine whether it could be used to treat disease. Current research is evaluating the safety of gene therapy; future studies will test whether it is an effective treatment option. Several studies have already shown that this approach can have very serious health risks, such as toxicity, inflammation, and cancer. Because the techniques are relatively new, some of the risks may be unpredictable; however, medical researchers, institutions, and regulatory agencies are working to ensure that gene therapy research is as safe as possible.

Pharmacological Gene Therapy

Pharmacological gene therapy is a new field that combines pharmacological therapy and gene therapy. It is used either to prevent a defective gene from producing its protein or to increase the concentration of normal protein produced in the body by insertion of DNA or RNA fragments. It can also be using to generate immunity from contagious disease, such as TB, via the process of DNA vaccination.

Gene Therapeutics can be used to treat such conditions as Cystic Fibrosis (via the addition of a normal CFTR gene), Hemophilia A or even some of the complications of AIDS. It uses a number of methods including: *Gene augmentation Targeted Inhibition* (using Antisense or antigene technology) *Cell Killing* (either direct or assisted) and *DNA vaccination.*

Ethical Issues Regarding Gene Therapy

Because gene therapy involves making changes to the body's set of basic instructions, it raises many unique ethical concerns. The ethical questions surrounding gene therapy include:

- How can 'good' and 'bad' uses of gene therapy be distinguished?
- Who decides which traits are normal and which constitute a disability or disorder?
- Will the high costs of gene therapy make it available only to the wealthy?
- Could the widespread use of gene therapy make society less accepting of people who are different?
- Should people be allowed to use gene therapy to enhance basic human traits, such as height, intelligence, or athletic ability?
- Current gene therapy research has focused on treating individuals by targeting the therapy to body cells, such as bone marrow or blood cells. This type of gene therapy cannot be passed on to a person's children. Gene therapy could be targeted to egg and sperm cells (germ cells), however, which would allow the inserted gene to be passed onto future generations. This approach is known as germline gene therapy.
- The idea of *germline gene therapy* is controversial. While it could spare future generations in a family from having a particular genetic disorder, it might affect the development of a fetus in unexpected ways or have long-term side effects that are not yet known. Because people who would be affected by germline gene therapy are not yet born, they cannot choose whether to have the treatment. Because of these ethical concerns, the Governments of different countries does not allow research units to be used for research on germline gene therapy in people.

Role of Nurses in Gene Therapy

Gene therapy is one of the complex medical procedure nurses have following responsibilities:

- Assess the patient's family, health and other related history
- Collect all the relevant gentic testing records
- Provide psychological support during gene therapy procedure
- Ensure that all the physical needs of individual are fulfilled
- Provide relevant information regarding gene therapy to individual and family
- Coordinate between the individual and genetic specialist

- Assist the genetic specialist in implementation of gene therapy procedure
- Regularly monitor individual for any adverse effect of the gene therapy
- Provide information and supportive services for individual and family
- Maintain all the records of patient related to gene therapy
- Provide regular evaluation and follow-up care.

THE EUGENIC MOVEMENT

Eugenics is a social philosophy, which advocates the improvement of human hereditary trails through various forms of intervention. Throughout history, eugenics has been regarded by its various advocates as a social responsibility, to create healthier and more intellectual people, to save resources, and lessen human suffering.

The term eugenics is often used to refer to movements and social policies influential during the early twentieth century. In the historical and broader sense, eugenics can also be a study of improving human genetic qualities. It is sometimes broadly applied to describe any human action whose goal is to improve the gene pool. Some form of infanticide in ancient societies, present day prenatal testing, preimplantation genetic testing, are referred as eugenics.

Eugenics was an international scientific, political and moral ideology and movement which was at its height in first half of the twentieth century and was largely abandoned after the Nazi Holocaust and its future associations with racism. Its advocates regarded it as a social philosophy for the improvement of human hereditary traits through various forms of intervention. Today it is widely regarded as a brutal movement which inflicted massive human rights violations on millions of people.

In India since ancient period, there are some of the social eugenic movements are practiced. For example, among many social groups marriages are avoided within close related subcastes and marriage is allowed outside the certain close related paternal and maternal subcastes. The eugenics movement arose in the 20th century as two wings of a common philosophy of human worth. Francis Galton, who coined the term eugenics in 1883, perceived it as a moral philosophy to improve humanity by encouraging the ablest and healthiest people to have more children. The Galtonian ideal of eugenics is usually termed positive eugenics. Negative eugenics, on the other hand, advocated culling the least able from the breeding population to preserve humanity's fitness. The eugenics movements in the United States, Germany, and Scandinavia favored the negative approach.

Purpose of Eugenic Movements

- To develop a genetically strong human population which is free from diseases and suffering.
- To improve the human hereditary through various interventions
- To improve human race, which is healthier, intelligent and more productive.

Types of Eugenic Movement

Eugenic movements are broadly classified into two categories:

- *Positive eugenics:*
  - It is aimed to encourage reproduction among the genetically advantaged people.
  - Possible approach include financial and political stimuli, targeted demographic analysis, *in vitro* fertilization, egg transplantation, and cloning to improve the genetic composition of the population by encouraging the carriers of desirable genotypes to assume the burden of parenthood.
  - Current positive eugenic movements are preimplantation genetic testing, prenatal testing and screening, premarital and preconception genetic counseling, genetic engineering, discouraging consangeous marriages.
- *Negative eugenics:*
  - It is aimed at lowering fertility among the genetically disadvantaged.
  - This includes abortion, sterilization and other methods of family planning. Hitler sought to improve the German race by killing the weak and defective. This was negative eugenics, but nobody in civilized world would improve the human race by these means. The people who

were suffering from serious hereditary diseases are sterilized or otherwise debarred from producing children.

- Other historical examples of negative eugenic movements are state sponsored discrimination, forced sterilization of person deemed genetically defective and the killing of institutionalized genetically affected disabled people.

However, developments in genetic, genomic, and reproductive technologies at the end of the 20th century have raised many new questions and concerns about what exactly constitutes the meaning of *eugenics* and what its ethical and moral status in the modern era.

GENETIC COUNSELING

In response to increasing knowledge of the role of genetics in health and disease; Reed proposed the term 'genetic counseling' in 1947, although giving of genetic advice and the transmission of certain traits were not new ideas.

'Genetic counseling is a communication process which deals with the human problems associated with the occurrence or the risk of occurrence of a genetic disorders in a family.'

In other words 'Genetic counseling is the process by which patients or relatives, at risk of an inherited disorder, are advised of the consequences and nature of the disorder, the probability of developing or transmitting it, and the options open to them in management and family planning in order to prevent, avoid or ameliorate it. This complex process can be seen from diagnostic (the actual estimation of risk) and supportive aspects'.

Genetic counseling is offered to people with genetic or inherited diseases and their families and to individuals (often children with birth defects or developmental delays) who are suspected of having a genetic condition. These services help families and their health care providers make informed decisions about their health care. In some cases, families use the information they get in a genetic evaluation to help them make reproductive decisions.

Purpose of Genetic Counseling

Genetic counselors provide supportive counseling to families, serve as patient advocates and refer individuals and families to community or state support services. counseling process involves an attempt by one or more appropriately trained person to help the individual or family:

- To comprehend the medical facts, including diagnosis, the probable course of the disorder and the available management.
- To appreciate the way hereditary contributes to the disorders and the risk of recurrence in specific relatives.
- To understand the options for dealing with the risk occurrence.
- To choose the course of action which seems appropriate to them in view of their risk and family goals and act in accordance with that decision.
- To make the best possible adjustment to the disorder in an affected family members and/ or the risk of recurrence of that disorder.

Beneficiaries of Genetic Counseling

- People who have a birth defect or genetic condition
- Parents who have had a child with a birth defect or genetic condition
- Parents who have a child with developmental delay, mental retardation or other problems with growth and development
- Women who have had three or more miscarriages or infertility from an unknown cause
- Pregnant women or couples considering having children in which:
  - The mother will be 35 years or older at the time of delivery
  - The couple are blood relatives (second cousins or closer)
  - Testing during the pregnancy indicated that the baby may have a birth defect or genetic condition
  - There is a family history of birth defects, mental retardation, or genetic disease
- People concerned they may have inherited a tendency to develop cancer
- People concerned that may have inherited a tendency to develop a neurologic condition, such as Huntington Disease (Huntington's Chorea)
- A person whose doctor or health care provider has recommended a genetic evaluation or genetic testing.

Phases of Genetic Counseling

- *Assessment phase:* This is the primary beginning phase of counseling in which following tasks are accomplished:
  - Initial interview with counselee and family for preparation of counselee for genetic counseling.
  - Collect family history, and other relevant histories, prepare and analyze predigree.
  - Carry-out primary assessment of counselee: physical examination, etc.
  - Considering potential diagnosis based on collected information.
- *Diagnostic phase:* In some cases, the goal of a genetic evaluation is to make a diagnosis of a particular genetic condition or syndrome. This is commonly the case when a child is born with multiple birth defects or problems with growth and development. In other cases, the diagnosis already is known, and the genetic counselor or geneticist probably will confirm the established diagnosis to proceed for next phases of the counseling. Therefore, this phase includes following steps:
  - Confirmatory or supplementing tests or procedure such as:
    - Chromosomal analysis
    - Biochemical tests
    - Molecular DNA testing
    - X-rays, biopsy
    - Linkage analysis
    - Developing testing
    - Dermatolography
    - Prenatal diagnosis
    - Immunological tests, etc.
  - Establishment of an accurate diagnosis.
- *Analysis phase:* This phase includes following tasks.
  - Literature search and review of information.
  - Consultation with other experts.
  - Compiling of information and determination of recurrence risk.
- *Communication phase:* This phase includes:
  - Communication of the results and risk to the counselee and to the family, if appropriate.

- Discussion of natural history of disorder, current treatment options and anticipatory guidance, if relevant.
- Discussion of options and review of questions.
- Assess the counselee's understanding about facts and relevant hereditary pattern, diagnostic and management options for disorder.
- All explanation should be culturally appropriate for counselee and appropriate for their educational.

- *Referral and support phase:* In this phase counselor offers following services:
  - Refer the individual to genetic specialist for further interventions, e.g. referral for prenatal diagnosis or treatment modalities for different disorders.
  - Support of decision made by counselee.
  - Psychological support should be provided throughout the process.
  - Follow-up and evaluation.

Role of Nurses in Genetic Counseling

Nurses work as members of a health care team and act as a patient advocate as well as a genetic resource to physicians. Genetic nurses are present at high-risk or specialty prenatal clinics that offer prenatal diagnosis, pediatric care centers, and adult genetic centers. Genetic counseling can occur before conception (i.e. when one or two of the parents are carriers of a certain trait) to adulthood (for adult onset genetic conditions, such as Huntington's disease or hereditary cancer syndromes). Following are the main role of a general genetic nurses have to accomplish during geentic counseling:

- Receive the client and family and make them comfortable in assessment room for genetic counseling.
- Obtain prenatal, family, and other health histories from individual and family.
- Conduct a primary physical examination and collect other relevant information.
- Identify families at risk, investigate the problems present in the family, interpret information about the disorder, analyze inheritance patterns and risks of recurrence and review available testing options with the family.

- Prepare and analyze a pedegree, to establish information about hereditary pattern.
- Provide psychological support to individual and family throughout the counseling.
- Collect other related information from individual and family, for example, any prior test report or documents.
- Obtain an informed written consent for any planned genetic test or intervention.
- Encourage the individual and family to ask question as much as they can understand about all aspects of disorder, about genetic testing, management, inheritance pattern and natural course of disorder.
- Provide all explanation about all the question related to genetic testing, treatment modalities and inheritance pattern of disorder, which should be culturally appropriate for counselee and appropriate for their educational level.
- Genetic nurses provide information and support to families who have members with birth defects or genetic disorders, and to families who may be at risk for a variety of inherited conditions.
- Establish a plan of care with the family and coordinate care with other health care professionals.
- Maintain privacy and confidentiality of all the information related to individual and family, only disclose the information as per individual's wish and permission.
- Provide the referal guidance to individual for genetic specialist for further interventions.
- Coordinate for available community resources to help individual and family to provide available help.
- Be available for the individual and family for any genetic services through the course of disorder.
- Ensure follow-up and supportive services to individual and family during entire course of need.

PHARMACOGENOMICS

Pharmacogenomics is the study of how genes affect a person's response to drugs. This is relativity new field combines pharmacology and genomics (the study of genes and their functions) to develop effective, safe medications and doses that will be tailored to a person's genetic make-up.

Many drugs that are currently available are 'one size fits all,' but they do not work the same way for everyone. It can be difficult to predict who will benefit from a medication, who will not respond at all, and who will experience negative side effects (called adverse drug reactions). Adverse drug reactions are a significant cause of hospitalizations and deaths. With the knowledge gained from the Human Genome Project, researchers are learning how inherited differences in genes affect the body's response to medications. These genetic differences will be used to predict whether a medication will be effective for a particular person and to help prevent adverse drug reactions.

The field of pharmacogenomics is still in its infancy. Its use is currently quite limited, but new approaches are under study in clinical trials. In the future, pharmacogenomics will allow the development of tailored drugs to treat a wide range of health problems, including cardiovascular disease, Alzheimer disease, cancer, HIV/AIDS, and asthma.

REVIEW QUESTIONS

Short-note Questions

1. Genetic counseling.
2. Legal and ethical issues of genetic services.
3. Gene therapy.
4. Role of a nurse in genetic counseling.
5. Normal Karyotype.
6. Role of Nurses in analysis of Genetic disorders.

Short-answer Questions

1. Name two methods for detection of genetic alterations.
2. Define genomics.
3. Karyotyping.
4. Mention any two recent methods to study chromosomes.
5. Mention two benefits of Human Genomic Project.

Multiple Choice Questions (MCQs)

1. **A picture showing the arrangement of a full set of human chromosomes is called ____.**
   a. Karyotype
   b. Genotype
   c. Phenotype
   d. None of the above

2. **Research from _____ is providing a new and better understanding of genetic contribution to disease.**
   a. Gene project
   b. Genetic project
   c. Human genome project
   d. Human genetic study

3. **Which of the following are the purposes of genetic testing Except?**
   a. Finding possible genetic diseases in unborn babies
   b. Finding carrier state of individual with the genetic disorder
   c. Finding out the antimicrobial sensitivity of microorganism
   d. Finding out the genetic disease in an adult with symptoms

4. **Which of the following may be considered as genetic testing?**
   a. Prenatal testing
   b. Carrier testing
   c. Preimplantation testing
   d. **All of the above**

5. **Which of the following may be considered as benefits of the genetic testing Expect?**
   a. Lifestyle adaptation
   b. Emotional, social and financial stress
   c. Future planning and life preparation
   d. Reproductive choice

6. **Which of the following is not a ethical issue in genetic testing?**
   a. Privacy
   b. Individual discrimination
   c. Informed consent
   d. Confidentiality

7. **When the Human Genome Project was completed?**
   a. 2002 b. 2003
   c. 2004 d. 2005

8. **Approximately, how many genes were identified in human DNA during the Human Genome Project:**
   a. 20,000–25, 000 b. 25,000–30,000
   c. 30,000–35,000 d. 35,000–40,000

9. **Which of the following one can be considered as an example of negative aspect of genomic era?**
   a. A woman found with mutation in BRCA2 gene may be benefited with tamoxifen
   b. A patient with hereditary hemochromatosis is suggested to avoid iron supplementation
   c. Every person carrying CFTR mutated gene will not develop cystic fibrosis
   d. Possibility of some of the genetic diseases treated through gene therapy

10. **Which of the following may be considered as vector of gene therapy?**
    a. Human artificial chromosome
    b. Adenoviruses
    c. Herpes simplex viruses
    d. All of the above

11. **Which of the following could be the beneficiaries of genetic counseling?**
    a. People who have a birth defect or genetic condition
    b. Parents who have a child with a birth defect or genetic condition
    c. Person with symptoms of congestive heart failure
    d. Pregnant women age 35 years of above

12. **Gene therapy is:**
    a. Method aim to cure genetic disorders
    b. Method to provide correct version of the defective gene
    c. Method to replace a defective gene with a healthy gene
    d. All of the above

13. The introduction of remedial gene to bone marrow cells comes under:

a. Germ line therapy
b. Somatic cell therapy
c. Both a and b
d. Corrective gene therapy

14. Introduction of healthy gene into cells, tissues or organs cultured *in vitro* and reimplanting back to the patient is referred as:

a. Germ line therapy
b. Somatic cell therapy
c. Ex-vivo therapy
d. In vivo therapy

15. Introduction of healthy gene at specific sites to displace the defective gene is referred as:

a. Germ line therapy
b. Somatic cell therapy
c. Both a and b
d. Corrective gene therapy

ANSWER KEY

1. a	2. c	3. c	4. d	5. b	6. b	7. b
8. a	9. c	10. d	11. c	12. d	13. b	14. c
15. d						

FURTHER READING

1. Allingham-Hawkins, Diane (2008-08-01). 'Successful Genetic Tests Are Predicated on Clinical Utility', Genetic Engineering & Biotechnology News (Mary Ann Liebert) 28 (14): 6, 9.
2. Amy Harmon. 'Insurance Fears Lead Many to Shun DNA Tests,' The New York Times, February. 24, 2008.
3. ANA: Comments on the HIPAA Regulations Submitted to the Department of Health and Human Services (February 17, 2000). http://www.nursingworld.org/gova/federal/agencieS/ dhhs/dhanacmt.htm
4. ANA: State Legislative Tracking of Telehealth Legislation. Washington, DC, ANA, 1998, 1999, 2000.
5. Andres LB, Fullarton JE, et al. Assessing Genetic Risks: Implications for Health and Society (TOM Report). Washington, DC, National Academy Press, 1994 .
6. Begley S, Decoding the Human Body. Newsweek April 10, 2000.
7. Bowles, BB Marteau TM. The future of genetic counseling: an international perspective. Nat Genetics 1999;22(2):133-7.

8. Colby JA. An analysis of genetic discrimination legislation proposed by the 105 Congress. American Journal of Law and Medicine 24:443, 466.
9. Cooper RA, Henderson T, Dietrich CL Roles of nonphysician providers as autonomous providers of patient care. JAMA 1998;280:795-802.
10. Cooper RA, Laud P, Dietrich CL. Current and projected workforce of nonphysician clinicians. JAMA 1998;280:788-94.
11. Fuetz-Harter SA. Nursing and the Law. Eau Claire, Wisconsin, Professional Education Systems, mc, 1993.
12. Haollowell C. Playing the Odds: Health Insurers Want to Know What's In Your DNA. Time Jan. 11, 1999.
13. Holtzman NA, Murphy PD, Watson MS, et al. 'Predictive genetic testing: from basic research to clinical practice'. Science (journal) 1997 278 (5338): 602–5.
14. Keim, Brandon. 'Genetic Discrimination by Insurers, Employers Becomes a Crime', Wired.com. Retrieved on 28 May 2008.
15. Kotval JS. Market-driven managed care and the confidentiality of genetic tests: The institution as double agent. Albany Law Journal of Science and Technology 39:1, 1998.
16. Mehlman MJ. How will we regulate genetic enhancement? Wake Forest Law Review 1999;34:671-714.
17. Roth RL, Jarquin JB, Palmer AJ. Confidentiality Issues Affecting Practitioners in Telemedicine: What Someone Else Does Not Know Could Hurt You. In Gosfield AG (ed): Health Law Handbook. St. Paul, MN, West Group, 1999.
18. Scanlon C. The legal implications of genetic testing. RN: 1998:61-65.
19. Schneider, KA. Counseling About Cancer: Strategies for Genetic Counselors. Massachusetts: Graphic Illusions, 1994.
20. Serbaroli FJ. Telemedine and the Internet. New York Law Journal 1999.
21. Swindler RN, Rothstein MA. Discrimination based on genetic information. Jurimetrics Journal: 1992;33:13.
22. Wakitsch DJ. New York's legal restrictions on the employer's collection and use of an employee's genetic information. Albany Law Journal of Science and Technology 1998;39:102.
23. Waller AA. Computers and Health Care Integration: Mapping the New Legal. Landscape. In Gosfield AG (ed): Health Law Handbook. Deerfield, IL, Clark, Boardman, Callagan, 1996.
24. Waller AA. Preparing for the complexities of administrative simplification under HIPAA. In Gosfield AG (ed): Health Law Handbook. St. Paul, MN, West Group, 1999.

Glossary

- *Adenine (A):* Nitrogenous base that forms a nucleotide when paired with thymine.
- *Allele:* Alternative form of gene's locus or location. A person can inherit different alleles from each parent.
- *Amino acid:* One of 20 different molecules used to form proteins.
- *Anticipation:* Worsening of a genetic condition in each succeeding generation, e.g., Kennedy's syndrome.
- *Autosomal dominant:* Mendelian inheritance pattern that requires only one affected gene for an individual to express the disease or trait (Huntington's disease).
- *Autosomal recessive:* Mendelian inheritance pattern that requires two affected genes for an individual to express the disease or trait, e.g. cystic fibrosis.
- *Autosome:* A nonsex chromosome composed of deoxyribonucleic acid (DNA) base pairs. Human beings have 22 pairs of autosomes.
- *Base pairs:* Combinations of nucleotides that are attracted to one another and held together by weak bonds; abbreviated as CG (cytosine/guanine) and AT (adenine/thymine).
- *Centromere:* Central region of a chromosome between p and q arms.
- *Chromatids:* Areas above and below a chrosome's centromere.
- *Chromosome:* A collection of genes arranged in the nucleus of the cell.
- *Chromosome disorders:* Clinical conditions resulting from variations in chromosomal structures rather than individual genes, e.g. Down syndrome, which is caused by an extra chromosome.
- *Cordon:* The three bases (triplet) in DNA that specify directions for one of the 20 different amino acids.

- *Cytosine (C):* Nitrogenous base that forms a nucleotide when paired with guanine.
- *Deletions:* Loss of a part of DNA possibly leading to disease e.g. early-onset familial Alzheimer's disease, e.g. achondroplasia penetrance is 100% meaning all persons with the affected gene will show symptoms.
- *Deoxyribose:* The sugar molecule found in the DNA nucleotide.
- *DNA double-stranded helix:* deoxyribonucleic acid, a double-stranded molecule consisting of base pairs of nucleotides adenine (A) and thymine (T) or guanine (G) held together by weak bonds.
- *Exons:* Part of DNA with directions for creating a specific protein.
- *Gene:* Segment of DNA in a chromosome that provides directions for heredity; made-up of a series of base pairs that encode for a protein, RNA molecule, or enzyme.
- *Gene expression:* Conversion of genetic information of DNA into protein; not all genes are expressed.
- *Genotype:* Genetic profile of an individual represented by base pair sequences.
- *Guanine (G):* Nitrogenous base that forms a nucleotide when paired with cytosine.
- *Heterozygous:* Inheriting two different forms of a particular gene (can be a carrier of a disease trait, such as cystic fibrosis).
- *Homozygous:* Inheriting the same form of a particular gene.
- *Imprinting:* Non-Mendelian inheritance mechanism that results in a disease phenotype in a child that varies depending on which parent (mother or father) had the affected gene. e.g. Prader-Willi syndrome if father's complement of chromosome 15 missing; Angelman's syndrome if the mother's missing.
- *Introns:* Part of DNA sequence that interrupts protein production.
- *Karyotype:* The map of paired chromosomes from a cell nucleus; allows visual inspection of the number, size and shape of each chromosome.
- *Kilobase (kb)* DNA unit of length equal to 1000 nucleotides.

- *Linkage:* Tendency of certain markers to be located near one another on a chromosome. Close proximity results in more frequent inheritance together.
- *Locus:* Position or location of a gene (segment of DNA) on a particular chromosome.
- *Meiosis:* Process of cell division that results in four daughter cells each with half of the parent cell chromosomes.
- *Messenger RNA (mRNA):* A segment of base pairs that acts as a template for replicating a sequence of DNA to make amino acids.
- *Mitochondrial DNA:* Genetic material found in the mitochondria (organelles that generate energy for the cell).
- *Mitosis:* Process of nuclear cell division that results in two daughter cells identical to each other and to the parent cell.
- *Mosaicism:* Different cell lines within an individual that are passed on through cell division and may eventually cause disease, e.g. neurofibromatosis.
- *Multifactorial:* Conditions that involve multiple gene products, i.e. proteins and environmental interaction.
- *Mutations:* Changes in deoxyribonucleic acid (DNA) that can be either harmful or harmless, e.g. BRCA I.
- *Nondisjunction:* Failure of a segment of chromosome to separate during meiosis.
- *Nucleotide:* Segment of DNA that includes a nitrogenous base (adenine, guanine, thymine, or cytosine) or in RNA (adenine, guanine, uracil, or cytosine) along with a phosphate molecule and a sugar molecule.
- *P-arms of a chromosome:* Short segment of a chromosome; used to define the location of a particular gene.
- *Penetrance:* Proportion of people with an affected gene who show symptoms, e.g. achondroplasia penetrance is 100% meaning all persons with the affected gene will show symptoms.
- *Phenotype:* Visible expression of the genetic make-up of an individual evident in physical appearance.
- *Polygenic:* Genetic conditions that result from more than one gene, e.g. Alzheimer's disease.

- *Polygenic disorder:* Complex genetic disorder resulting from more than one allele or more than one gene e.g. heart disease, diabetes, some cancers.
- *Polymorphisms:* Common variations in DNA structure (not disease causing).
- *Polymorphisms:* Common variations in DNA structure.
- *Proteins:* Substances used to regular body structure and functioning; made-up of amino acids determined by the DNA in genes that code for specific proteins.
- *Q-arms of a chromosome:* Long segment of a chromosome; used to define the location of a particular gene.
- *Ribonucleic acid (RNA):* A structure in the cell nucleus and cytoplasm that assists with protein synthesis and chemical activities.
- *Ribose:* The sugar molecule found in the RNA nucleotide.
- *Ribosome:* Protein manufacturing structure in cells; 'reads' messenger RNA and creates protein based on sequence of base pairs.
- *Sex-linked transmission:* Mendelian inheritance pattern that requires an affected gene on one of the sex chromosomes (X or Y) for an individual to express the disease or trait, e.g. hemophilia.
- *Sex chromosomes:* Pair of chromosomes that is usually found as either two X chromosomes (female) or an XY combination (male), which determines the sex of the fetus.
- *Single gene disorder:* Genetic disorder resulting from one allele, e.g. Duchenne's muscular dystrophy, sickle cell disease.
- *Thymine (T):* Nitrogenous base that forms a nucleotide when paired with adenine.
- *Transcription:* Synthesis of RNA from DNA, the first step in gene expression.
- *Translation:* Process of directing protein syntheses based on the code contained in messenger RNA.
- *Translications:* Parts of a chromosome being interchanged, e.g. Prader-Willi syndrome.
- *Trinucleotide repeats:* Non-Mendelian inheritance evidenced by copies of the same three nucleotides, e.g. fragile X syndrome.
- *Variable expressivity:* Differences in severity of a disorder among people, e.g. in neurofibromatosis.

Index

Page numbers followed by *f* refer to figure and *t* refer to table.

D

E

F

N

O

Q

R

S

T

U

V

W

X

Y

Z